Standards for Ocular Toxicology and Inflammation

Brian C. Gilger • Cynthia S. Cook
Michael H. Brown
Editors

Standards for Ocular Toxicology and Inflammation

Springer

ACVO
AMERICAN COLLEGE OF VETERINARY OPHTHALMOLOGISTS

Editors
Brian C. Gilger
Department of Clinical Sciences
North Carolina State University
Raleigh, NC, USA

Cynthia S. Cook
Veterinary Vision
San Francisco, CA, USA

Michael H. Brown
Veterinary Ophthalmology Services, Inc.
Little Falls, NJ, USA

Endorsed by the American College of Veterinary Ophthalmologists (ACVO)

ISBN 978-3-030-08687-9 ISBN 978-3-319-78364-2 (eBook)
https://doi.org/10.1007/978-3-319-78364-2

This Springer imprint is published by the registered company Springer Nature Switzerland AG
The registered company address is: Gewerbestrasse 11, 6330 Cham, Switzerland

Preface

This book was developed and is endorsed by the Pharmaceutical/Toxicology Committee of the American College of Veterinary Ophthalmologists (ACVO), whose membership consists of board-certified veterinary ophthalmologists with interest and experience in the pharmaceutical and toxicology industry.

The mission of the ACVO pharmaceutical/toxicology committee is to increase awareness of the pharmaceutical industry and contract research organizations (CROs) about the specialty of veterinary ophthalmology, to protect the public by encouraging participation of trained veterinary ophthalmologists in studies of investigational drugs and devices, and to establish standards for ophthalmic examinations in pharmaceutical and toxicological studies. This book is being developed to assist in this mission, especially to develop a standard for conducting ophthalmic studies.

This book is a consensus document to provide standards and harmonization for procedures, terminology, and scoring schemes for ocular toxicology studies. This information will be used by industry, pharmaceutical companies, and government agencies to help improve the drug development process and to reduce and refine the use of animals in research.

The purpose of Chap. 1 is to review laboratory animal ophthalmic examination procedures and techniques as it pertains to the pharmaceutical industry and preclinical research studies and to develop standards for the conduct of these examinations.

In Chap. 2, the authors provide harmonized protocols for commonly performed ophthalmic procedures in laboratory animals, including techniques such as intracameral, intravitreal, subconjunctival, retrobulbar, and subretinal injections, to assist in development of institutional standard operating procedures (SOP) documentation. Having similar protocols and SOPs among researchers and institutions will allow better comparison between studies, more efficient use of animals, and enhance the quality of ocular research.

The goal of Chap. 3 is to provide a consensus for the harmonization of preclinical terminology for ultimate adoption for studies submitted to the United States Food and Drug Administration (FDA) and other global regulatory agencies. Provided is a list of terminology for each anatomical section of the eye with definitions, synonyms, and justification for the descriptive-based terminology recommended for the harmonization process, including a number of representative lesion images.

Chapter 4 provides incidence data on spontaneous ophthalmic abnormalities in the most commonly used species compiled from CROs in North America. This data will allow differentiation between test article related ocular findings and background incidental lesions and thus enhance interpretation of ophthalmic findings, improve speed of drug development, reduce the number of studies that need to be repeated, and reduce the overall number of animals used in toxicology research and drug development.

Chapter 5 provides a comprehensive review of the approaches and methods used to perform clinical ocular scoring of the ocular anterior and posterior segment in laboratory animals in toxicologic and preclinical drug development studies. Following this review, there is an introduction of an enhanced scoring scheme modified from previous systems to improve the applicability and predictive value of clinical observations made in support of modern preclinical ocular drug and device development programs.

ACVO diplomates act as consultants to sponsoring pharmaceutical companies or CROs in performing ophthalmic examination of animals. These studies are designed to evaluate the potential for ocular toxicity or other adverse effects arising from the systemic, topical, or other administration of drugs or compounds, the application of medical devices, or certain surgical procedures. The ACVO recognizes that insuring public safety is the goal of such studies and that diplomates of the ACVO have unique training and experience in ophthalmology in a variety of animal species that make them exceptionally qualified for conducting ophthalmic examinations in such studies. A diplomate of the American College of Veterinary Ophthalmologists (Diplomate, ACVO), in addition to being a licensed veterinarian, has completed a minimum of 3–5 years of postgraduate specialty training in veterinary ophthalmology. This training encompasses the diagnosis and treatment of eye conditions in a variety of animal species, including those commonly used in toxicological testing. The ACVO is the only credentialing body in North America that supervises the training and certification of those qualified to perform ophthalmic diagnosis in animals. Sponsors engaging the services of a CRO must be advised of the participation, or lack thereof, by veterinary ophthalmologists and the potential limitations that may arise if such studies do not involve veterinary ophthalmologists.

The ACVO recommends that, to ensure the highest quality of toxicological testing, ACVO diplomates be used exclusively for study design, ophthalmic examinations of treated animals, and evaluation of study results in pharmacologic and toxicologic testing.

The authors of this book thank the ACVO for their support and Springer Scientific for developing this book.

Raleigh, NC, USA — Brian C. Gilger
San Francisco, CA, USA — Cynthia S. Cook
Little Falls, NJ, USA — Michael H. Brown

Contents

Chapter 1
Standards for Conducting Ophthalmic Examinations in Laboratory Animals

David A. Wilkie, Brian C. Gilger, and Joshua T. Bartoe

Abstract Ocular toxicology pertains to toxicological effects on the eye of drugs administered topically, periocularly, intraocularly, or systemically. The ophthalmic examination is able to provide detailed in-life information and is used in combination with clinical observations, clinical pathology, and histopathology to assess potential toxicologic effects. The ophthalmologist must be familiar with the wide range of species used in the field of toxicology, be familiar with the anatomic variations associated with these species, be able to differentiate an inherited or a breed-related finding from a study-related effect, be competent with the required ophthalmic equipment, and be capable of examining this wide range of animals.

Keywords Laboratory animal · Examination · Ophthalmology · Ocular toxicology · Standards

Introduction

The purpose of this chapter is to discuss laboratory animal ophthalmic examination procedures as it pertains to the pharmaceutical industry and preclinical research studies. The industries of interest include contract toxicology laboratories and researchers in an academic environment that may require the expertise of a board-certified veterinary ophthalmologist.

Contract research organizations (CROs) evaluate products for pharmaceutical and agricultural use and are governed by Food and Drug Administration (FDA) and Environmental Protection Agency (EPA) guidelines. In addition, they may test cosmetics, contact lenses and associated materials, intraocular devices, and a host of other products that might have an ocular use, contact the eye, or be applied topically

Endorsed by the American College of Veterinary Ophthalmologists (ACVO).

D. A. Wilkie · B. C. Gilger (✉) · J. T. Bartoe
Department Chair, Department of Veterinary Clinical Sciences, The Ohio State University, Columbus, OH, USA
e-mail: bgilger@ncsu.edu

B. C. Gilger et al. (eds.), *Standards for Ocular Toxicology and Inflammation*,
https://doi.org/10.1007/978-3-319-78364-2_1

or be inhaled, ingested, or injected. The evaluation of potential drug effects and toxicity must integrate the disciplines of pharmacology, toxicology, pathology, and ophthalmology [1]. Toxicology studies conducted for regulatory purposes need to be conducted in compliance with good laboratory practice (GLP). All personnel, including the consulting ophthalmologist, involved in animal studies will be expected to be familiar with GLP and will usually be required to take annual GLP-refresher courses.

Systemic and ocular toxicity studies require evaluation of both systemic toxicity using clinical observations, body weight, and clinical and histologic pathology and ocular toxicity using detailed ophthalmic examinations [1]. The eye, as it pertains to toxicology, can be considered in one of three ways. With respect to undesirable ophthalmic toxicologic effects, the ophthalmologist is concerned with (1) undesirable ocular effects when the eye is the target organ of interest with the drug of interest applied to the eye, (2) undesirable systemic effects associated with an ocularly applied agent, and (3) undesirable ocular effects from an agent applied in a systemic manner (oral, dermal, injection, inhalation) with resulting ocular effects [2–5]. In addition to drug effects, animals may be used to evaluate the effects and side effects of a procedure or device. With regard to the eye, this may include evaluation of a new intraocular device such as an intraocular lens or viscoelastic agent or evaluation of a new surgical procedure.

The eye, because of its large blood flow by organ weight, makes it a prime target for various systemic toxicities. In addition to the adnexal structures, vascularized intraocular structures include the retina and uveal tissues (iris, ciliary body, and choroid) [6]. The transparent nature of the eye and the ability to visualize arteries, veins, and neural tissue make the eye an organ where toxicities may be readily detectable. This makes the eye unique in that it is possible to conduct a detailed assessment during the in-life portion of a study [1].

This chapter will emphasize the routine ophthalmic examination of laboratory animals. It will also provide information on more advanced ophthalmic diagnostic tools that are becoming more commonplace in the area of ocular toxicology.

Routine Examination

Prior to study initiation, the ophthalmologist should review all ophthalmic procedures, discuss with the study director and/or sponsor any issues or concerns with the study design or the examination procedures, and then follow standard operating procedures (SOPs) when conducting their examinations. It is the position of the American College of Veterinary Ophthalmologists (ACVO), that in order to ensure public safety that the status of Diplomate of the ACVO is the minimum qualification for performing these ocular examinations and assessment of findings in a laboratory animal study that is intended to support applications to the FDA (or other similar regulating agencies) for entry into human clinical trials. Evaluation of toxicological effects of pharmaceutical agents involves assessment by a number of personnel, many of which are board-certified specialists, including pathologists, cardiologists, and others in addition to ophthalmologists. Sponsors engaging the services of a CRO must be advised of the participation of veterinary ophthalmologists and the potential limitations and liability that may arise if such studies do not involve veterinary ophthalmologists.

A board-certified veterinary ophthalmologist is uniquely qualified to consult in the development of the experimental design (including the species selected, appropriate diagnostic tests, and frequency of exams) and the assessment of ocular effects of test materials being evaluated. Coordination between the testing agency and the veterinary ophthalmologist is essential throughout the process, including protocol development, establishing SOPs, and the identification and assessment of ocular findings. If ocular abnormalities are identified, communication between the ophthalmologist, study director, and the pathologist will allow correlation of clinical and histopathologic findings.

The components of an ophthalmic examination may vary depending on the species involved and the specific objective of the study. However, if the purpose of such a study is to screen for adverse effects on any ocular tissue including, at a minimum, the adnexal structures (eyelids and conjunctiva), anterior segment (cornea, anterior chamber, iris, and lens), and posterior segment (vitreous and fundus), the following must be included:

1. Pharmacologic pupillary dilation
2. Darkened ambient light conditions
3. Indirect and/or direct ophthalmoscopy
4. Slit-lamp biomicroscopy

Additional procedures may be included depending on the objective of the examination. These may include, but are not limited to, corneal staining, corneal aesthesiometry, pachymetry, tonometry, fundus photography, fluorescein angiography, optical coherence tomography (OCT), and electrophysiological assessment of the visual system (e.g., electroretinography, multifocal electroretinography, visual evoked potentials). Topical anesthesia, sedation, or general anesthesia may or may not be required depending on the species, the procedure being performed, and individual animal.

The routine ophthalmic examination for all animals used in toxicologic studies should begin with the minimum database of the results of examinations using both slit-lamp biomicroscopy and indirect ophthalmoscopy. Regardless of the species of interest, these two examination techniques are essential to ensure an accurate and complete examination of both the anterior and posterior segments of the eye. Together these two examinations must, at a minimum, include evaluation of the adnexal structures (eyelids and conjunctiva), anterior segment (cornea, anterior chamber, iris, and lens), and the posterior segment (vitreous and fundus).

Ophthalmic examinations should be conducted on eyes that have been pharmacologically dilated and should be performed in a darkened examination room. While some have advocated the use of 10% phenylephrine HCl to aid in dilation of rodents [7, 8], this is generally not required. Pharmacologic dilation is most commonly performed using tropicamide at a concentration of 0.5% for rodents and 1% for larger mammals. The ophthalmologist should be familiar with the length of time required to achieve mydriasis and the duration of the mydriasis for the species being examined. In general, 10–15 min is the minimum time required to achieve acceptable mydriasis, and this may be slightly longer in heavily pigmented eyes. The duration of mydriasis is directly related to the amount of intraocular melanin. In albinotic rodents, mydriasis will last no more than 1 h, while in a pigmented eye of a dog or primate, the effect will persist for 3–5 h. This information is important, so the ophthalmologist knows when to begin dilation and how many animals should be dilated at one time. The latter will depend on how many animals the ophthalmologist can examine in a given time period. For the basic examination, slit-lamp biomicroscopy and indirect ophthalmoscopy, animals are either manually restrained (rodent, dog, rabbit, pig, guinea pig, cat) or sedated or anesthetized (primates). Rats and mice may be held in a dose-hold and presented to the ophthalmologist with their heads restrained. Some ophthalmologists prefer the eyes to be slightly proptosed in rodents. Dogs and rabbits are most often examined on a table. Rabbits seem to do best if there is a towel on the table as this decreases their movements and may provide some comfort. Alternatively, some ophthalmologists prefer to use restraint bags for rabbits and cats to minimize movement during the examination. For rabbits, the ophthalmologist should be seated slightly below the level of the restraint table to allow easy visualization of the rabbit's optic nerve and retinal vasculature which are located in the superior fundus. For dogs, the examiner may be seated or standing. Since primates will be usually anesthetized or heavily sedated, they may be manually restrained or placed on an examination table. If more extensive examinations such as electrodiagnostic testing or OCT are necessary, sedation or anesthesia may be required regardless of the species.

Additional examination procedures such as direct ophthalmoscopy, corneal staining, tonometry, pachymetry, fluorescein angiography, photographic documentation (anterior or posterior segment), electrodiagnostic testing, ultrasonography, OCT, and other tests may be indicated depending on the study and toxicologic effects of interest. If any of these additional tests are required, the order in which tests are performed and when to perform pupil dilation must be considered. For example, determination of intraocular pressure (IOP) should be performed prior to pupil dilation. In addition, if repeated IOP measurements are required during a study, they should be performed at the same time of day to avoid diurnal pressure fluctuation and performed preferably by the same individual to limit interobserver variation. When possible, examination of the cornea, including fluorescein staining, should be performed prior to procedures that may result in corneal changes as a result of corneal contact (pachymetry, tonometry) or the use of topical anesthesia. If sedation is required for the ophthalmic examination, then consideration must be given to dosing and feeding schedules, clinical observations, and clinical pathology sampling. Finally, from an animal well-being standpoint, a balance must be struck between multiple procedures performed on the same day as compared with multiple repeated days requiring sedation [1].

Animals will be most commonly identified by tattoo, ear tag, or microchip. If a tattoo or ear tag is used, the animal handler will need to have enough light during the examination to read the identification to ensure accurate data collection. This may be provided by a separate light source elsewhere in the examination room or if possible by performing the ophthalmic examinations in a darkened anteroom allowing the handlers to keep the main animal room lights on. When identified by microchip, a computer scanner will allow animal identification to be linked to the computer program for data entry. To ensure accuracy, each animal must be identified to both the ophthalmologist and the data entry person at the time of the examination. The data entry person must verify that the animal being examined and the animal for which the data are being entered correspond.

Depending on the compound being evaluated and the SOP, the ophthalmologist will be expected to wear shoe covers, a lab coat or surgical scrubs, and gloves at a minimum and may be required to wear a Tyvek® suit, surgical cap, mask, and occasionally a respirator. When working with nonhuman primates (NHP), annual testing for tuberculosis (TB) using a TB intradermal PPD skin test or the new QuantiFERON®-TB blood test will generally be required of all personnel including the ophthalmologist.

The ophthalmologist must be familiar with what is normal for the species being examined and what are the common spontaneous abnormalities for that species, age of animal, and breed/strain (see Chaps. 3 and 4). Normal differences in albino vs. pigmented eyes and characteristics of species-specific retinal vasculature patterns (holangiotic vs. merangiotic vs. paurangiotic vs. anangiotic) should be well known to the ophthalmologist. The presence or absence of a tapetum lucidum and whether the animal has a fovea should be considered. In addition, the examination techniques to be used, type of biomicroscope and indirect ophthalmoscope, diameter and diopter strength of the indirect lens, and number of animals that can be examined in an hour must be understood. The role of the veterinary ophthalmologist is to perform a pretest examination designed to identify those animals not ideally suited to the study due to presence of pre-existing ocular changes and to establish a baseline database to which comparisons of interim and terminal findings can be made. Animals are then subsequently examined one or more times during the study, at termination of the study and possibly in a recovery phase depending on the study duration and design. Typically, studies are divided into acute, subacute, subchronic, and chronic depending on the study duration. The ophthalmologist must then interpret findings in light of the species examined, pretest data, compound evaluated, additional study procedures performed (anesthesia, orbital blood collection), and dose group outcome.

Since most laboratory studies involve a significant number of animals, organization and efficiency are essential. In general, most canine, primate, swine, feline, and rabbit studies involve 40–60 animals, while rats and mice may involve 250–1500 animals in a single study. An individual ophthalmologist generally requires 2–3 animal handlers, a data entry person, and in studies over 250 animals 1–2 individuals to go ahead of the animal handlers to dilate the pupils. For efficiency, an animal should be in front of the ophthalmologist at all times. The ophthalmologists' findings are reported verbally to the data entry individual who then either enters it into a computer program or records on a paper for later entry into a computer database. These data are then verified at the end of the examination, and both the ophthalmologist and data entry individual date and initial the accuracy of the report.

When an ophthalmic abnormality is observed, it must be characterized with respect to diagnosis, location, and severity. Depending on the laboratory, some will use a standardized scheme for recording of clinical observations such as Provantis® that has a set of preloaded ophthalmic terms for organ location (cornea, lens, iris, etc.), clinical signs/diagnosis (opacity, coloboma, degeneration, hemorrhage, etc.), specific location (cortex, nucleus, tapetal, anterior, posterior, etc.), and severity (slight, moderate, severe). Other CROs may have their own in-house computer or paper-based recording system. The ophthalmologist should be familiar with each laboratory's recording system and terminology to be consistent both within and between studies. See Chap. 3 for terminology harmonization designed to streamline and allow easy comparisons across the industry. When an abnormality is observed, correlation between dose groups is important when evaluating the incidence and severity of lesions so that any association with the test article can be assessed [1]. While it would be best if animals were examined out of dosing order so as to mask the ophthalmologist with respect to dose group being examined, this is often not possible given the way animals are housed and entered into the data collection system.

The ophthalmologist should also have a standardized scoring or grading scheme to assign a severity to any abnormalities seen. In general, a grading scheme of slight, moderate, and severe/marked is most common. When using this grading scheme for the transparent media (cornea, aqueous humor, lens, and vitreous humor), a grading of slight would imply a lesion that does not obstruct visualization of the deeper tissues past the lesion, a moderate grade implies a lesion that interferes with but does not fully obstruct the view of the tissues deep to the lesion, and a severe/marked lesion fully obstructs the view of structures deep to the lesion. The reader is directed to Chap. 3 (Harmonization of Lesion Nomenclature) for updated information on lesion descriptions.

For studies involving topical ophthalmic application of a drug or an ocular/intraocular device, a more specific detailed biomicroscopic examination protocol with standardized scoring or grading criteria is frequently used. The reader is directed to Chap. 5 (Standard Ocular Irritation/Inflammatory Scoring: Anterior and Posterior Segments) for more information on ocular inflammatory scoring criteria.

Slit-Lamp Biomicroscopy

Slit-lamp biomicroscopy is used to examine the ocular anterior segment including the eyelids, conjunctiva, third eyelid, tear film, cornea, anterior chamber, iris, lens, and anterior vitreous humor. Biomicroscopy provides a magnified view of the living eye using a light that can be varied in intensity, width, height, and color. In general, for laboratory animals, this is performed using a handheld slit lamp of the ophthalmologist's preference. The slit lamp used for routine examination should be portable, lightweight, and easy to use on a variety of species. The two most common portable slit lamps used for laboratory animals are the Zeiss HSO-10 and the Kowa SL-15 or SL-17 (Fig. 1.1). The Zeiss HSO-10 provides a 12× magnification with a

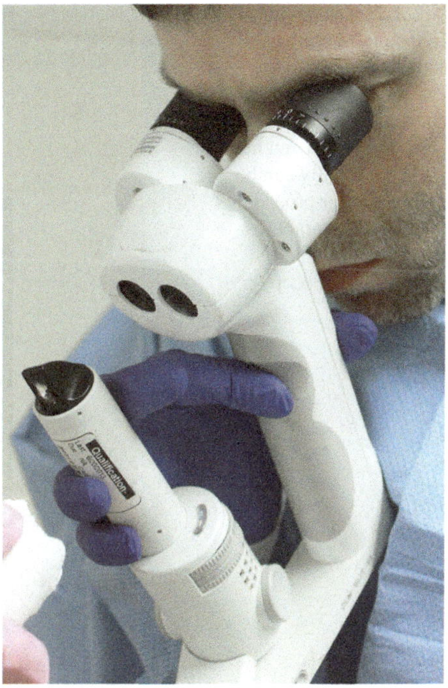

Fig. 1.1 A Kowa SL-15 handheld slit lamp is battery-powered and portable. As with the Zeiss HSO-10, they are suited for use in all laboratory animal species

125 mm working distance and is both lightweight and easy to use on all species. The Kowa SL-15 has either a 10× or 16× magnification with a 100 mm working distance. Unlike the Zeiss, the Kowa works from a battery pack. Both have fixed slit widths (0.15 and 0.75 mm Zeiss; 0.1, 0.2, and 0.8 mm Kowa), and both have a cobalt blue filter for visualization of fluorescein staining. If higher magnification or photographic documentation is required, a table-mounted slit lamp may be used (Fig. 1.2). Table slit lamps provide higher-quality optics, increased magnification, and variable width and height of the slit beam and with additional attachments can allow for photographic documentation, gonioscopy, or specular microscopy. Table slit lamps are however significantly more expensive, less portable, and more difficult to use on a large number of animals or un-sedated animals.

The slit lamp performs two major functions. First, it provides magnification for a more detailed examination of the eye. Second, it makes use of an aperture, decreasing the beam of light to a slit allowing an optical cross section of the eye to be obtained (Figs. 1.3 and 1.4). This allows precise localization of the depth of a lesion and allows visualization of subtle changes that cannot be seen with full illumination (Figs. 1.5, 1.6, 1.7, 1.8, and 1.9). The term for this type of illumination and examination is an optical section, and it is the most common method of biomicroscopic examination. Using a narrow slit beam, a highly magnified optical section of the eye is obtained. The direction of the slit beam may be varied so that the structures may be viewed using either direct illumination or by retroillumination [1]. This allows the examiner to detect and localize, with respect to depth, abnormalities in the ante-

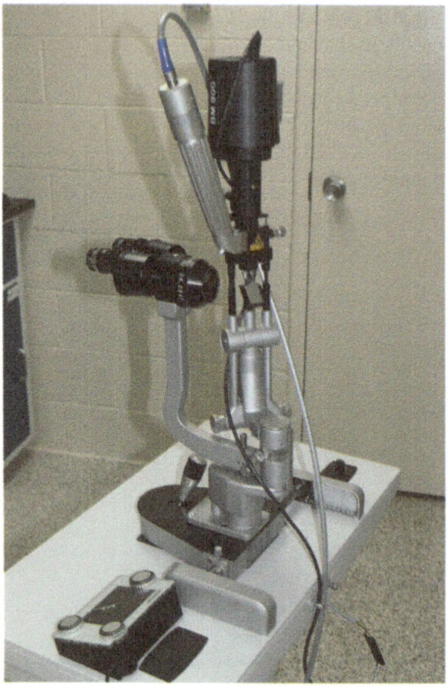

Fig. 1.2 Haag-Streit BM 900 table-mounted slit lamp. This provides excellent optics, higher magnification, and variable slit beam width and height and additionally can be used for other procedures such as photographic documentation and specular microscopy

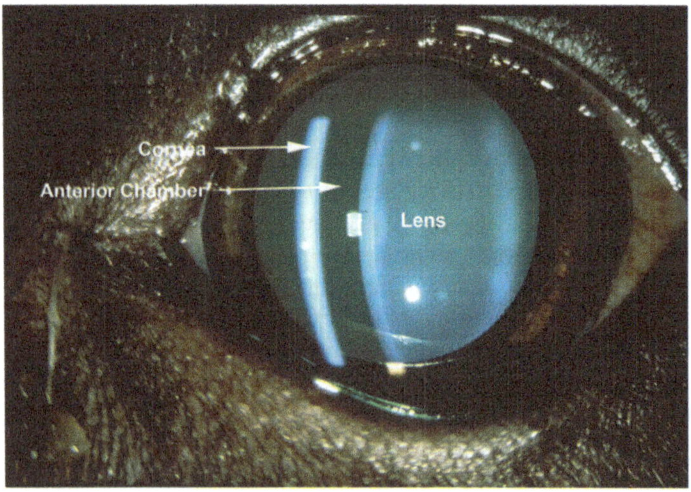

Fig. 1.3 A normal slit-lamp examination using the technique of optical section to examine the anterior segment of a normal Beagle

rior segment of the eye. For example, a corneal lesion can be localized to superficial, stromal, or endothelial; aqueous humor opacities such as cells, flare, or hemorrhage are detectable and quantifiable, and lesions of the lens may be localized to anterior, posterior, and equatorial and further to capsular, cortical, or nuclear. Interpretation

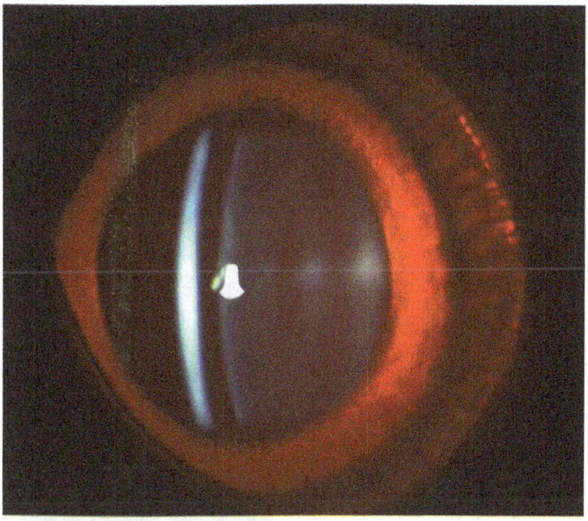

Fig. 1.4 A normal slit-lamp examination using the technique of optical section to examine the anterior segment of a normal New Zealand white rabbit

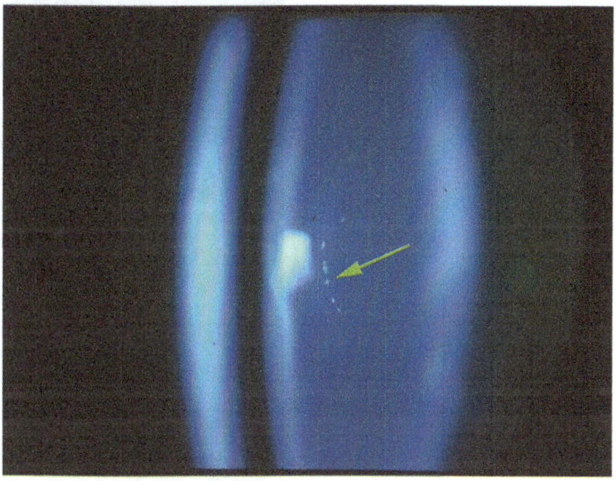

Fig. 1.5 Multiple anterior cortical suture opacities/cataracts are noted (arrow) in a Beagle on pretest examination

of the findings on slit-lamp biomicroscopy requires extensive knowledge of normal biomicroscopic anatomy as well as background lesions that occur as incidental findings in the species and strain being examined [1].

Indirect/Direct Ophthalmoscopy

Indirect ophthalmoscopy is the preferred technique of choice for routine screening of the posterior segment in all laboratory animal species. Indirect ophthalmoscopy provides a binocular, inverted, and reversed aerial image with a wide field of view. It requires an indirect headset and a condensing lens. Once perfected, the technique of indirect examination also allows for a more rapid examination of the entire

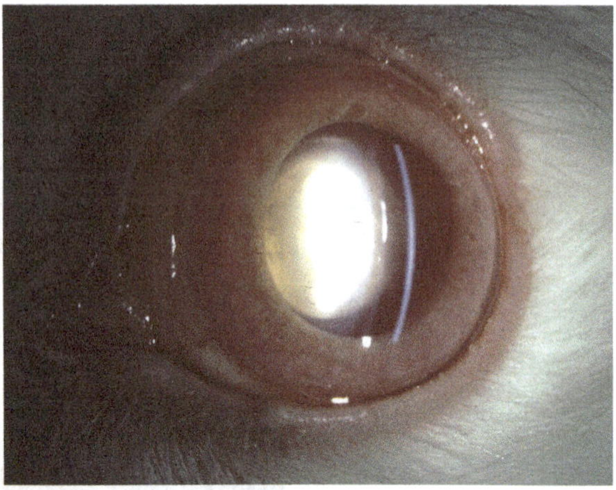

Fig. 1.6 An immature, nuclear cataract noted in a New Zealand white rabbit on pretest examination

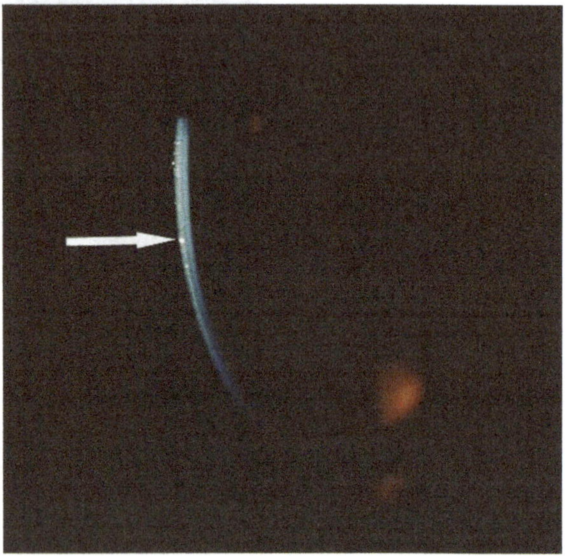

Fig. 1.7 Multifocal, corneal anterior stromal opacities (arrow) observed as a treatment-related effect in high-dose Beagles during a chronic study

posterior segment as it provides a wider panoramic field of view, allowing the examiner to evaluate more animals, more accurately in a shorter period of time. The indirect headset of choice should be lightweight, comfortable, and easy to manipulate out of the way with one hand and have a small pupil setting. The ease of manipulation will allow the examiner to move efficiently between indirect and biomicroscopic examination techniques. While several excellent choices are available, the Keeler All Pupil® is very portable (Fig. 1.10). Alternatively, the Heine indirect ophthalmoscope also offers excellent optics and can be fitted with a portable power supply. The indirect condensing lens of choice varies by species examined and by the examiners' choice. In general, a 2.2 Volk Pan Retinal or 28–30 diopter lens works well for routine screening examination of most larger species,

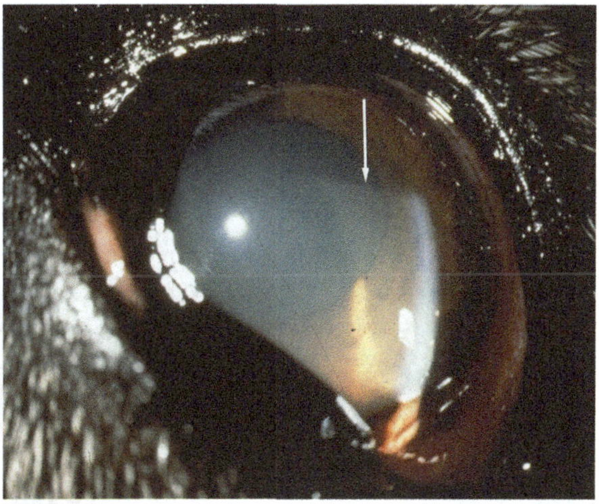

Fig. 1.8 Aqueous flare is noted in the anterior chamber as a cloudiness (arrow) in the normally transparent aqueous humor

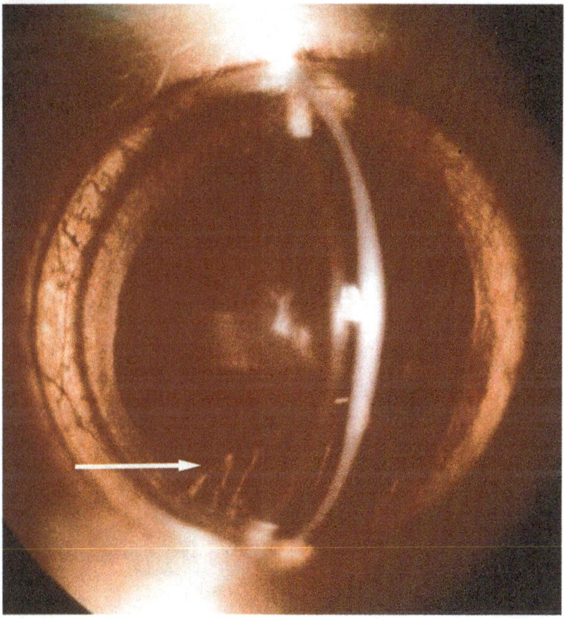

Fig. 1.9 A Sprague-Dawley rat with several persistent pupillary membranes (arrow) noted on pretest examination

and a 28, 40, or 60 diopter lens works best for rats and mice. The addition of a 20 diopter and/or a 15 diopter lens may be advised for higher magnification of the fundus in the canine and to examine the fovea and optic nerve in greater detail in NHP. Alternately, a direct ophthalmoscope (Fig. 1.11) can be used to examine the optic nerve head and fovea in NHP, but given its small field and monocular view, it may be less than optimal. In addition, when performing direct ophthalmoscopy, significant opacity of the cornea, aqueous, lens, or vitreous will severely impair or prevent visualization of the posterior segment. Lastly, the use of a direct

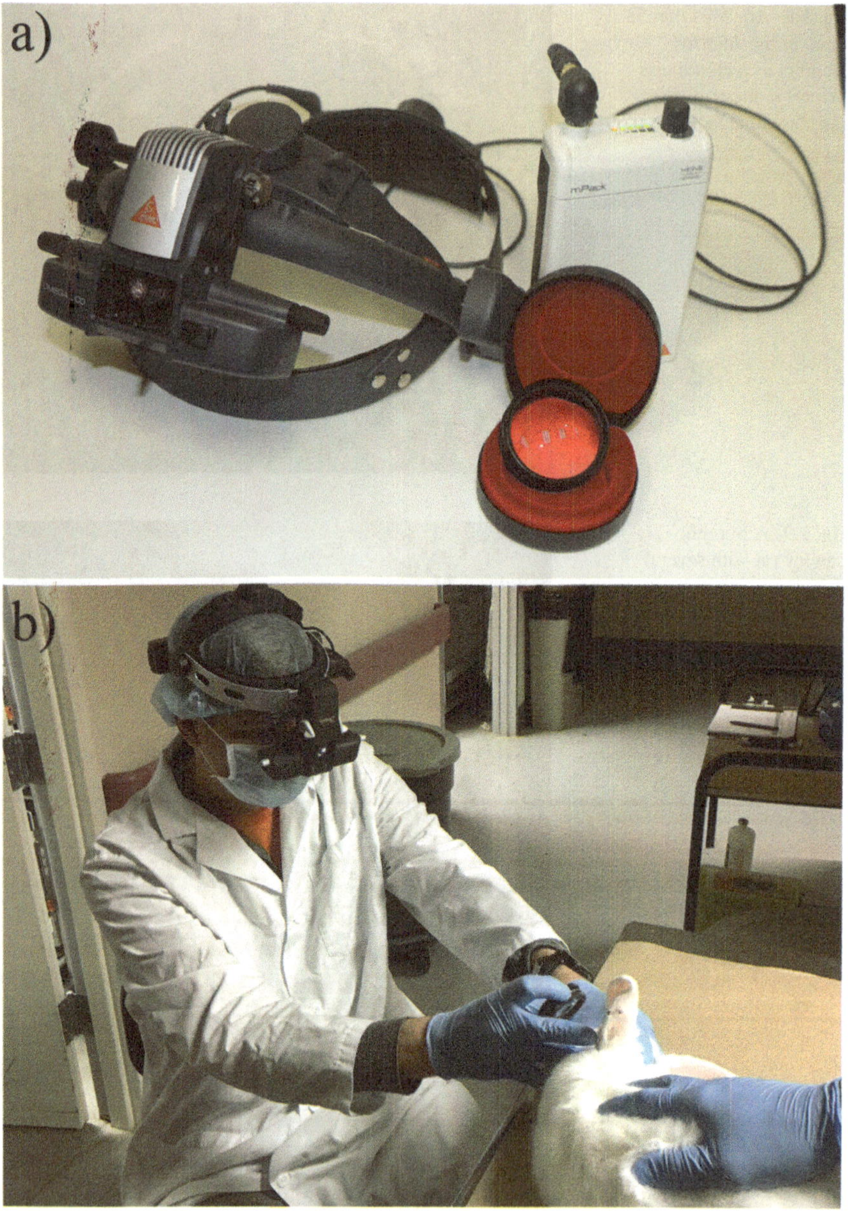

Fig. 1.10 (**a**) The Heine Omega 500 indirect ophthalmoscope and 28D Volk lens. (**b**) The Keeler All Pupil® Vantage indirect ophthalmoscope and 28D Volk condensing lens for examination of the ocular fundus in a New Zealand white rabbit

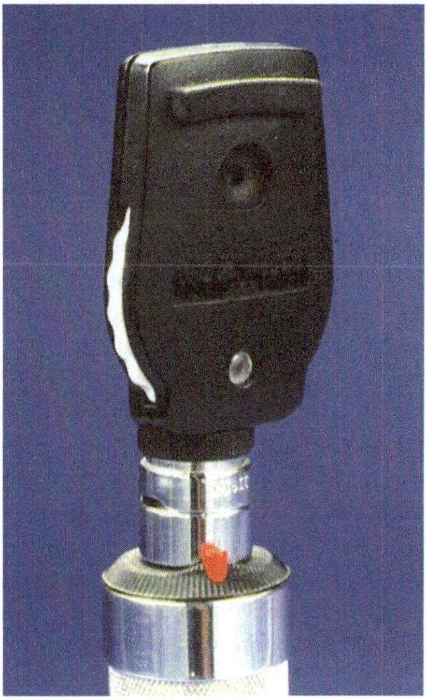

Fig. 1.11 A Welch-Allyn direct ophthalmoscope

ophthalmoscope requires the examiner to be in very close proximity to the animal's face which may present a safety concern when working with NHP due to infectious disease transmission and possible arousal from sedation.

Prior to indirect ophthalmoscopy, a short-acting mydriatic agent is required to dilate the pupil. Tropicamide 0.5–1.0% is the mydriatic of choice. When performing indirect ophthalmoscopy, the examiner remains at arm's length and places the condensing lens just anterior to the cornea. This technique is used to examine the posterior vitreous, optic nerve, retinal vasculature, retina, and choroid. In addition, opacities of the clear media (cornea, aqueous, lens, and vitreous humor) are readily detectable using retroillumination. Given the wide variety of laboratory animals, the examiner must be familiar with the variation of normal anatomy and species differences. The retinal vasculature will vary with the species: anangiotic (guinea pig), merangiotic (rabbit), and holangiotic (rodent, dog, pig, NHP). The pigmentation of the retinal pigment epithelium (RPE) and the choroid vary between albinotic, subalbinotic, and pigmented animals of the same species (mouse, rat, rabbit, dog, etc.). Some species such as the dog will have a tapetum lucidum located in the superior choroid, but this can be absent in color dilute or lemon beagles or young dogs in which the tapetum has not yet developed. Finally, NHP are foveated, and this region must be examined carefully for abnormalities.

Additional techniques to evaluate the retina may include fluorescein angiography, OCT, confocal scanning laser ophthalmoscopy, fundus photography, and electrodiagnostic testing. When these tests are used correctly and in combination, they can provide additional en face, cross-sectional, and functional information of the retina that may then be correlated with histopathology.

Pretest Examination

Prior to study initiation, a pretest ophthalmic examination should be performed on all study animals. This is done for two reasons. The first is to eliminate from study any animals with current significant or potentially progressive ophthalmic abnormalities. The second is to establish a baseline of ocular findings to compare to as the study progresses and subsequent ophthalmic examinations are performed. Examples of pretest abnormalities that should automatically result in an animal's elimination from the study would include all ocular findings with a severity score of moderate or higher and all abnormalities that currently prevent, or may prevent if progressive, complete examination of intraocular structures. Examples of ocular findings that may be progressive during the course of the study and should result in elimination include cataract, intraocular hemorrhage, uveitis, and any other findings that may result in progressive opacification and interfere with a complete ophthalmic examination on subsequent examinations.

Common background abnormalities will vary by species and are described in detail in Chaps. 3 and 4. Whenever possible, animals with ocular abnormalities are eliminated from inclusion in the study. However, some abnormalities are so common as to preclude elimination. The most common example of this would be corneal dystrophy in the rat and mouse. The prevalence of corneal dystrophy varies by stain, age, and sex of the rat. Please see Chap. 4 (Spontaneous Incidence of Ocular Abnormalities in Laboratory Animals) for more information on incidence of spontaneous common ocular abnormalities in laboratory animals.

Additional Ophthalmic Diagnostic Procedures

There are numerous noninvasive ophthalmic diagnostic techniques that, depending on the tissue of interest, can provide both structural and functional information of both the anterior and posterior segments of the eye. Some of the more common techniques are discussed below, and a more detailed discussion of these and additional techniques as they apply to toxicologic, ophthalmic research and clinical application have recently been published [7, 9].

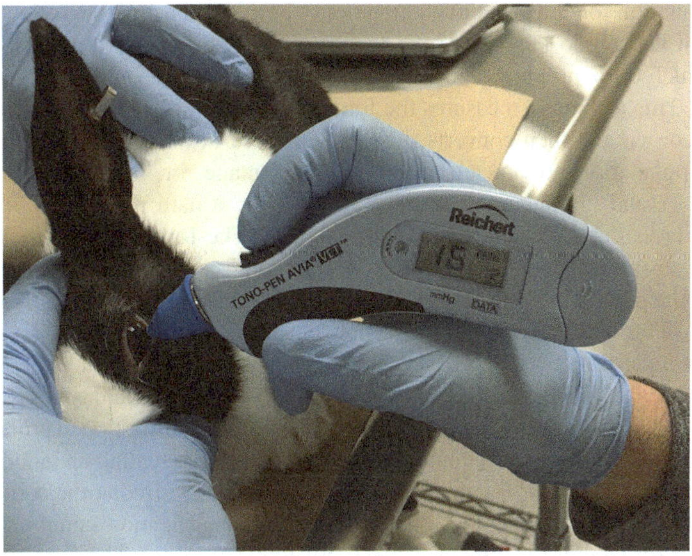

Fig. 1.12 A Tono-Pen AVIA Vet® being used to estimate intraocular pressure in a Dutch Belted rabbit

Tonometry

Tonometry is used to obtain an indirect measurement of the intraocular pressure (IOP). There are several methods including indentation, applanation, and rebound tonometry utilized in commercially available handheld devices sufficiently portable to be used by a consulting veterinary ophthalmologist. Of these, indentation tonometry, utilizing the Schiotz tonometer, would be considered inaccurate and unreliable in many of the species commonly encountered at CROs and so should not be used for ocular toxicology studies. As many tonometers were originally designed for the human cornea, readings in animals may be slightly inaccurate, but provided the same tonometer is used throughout a study by the same examiner, the changes in IOP that occur on study will be valid [8, 10–12].

The IOP in most laboratory animals will range between 12 and 25 mmHg, and there should be ≤5 mmHg difference between both eyes. The IOP can be affected by restraint techniques, animal stress, diurnal or circadian rhythm eye position, sedation or anesthesia, corneal thickness, and several other variables [8, 13]. If possible, the IOP should be obtained for all animals at the same general time of day throughout the study and by the same examiner, using the same tonometer, same handling personnel, and the same technique each time. Determination of IOP should be performed prior to pharmacologic dilation. When IOP is a critical aspect of a study, it is also advisable for the animals to be acclimatized to both the procedure and restraint techniques prior to study initiation.

Applanation tonometry is most commonly performed using the Tono-Pen XL®, Tono-Pen Vet®, Tono-Pen AVIA®, or pneumotonograph. It requires topical anesthesia of which 0.5% proparacaine is the most common topical ophthalmic anesthetic selected. This technique measures the force required to applanate or flatten a given area of cornea and then converts this applied force into an IOP value in mmHg. Some applanation tonometers have the advantage of being self-calibrating (Fig. 1.12), and the pneumotonograph can provide a hard paper copy for record keeping, both ideal characteristics for a GLP study. The Tono-Pen XL and Tono-Pen Vet® obtain four independent readings, average the readings, and display both the IOP and the percent error indicating the variability between the individual readings. The Tono-Pen AVIA® obtains ten independent readings and reports IOP and variability as a percent confidence. For the Tono-Pen XL®, the percent error should be <5%, and for the Tono-Pen AVIA®, the percent confidence should >95%.

Rebound tonometry determines IOP by firing a small plastic-tipped probe against the cornea. The probe then rebounds back into the device creating an induction current from which the IOP is calculated. The probe must be fired at the cornea in the horizontal position, parallel to the floor to be accurate. The most common rebound tonometer for laboratory animals is the Tonovet® (Fig. 1.13a). The Tonovet® is specifically calibrated for the dog, cat, and horse, but it has been used reliably in other species. The TonoLab tonometer is specifically designed and calibrated for use in mice and rats (Fig. 1.13b). The Tonovet and TonoLab tonometers have the advantage of not requiring topical anesthesia and seem to obtain the IOP more easily than the Tono-Pen® in many laboratory animals including the dog, rabbit, and rat. Its disadvantage is that it cannot be self-calibrated prior to use. Like the Tono-Pen® and the Tonovet®, it also averages six readings and gives an indication of percent error using a bar at the left of the IOP value. There should be no error bar, or the bar should be at the left lower corner of the screen for a reading to be acceptable.

Regardless of the tonometer used, typically a minimum of 2–3 final averaged readings per eye should be obtained and recorded. As all tonometers except the pneumotongraph, give only digital readouts, the IOP must be either hand recorded or entered into a computer database as no permanent record is created by the device.

Pachymetry

Pachymetry is the noninvasive evaluation of corneal thickness. It is most commonly performed with use of a contact ultrasound device specifically designed for this purpose (e.g., the PachPen®) (Fig. 1.14), but the corneal thickness measurement can also be obtained by high-resolution ultrasonography or OCT. Pachymetry allows evaluation of subtle changes in corneal thickness prior to the appearance of clinically detectable corneal edema on biomicroscopy. The corneal thickness varies between species but also varies by region of the cornea (axial vs. peripheral). As a result of the regional variation, readings must be obtained from the same region of the cornea, usually axially, at each time point.

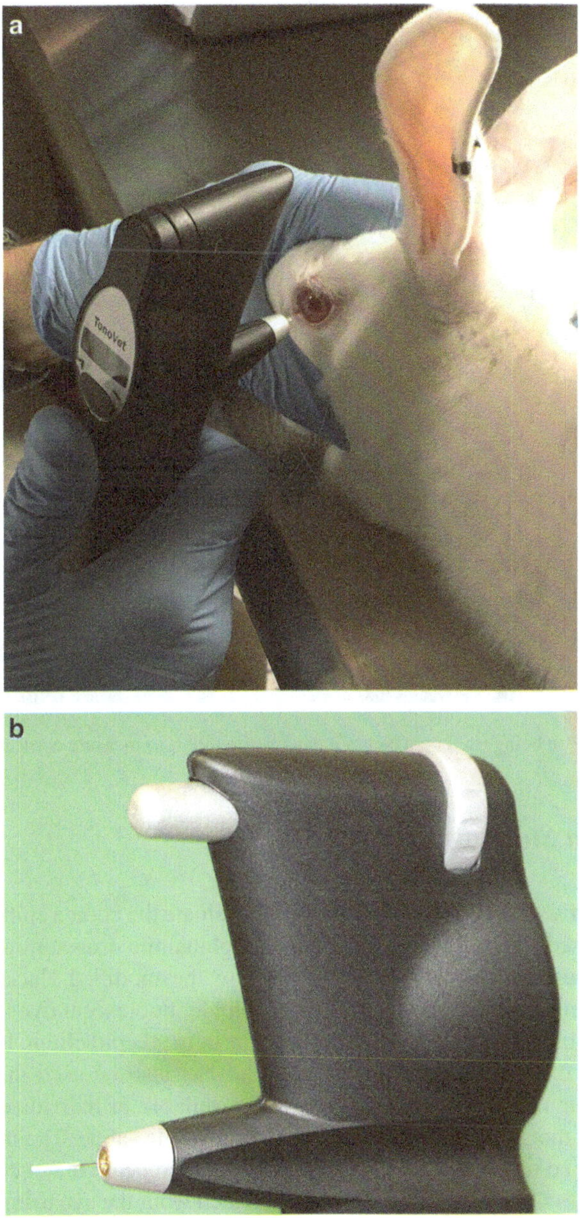

Fig. 1.13 (*Top*) The Tonovet® rebound tonometer being used to estimate intraocular pressure in a New Zealand white rabbit. (*Bottom*) The small tip of the TonoLab tonometer is useful for measuring intraocular pressure in rodents

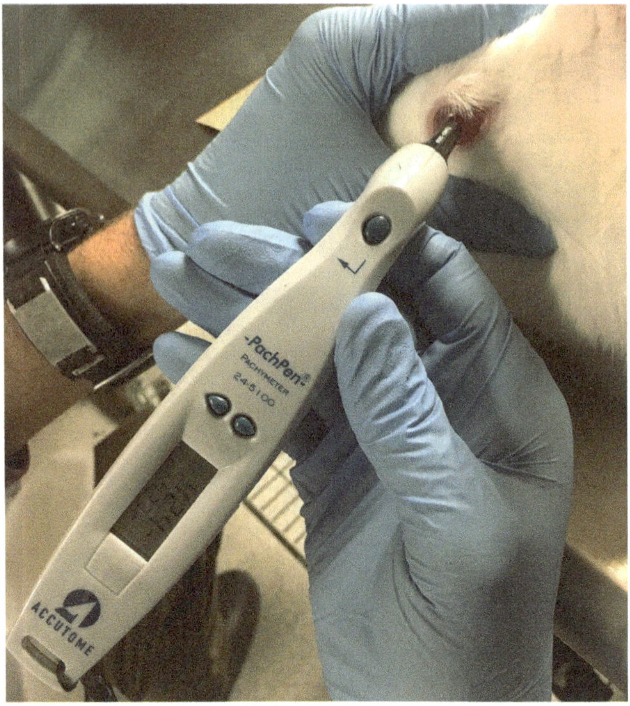

Fig. 1.14 PachPen being used on a New Zealand white rabbit to measure corneal thickness

Fluorescein Staining

Application of sodium fluorescein solution to evaluate the cornea epithelial integrity is routinely used on studies involving topical ophthalmic drug administration, contact lens evaluation, and other studies that use the modified Hackett-McDonald scoring system [14]. Fluorescein is a water-soluble, fluorescent dye that is retained by the hydrophilic corneal stroma but not by the corneal epithelium. It is used to aid identification of corneal epithelial defects and can also be used in evaluation of precorneal tear film retention. Fluorescein is available in individual impregnated strips that are moistened at the time of use using sterile saline. The moistened strip is gently applied to the dorsal bulbar conjunctiva taking care to not contact the cornea. The excess fluorescein is then gently irrigated from the eye using a gravity-fed stream of saline rather than a forced high-velocity stream. Alternatively, fluorescein strips can be placed in a plastic syringe and filled with a predetermined volume sterile saline to create a solution of known fluorescein concentration and then dripped on the cornea. The cornea is examined by the ophthalmologist using a biomicroscope and the cobalt blue filter to excite the fluorescein, should any remain following irrigation.

Photographic Documentation

Ophthalmic photography may be used to demonstrate a lack of change in an area like the fundus, to document abnormalities or to monitor progression of a lesion. Serial photographs taken at various time points during a study will allow comparison to accurately establish whether an abnormality is static or progressive. As photography adds additional time, cost, and animal stress, it is not routinely performed on all studies. Rather it is in a study protocol as an option to be used to document a lesion when observed or for studies where abnormalities are more likely to occur, such as with an intraocular implant or for intravitreal or subretinal injection studies.

Ophthalmic photography can be divided into external and intraocular. External photography can be performed using a standard SLR digital camera with a macro lens or with a digital Kowa Genesis-D fundus camera with the diopter settings adjusted to allow external and anterior segment imaging. Photography of the posterior segment requires some type of fundus camera and the digital Kowa

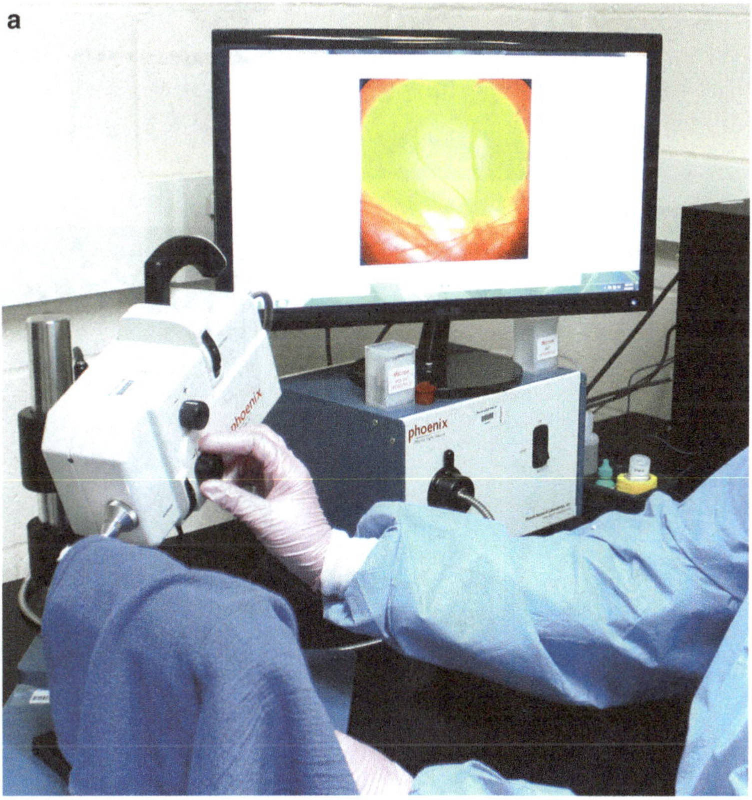

Fig. 1.15 Fundus cameras that can be used on laboratory animals: (**a**) Micron IV—for rodents. (**b**) RetCam Shuttle—large animals. (**c**) Micron X—large animals

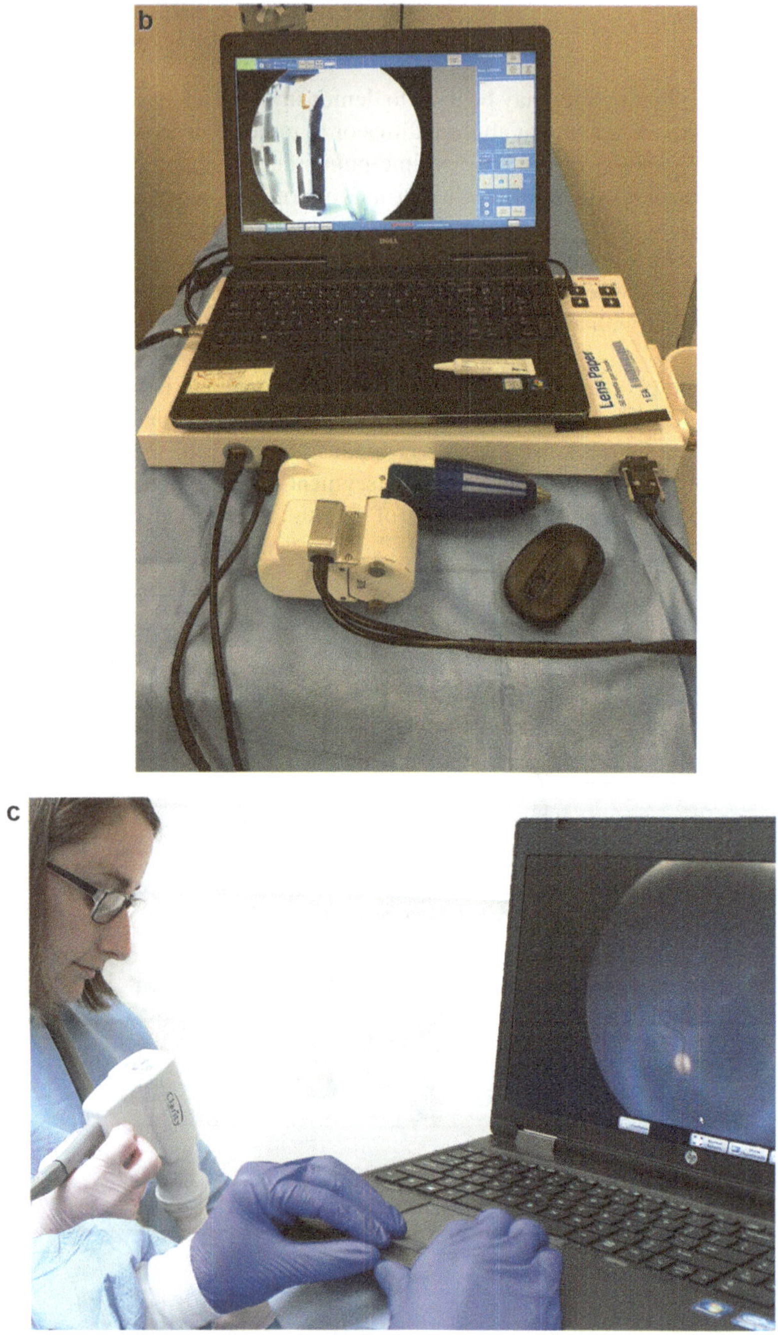

Fig. 1.15 (continued)

Genesis-D camera, RetCam, or Phoenix Micron IV and Micron X are suitable for most routine laboratory animal photography (Fig. 1.15). These cameras can be adapted for indirect ophthalmic photography, rodent fundus photography, and fluorescein angiography. In addition, alternate methods for fundus photography in small rodents have been described. The advantages of fundus photography are the ability to have a permanent stored record to compare potential study-related findings and, if indicated, to obtain an independent review by another ophthalmologist [9].

When obtaining photographs, the magnification and illumination settings should be standardized for all images. In addition, the eyes (left vs. right) should be photographed in the same order, and all photographs should be accompanied by an animal identification photograph, and a photographic log should be maintained as part of SOP.

Fluorescein Angiography

Fluorescein angiography is used to evaluate the vascular integrity of the intraocular arteriolar and venous vasculature. While it is most commonly used for examination of the retinal and choroidal vessels, it can be applied to iris vasculature as well. It is most frequently used in toxicology studies to evaluate a compound's effect on neovascularization. It has been applied to various laboratory animals with 10% sodium fluorescein most commonly used but with the use of indocyanine green also described [15–24].

The technique of fluorescein angiography requires sedation or anesthesia and pupil dilation [22]. The light excitable compound, fluorescein, is injected intravenously, and a series of timed images of the tissue of interest (chorioretinal, iris) are obtained. Complications associated with fluorescein injection may include extravasation and tissue irritation, vomiting, and anaphylaxis. An excitation filter (490 nm) and a barrier filter (520–520 nm) must be used on a fundus camera that is capable of taking multiple, rapid sequenced images. The Kowa Genesis-Df, RetCam Shuttle, Phoenix Micron X, and Heidelberg Spectralis cSLO are designed for fluorescein angiography and are portable (Fig. 1.15). Prior to injection, a baseline color image is obtained, and then sequential images are taken every 20 s. As the fluorescein fills the chorioretinal vasculature, various phases of vascular filling are described. They include the pre-arteriolar, retinal arteriolar, capillary, early venous, late venous, and recirculation. Abnormalities noted on fluorescein angiography may include vascular anomalies (aneurysms, neovascularization), blocked fluorescence, leakage of fluorescein, hypofluorescence, and hyperfluorescence.

Electroretinography/Visual Evoked Potential

Depending on the toxicologic study and the specific aspect of the visual system that may be affected, there are various electrophysiologic tests that are available to evaluate the retina and visual pathways. Electroretinography (ERG) is the measurement of the electrical potential generated by the retina when stimulated by light. The standard ERG is a full-field stimulation that provides information about the retina as a whole and is a mass response of the retinal pigment epithelium, photoreceptors, and inner retina [7]. For localized retinal evaluation, the multifocal electroretinogram (mfERG) and for evaluation of macular ganglion cells the pattern reversal electroretinogram (PERG) are indicated [7]. To evaluate the entire visual pathway from the retina to the visual cortex, a visual evoked potential (VEP) is the technique of choice [7]. Of these tests, the full-field ERG is most common for preclinical toxicologic testing. The ERG provides a noninvasive means of repeatedly assessing retinal function that in combination with indirect ophthalmoscopy and histology provide integrated assessment of retinal anatomy and function.

The ERG should be conducted in a standardized manner following pupil dilation, and there are internationally recognized protocols developed for human and canine ERGs that can serve as a study design guide [25, 26]. The conditions for obtaining a full-field ERG must be consistent with respect to room illumination, dark adaptation, flash intensity and frequency, and sedation or anesthetic used and dosage. Discussion of these details and protocols is provided elsewhere and is beyond the scope of this chapter [7, 25, 26].

Optical Coherence Tomography

Optical coherence tomography is a high-resolution, noninvasive imaging technique that can provide a real-time cross-sectional image of ocular structures, most commonly retina and optic nerve, at an axial resolution of 2–10 um [1, 27–29]. It can also be used to image the anterior segment of the eye. Like many advanced imaging techniques, it requires sedation or anesthesia, pupil dilation, and specialized equipment. When imaged by OCT, all individual retinal layers can be seen and their thickness measured to allow a quantitative and repeated evaluation over time. The optic disc can be measured with respect to the cup area, disc area, cup diameter, disc diameter, and rim area [28]. Evaluation of the anterior segment by OCT provides structural information of the cornea, anterior chamber, iris, and iridocorneal angle without the need for corneal contact as is required for ultrasound biomicroscopy (UBM) [28]. It also provides greater axial resolution than that provided by UBM [28]. The use of OCT in laboratory animals has been well described in a variety of species, and its use is increasing in animal models of human disease and preclinical trials [29, 30].

A recent advancement, spectral-domain OCT (SD-OCT), uses nonmechanical technology and is significantly faster than traditional OCT or time-domain OCT (TD-OCT) [30, 31]. SD-OCT simultaneously measures multiple wavelengths of

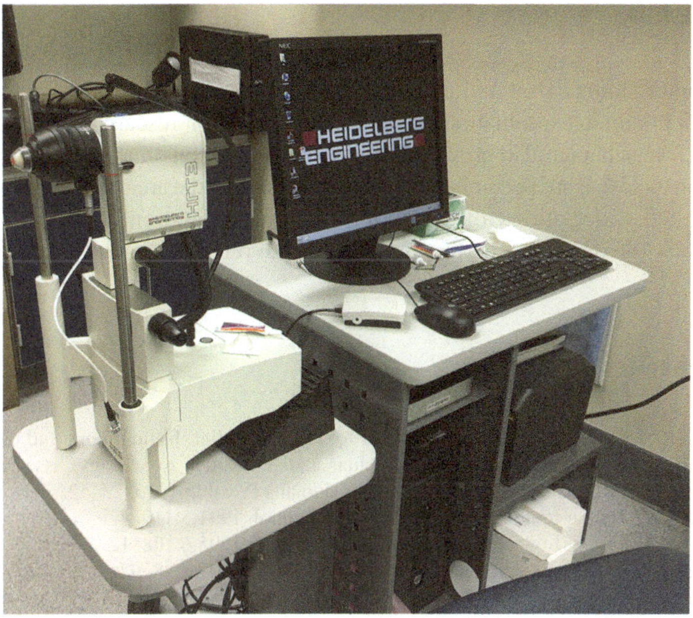

Fig. 1.16 Heidelberg Retina Tomograph (with Rostock Corneal Module) for imaging and analysis of the corneal endothelium

reflected light across a spectrum, hence the name spectral-domain. SD-OCT is 100 times faster than TD-OCT and acquires 70,000 + A-scans per second. The increased speed and number of scans translates into higher resolution.

Specular Microscopy

Specular microscopy provides in vivo, noninvasive imaging of the corneal endothelial cells [9, 32]. It can be performed using a contact or noncontact method. Once visualized, the corneal endothelial cells can be evaluated with regard to cell morphology and can be quantified as to the number of cells per mm [2]. Normal corneal endothelial cells are regular in arrangement and hexagonal in shape. Cells are evaluated for cell density, pleomorphism, and polymegethism. As cell counts vary by age of the animal and region of the cornea, these variables must be standardized using animals of the same age and examining the axial cornea. Animals must be sedated or anesthetized to obtain an accurate image, and automated systems are available that simplify the technique. FDA guidelines for specular microscopy in human clinical trials have been established, and these can be used as a starting point for preclinical study design [32]. Another option is to use an in vivo, high-resolution confocal microscope (Heidelberg Retina Tomograph with Rostock Corneal Module) for imaging and analysis of the corneal endothelium (Fig. 1.16).

Conclusion

This chapter summarized and emphasized the proper methods and techniques for routine ophthalmic examination of laboratory animals in research settings, such as at CROs. This chapter also provided overview information on advanced ophthalmic diagnostic tools that are becoming more commonplace in the area of ocular toxicology. For detailed descriptions of techniques and interpretation of these advanced diagnostics, please review pertinent articles in the reference list.

References

1. Munger RJ, Collins M. Assessing ocular toxicity potential: basic theory and techniques. In: Weir AB, Collins M, editors. Molecular and integrative toxicology: assessing ocular toxicology in laboratroy animals. New York: Humana Press; 2013. p. 23–52.
2. Novack GD. Ocular toxicology. Curr Opin Ophthalmol. 1994;5:110–4.
3. Novack GD. Ocular toxicology. Curr Opin Ophthalmol. 1995;6:108–12.
4. Novack GD. Ocular toxicology. Curr Opin Ophthalmol. 1997;8:88–92.
5. Santaella RM, Fraunfelder FW. Ocular adverse effects associated with systemic medications: recognition and management. Drugs. 2007;67:75–93.
6. Bill A. Blood circulation and fluid dynamics in the eye. Physiol Rev. 1975;55:383–417.
7. Ver Hoeve JN, Munger RJ, Gourley IM, et al. Emerging electrophysiological technologies for assessing ocular toxicity in laboratory animals. In: Weir AB, Collins M, editors. Molecular and integrative toxicology: assessing ocular toxicology in laboratroy animals. New York: Humana Press; 2013. p. 123–57.
8. Pereira FQ, Bercht BS, Soares MG, et al. Comparison of a rebound and an applanation tonometer for measuring intraocular pressure in normal rabbits. Vet Ophthalmol. 2011;14:321–6.
9. Nork TM, Rasmussen CA, Christian BJ, et al. Emerging imaging technologies for assessing ocular toxicity in laboratory animals. In: Weir AB, Collins M, editors. Molecular and integrative toxicology: assessing ocular toxicology in laboratroy animals. New York: Humana Press; 2013. p. 53–121.
10. Kontiola AI, Goldblum D, Mittag T, et al. The induction/impact tonometer: a new instrument to measure intraocular pressure in the rat. Exp Eye Res. 2001;73:781–5.
11. Goldblum D, Kontiola AI, Mittag T, et al. Non-invasive determination of intraocular pressure in the rat eye. Comparison of an electronic tonometer (TonoPen), and a rebound (impact probe) tonometer. Graefes Arch Clin Exp Ophthalmol. 2002;240:942–6.
12. Danias J, Kontiola AI, Filippopoulos T, et al. Method for the noninvasive measurement of intraocular pressure in mice. Investig Ophthalmol Vis Sci. 2003;44:1138–41.
13. Rowland JM, Potter DE, Reiter RJ. Circadian rhythm in intraocular pressure: a rabbit model. Curr Eye Res. 1981;1:169–73.
14. Hackett RB, McDonald TO. Ophthalmic toxicology and assessing ocular irritation. In: Marzulli FN, Maibach HI, editors. Dermatotoxicology. 5th ed. Washington, DC: Hemisphere Publishing Corp; 1996. p. 749–815.
15. DiLoreto D Jr, Grover DA, del Cerro C, et al. A new procedure for fundus photography and fluorescein angiography in small laboratory animal eyes. Curr Eye Res. 1994;13:157–61.
16. Satoh T, Yamaguchi K. Ocular fundus abnormalities detected by fluorescein and indocyanine green angiography in the Royal College of Surgeons dystrophic rat. Exp Anim. 2000;49:275–80.

17. Herren JI, Kunzelman KS, Vocelka C, et al. Angiographic and histological evaluation of porcine retinal vascular damage and protection with perfluorocarbons after massive air embolism. Stroke. 1998;29:2396–403.
18. Gelatt KN, Henderson JD, Steffen GR. Fluorescein angiography of the normal and diseased ocular fundi of the laboratory dog. J Am Vet Med Assoc. 1976;169:9.
19. Ninomiya H, Kuno H, Inagaki S. Vascular changes associated with chorioretinal and optic nerve colobomas in rats (Crj: CD(SD), IGS). Vet Ophthalmol. 2005;8:319–23.
20. Kommonen B, Koskinen L. Fluorescein angiography of the canine ocular fundus in ketamine-xylazine anesthesia. Acta Vet Scand. 1984;25:346–51.
21. Narfstrom K. Progressive retinal atrophy in the Abyssinian cat. Clinical characteristics. Investig Ophthalmol Vis Sci. 1985;26:193–200.
22. Gasthuys F, Pollet L, Simoens P, et al. Anaesthesia for fluorescein angiography of the ocular fundus in the miniature pig. Vet Res Commun. 1990;14:393–402.
23. Hyvarinen L, Flower RW. Indocyanine green fluorescence angiography. Acta Ophthalmol. 1980;58:528–38.
24. Flower RW. Injection technique for indocyanine green and sodium fluorescein dye angiography of the eye. Investig Ophthalmol. 1973;12:881–95.
25. Ekesten B, Komaromy AM, Ofri R, et al. Guidelines for clinical electroretinography in the dog: 2012 update. Doc Ophthalmol. 2013;127(2):79–87.
26. Marmor MF, Fulton AB, Holder GE, et al. ISCEV Standard for full-field clinical electroretinography (2008 update). Doc Ophthalmol. 2009;118:69–77.
27. Fujimoto JG, Pitris C, Boppart SA, et al. Optical coherence tomography: an emerging technology for biomedical imaging and optical biopsy. Neoplasia. 2000;2:9–25.
28. Gabriele ML, Wollstein G, Ishikawa H, et al. Optical coherence tomography: history, current status, and laboratory work. Investig Ophthalmol Vis Sci. 2011;52:2425–36.
29. McLellan GJ, Rasmussen CA. Optical coherence tomography for the evaluation of retinal and optic nerve morphology in animal subjects: practical considerations. Vet Ophthalmol. 2012;15(Suppl 2):13–28.
30. Huber G, Beck SC, Grimm C, et al. Spectral domain optical coherence tomography in mouse models of retinal degeneration. Investig Ophthalmol Vis Sci. 2009;50:5888–95.
31. Fleckenstein M, Charbel Issa P, Helb HM, et al. High-resolution spectral domain-OCT imaging in geographic atrophy associated with age-related macular degeneration. Investig Ophthalmol Vis Sci. 2008;49:4137–44.
32. McCarey BE, Edelhauser HF, Lynn MJ. Review of corneal endothelial specular microscopy for FDA clinical trials of refractive procedures, surgical devices, and new intraocular drugs and solutions. Cornea. 2008;27:1–16.

Chapter 2
Standard Operating Procedures for Common Laboratory Animal Ocular Procedures

Brian C. Gilger, Joshua T. Bartoe, J. Seth Eaton, and Ryan Boyd

Abstract In this chapter, we provide a basis for researchers, contract research laboratories, or other investigators to develop harmonized protocols for commonly performed ophthalmic procedures in laboratory animals and to assist in development of institutional standard operating procedure (SOP) documentation. Having similar protocols and SOPs among researchers and institutions will allow better comparison between studies and more efficient use of animals and enhance the quality of ocular research overall. The chapter is organized by procedure and animal species, including techniques such as intracameral, intravitreal, subconjunctival, retrobulbar, and subretinal injections.

Keywords Standard operating procedures · Laboratory animal · Ophthalmology · Ocular toxicology

Introduction

The goal of this chapter is to establish guidelines and provide a basis for researchers, contract research laboratories, or other investigators to develop harmonized protocols for commonly performed ophthalmic procedures in laboratory animals. This chapter can also be the start of developing institutional standard operating procedure (SOP) documentation. Having similar protocols and SOPs among

---

Endorsed by the American College of Veterinary Ophthalmologists (ACVO).

B. C. Gilger (✉)
Department of Clinical Sciences, North Carolina State University, Raleigh, NC, USA
e-mail: bgilger@ncsu.edu

J. T. Bartoe · R. Boyd
MPI Research, Mattawan, MI, USA
e-mail: joshua.bartoe@mpiresearch.com; ryan.boyd@mpiresearch.com

J. S. Eaton
Ocular Services On Demand (OSOD), LLC, Madison, WI, USA

B. C. Gilger et al. (eds.), *Standards for Ocular Toxicology and Inflammation*,
https://doi.org/10.1007/978-3-319-78364-2_2

researchers and institutions will allow better comparison between studies and more efficient use of animals and enhance the quality of ocular research overall. The chapter will be organized by procedure, and within each section is a description of how the technique differs among species used, where applicable. Furthermore, appropriate institutional animal use and monitoring should be obtained prior to initiating any study, and all studies should be conducted in adherence to the Association for Research in Vision and Ophthalmology Statement for the Use of Animals in Ophthalmic and Vision Research.

Aqueocentesis/Intracameral Injection

Intracameral (IC) injection (injection into the anterior chamber) is an increasingly utilized technique for administration of drugs or therapeutic devices to the anterior segment. Intracameral dosing can provide high concentration of a drug within the aqueous humor and adjacent structures, though residence time may be very brief due to turnover of aqueous humor [1]. Sustained-release IC implants are being investigated to enhance the delivery and efficacy of such drugs at their intended sites in the anterior segment [2, 3]. Possible complications of IC injection, however, include infectious endophthalmitis, cataract formation, and toxicity to local tissues including the corneal endothelium. When performing IC injections in animal models, the depth of the anterior chamber must also be considered as the narrow anterior chamber depth of some species may preclude administration of a certain volume or may not accommodate a solid injectable implant. For this reason, this route of drug administration is not commonly performed in mice and rats whose anterior chamber depths are comparatively narrow (0.45 and 0.71 mm, respectively) [4].

Aqueocentesis (AC) uses a very similar technique to IC injection, except that aqueous humor is removed. This is most commonly performed in laboratory animals to allow analysis of aqueous humor constituents (e.g., cytokines) or for drug analysis in pharmacokinetic studies. The procedure for IC injection or AC is similar in most laboratory species including rabbits, dogs, pigs, and nonhuman primates (NHPs). Prior to injection, animals should be anesthetized as appropriate for that species (Table 2.1). The pupils are dilated with 1% tropicamide HCL and 10% phenylephrine HCL, followed by application of a topical anesthetic such as 0.5% proparacaine HCL. A full aseptic ocular surface preparation should be performed using 5% betadine solution. Rabbits, dogs, and pigs are placed in lateral recumbency, and NHPs are placed in dorsal recumbency, adjacent to the edge of the operating table. The injector's wrists should be stabilized on the table edge or with towels or sandbags on either side of the animal's head. It is preferred that the injector use magnification, either with an operating microscope or 3.5 to 5× magnifying loupes. After the animal is positioned, a sterile, fenestrated drape may be placed over the animal and the eye. Only sterile instruments should be used to perform the IC injection. A wire eyelid speculum (or other suitable self-retaining speculum) is placed to provide adequate exposure of the eye. The eye is irrigated with sterile

Table 2.1 Anesthetics for laboratory animal species

Species	Injectable anesthetic	Dose	Inhalant anesthetics	Dose (%)
Mice/rats	Ketamine/xylazine Ketamine/dexmedetomidine	40–100 mg/kg/5–10 mg/kg IM or IP 50–75 mg/kg/0.25–1 mg/kg IP	Isoflurane	1–2
Rabbits	Ketamine/xylazine	25–50 mg/kg IM/5–10 mg/kg	Isoflurane	1–5
Dogs	Tiletamine/zolazepam (Telazol)	6.6–13.2 mg/kg IM	Isoflurane	1–3
Pigs	Tiletamine/zolazepam (Telazol)	1–6 mg/kg IM	Isoflurane	1–3
Primates	Ketamine/dexmedetomidine	5–10 mg/kg/0.01–0.02 mg/kg IM	Isoflurane	1–3

IM intramuscularly
IP intraperitoneal

saline or balanced salt solution (BSS). Intracameral injections are most easily performed using a dorsal or dorsotemporal approach, and the limbus should be fixated at a location immediately adjacent to the intended site of needle entry. Needle selection will depend on the properties of the injectate; however, the largest needle gauge of needle recommended for IC injection in large animals is a 27 g. Needles must be sharp to minimize the need for use of excessive force when introducing the needle as excessive force may result in uncontrolled globe entry and trauma to the corneal endothelium, iris, or anterior lens capsule. The needle insertion point should be in the peripheral clear cornea, approximately 1 mm anterior to the point of limbal fixation. The needle is introduced into the anterior chamber with its bevel facing upward (anterior), along a plane anterior to and parallel to the iris face. Once the needle is securely within the central/paracentral anterior chamber, the test article is slowly injected (or aqueous humor slowly withdrawn when performing AC). The needle is left in place for approximately 30 s to allow distribution of material and lessen reflux from the needle track; then the needle is slowly withdrawn. Immediately following removal of the needle, a sterile cotton-tipped applicator or ophthalmic surgical sponge is used to tamponade the needle insertion site. Following tamponade, a drop of broad-spectrum antibiotic can be administered topically to reduce the risk of postinjection endophthalmitis. Any adverse effects observed at the time of dosing or immediately thereafter should be recorded.

An injection volume of ≤50 uL is recommended in all species, as egress of the injectate from the needle insertion site will increase as the intraocular pressure elevates as dose volume administered increases. In rabbits, the cornea is comparatively thinner and biomechanically softer than in the human [5]. Therefore, egress of the injectate is more likely in this species, and postinjection tamponade should be performed for at least 30 s. Approximately 100 uL of aqueous humor can be safely aspirated from the eye of a rabbit, dog, or NHP (e.g., macaques). All AC, no matter how atraumatic, will result in 24–72 h of inflammation including the development of aqueous flare and hypotony [6–8]. Therefore, study protocols that require AC, especially repeat procedures, must be controlled for the development of postinjection uveitis.

Intravitreal Injection/Vitreocentesis

Intraocular injections of medications, especially intravitreal (IVT) injections, are routinely performed in human medicine to treat diseases of the ocular posterior segment. Direct IVT injection provides a high concentration of drug to the target tissue (e.g., choroid, retina, optic nerve) and bypasses nearly all ocular barriers. Reviews of the ocular pharmacokinetics and distribution of a variety of drugs have been published [9–12]. Furthermore, aspiration of vitreous humor (vitreocentesis) can be used in pharmacokinetic studies or for collection of vitreous samples for diagnostic testing (e.g., cytology and culture/sensitivity). However, IVT injections are subject to complications such as hemorrhage, postinjection endophthalmitis, cataract formation, elevated intraocular pressure, and local drug toxicity [13]; and aspirations, particularly when repeated, may carry similar risks for hemorrhage, endophthalmitis, and cataract formation, as well as structural damage to the retina (e.g., detachment). Despite these complications, there is increasing interest in the use of IVT injection therapy in many animal models, and therefore, the review of the procedure for common laboratory animal species is described, including their similarities and differences.

Mouse

Following general anesthesia (1–2% isoflurane or other suitable inhalant or injectable anesthetic) and dilation of pupils with 0.5% tropicamide and 2.5% phenylephrine, the animal is placed under an operating microscope, on a heating pad at 37 °C, and the eyes moistened with artificial tears [14]. A microscope coverslip can be placed on the cornea to improve the visibility of the fundus. The conjunctiva is removed at the location of the injection, and a scleral hole is made 2 mm posterior to the superior limbus using a sterile 30-G needle which is inserted 1.5 mm into the vitreous [15] at a 45° injection angle [14] and the position visualized in the vitreous via the operating microscope. This needle is removed, and through the previously made hole, a 33-G blunt-end needle is inserted 1.5 mm into the eye, and 1–2 uL of drug is injected slowly (i.e., 0.1 μL/s) [15]. Following injection, the needle can be left in place for up to a minute to minimize reflux and a topical antibiotic given for infection prophylaxis. Following injection, it is important to examine the eye (ophthalmoscopy ± optical coherence tomography [OCT]) for presence of drug in the vitreous and any complications (e.g., lens injury, hemorrhage, retinal damage).

Rat

The technique for IVT injection in the rat is similar to the mouse, except that larger volumes of injection (2–5 uL) can be performed [16–18]. Following general anesthesia and placement under an operating microscope, a sclerotomy is made 1–2 mm posterior to the superior-temporal limbus, and a 30-G Hamilton bevel-tip syringe needle is inserted into the vitreous at about a 45° angle to avoid contact with the lens. The injection is then made and the needle slowly withdrawn [17, 18]. Following injection, the eye should be inspected for presence of drug or complications, followed by application of a topical prophylactic antibiotic [18].

Rabbit

The rabbit is the most common species for which preclinical IVT injections are performed [9]. This is likely because the eye size and vitreous volume are large enough to minimize potential ocular damage commonly seen in mice following IVT injection, e.g., lens trauma. Unlike rodents, the lens-to-globe size ratio is smaller allowing a larger vitreous volume for injection. The lens-to-globe ratio, however, is larger than that seen in dogs, pigs, and primates; therefore, careful injections with avoidance of the lens injury during injection is important (Table 2.2). Furthermore, pharmacokinetic parameters in the human and rabbit eye correlate well and have comparable absolute values, despite some anatomical differences [9]. Therefore, the rabbit is commonly used for evaluation of IVT therapies in preclinical studies.

Prior to injection, rabbits should be anesthetized, such as with the use of intramuscular injection of ketamine and xylazine (25–50 mg/kg and 5–10 mg/kg, respectively) or inhalation of isoflurane (1–5%). As a caution, rabbits should be monitored closely when masked or in an induction chamber. Rabbits dislike the smell of isoflurane and may hold their breath for a duration sufficient to cause hypoxia and risk death. Following induction of general anesthesia, the eye to be injected is thoroughly irrigated with 5% betadine solution, allowing a 30s contact time for lid mar-

Table 2.2 Relative size of the anterior and vitreous chambers in common laboratory animals

	Mice	Rat	Rabbit	Dog	Pig	Primate (cynomolgus)
Anterior chamber depth (mm)	0.45	0.71	2.8	3.8 ± 0.1	2.13 ± 0.22	2.79 ± 0.27
Anterior chamber volume (μL)	4.4–5.9	13.6	287	770 ± 24	300	90–110
Vitreous thickness (mm)	0.59–0.71	1.4–1.5	7.1 ± 0.45	8.5	–	11.25 ± 0.51
Vitreous volume (μL)	5.3	13.4–13.6	1060	1700	2000–2700	1800–2000

gins and conjunctiva at the site of injection, and then irrigated with sterile 0.9% saline [19, 20]. The pupils are dilated with 1.0% tropicamide and 10% phenylephrine, followed by application of a topical anesthetic, such as 0.5% proparacaine HCL. The rabbit is placed in lateral recumbency approximately 5 cm from the edge of the table with forehead of the rabbit parallel to the edge. It is preferable that the person performing the injection or aspiration uses magnification, such as an operating microscope or 3.5 to 5× magnifying loupes. Following positioning of the rabbit, a sterile drape with a 2 cm diameter circular hole may be placed over the rabbit and eye. Sterile instruments are used to make the injection or aspiration. A wire lid speculum or other suitable lid speculum for the rabbit is placed to ensure adequate exposure of the eye. The limbus of the eye is grasped with small forceps, such as scleral fixation forceps or 0.3 mm Colibri forceps to stabilize the globe. For superior injections, the superotemporal or superomedial limbus is stabilized with the forceps; for inferior injections, the globe is stabilized at the inferior medial or lateral limbus, and the globe is then rotated superiorly to expose the injection site. Globe rotation may not be required for superior injections. Following globe stabilization and rotation, if required, the injection can be made. Depending on the injection material, the largest gauge of needle that can be used without substantial leakage or ocular damage is a 25-G needle. It is preferable that a 27 or smaller needle be used. Furthermore, the needles must be very sharp, because dull needles require greater force for insertion through the sclera which increases the chance for lens contact and other trauma. Whether the needle placement is superior or inferior, the insertion point is approximately 1.5–2.0 mm posterior to the limbus. This location is chosen to allow entry into the vitreous through the pars plana and avoid the ciliary processes and peripheral retina. A good landmark is just anterior to the insertion of the rectus muscle (superior or inferior). The needle should be directed toward the posterior pole at a relatively steep angle to the globe to avoid the lens. The bevel of the needle routinely is positioned anteriorly, but depending on the desired location of the injectate, the bevel can be positioned in any direction as long as it has a consistent positioning for all injections. An injection of up to 50 uL of volume can be made without substantial increase of the intraocular pressure. Injection volumes of up to 100 uL are possible, but adverse effects of this volume will depend on the drug and vehicle administered. Alternatively, larger volumes can be administered via two smaller injections, separated by approximately 10 min to allow for normalization of IOP. When aspiration is being performed, a volume of no more than 25 uL should be removed. Following removal of the test article or aspiration, the needle is slowly withdrawn. Once removed, a sterile swab or cellulose sponge should be placed over the injection site to temporarily tamponade the site and minimize leakage. This swab should be used for 10–30 s, with longer times used with larger needle sizes. Following swab removal, a drop of a topical antibiotic may be given to help prevent endophthalmitis [21] although use of a prophylactic antibiotic is not thought to prevent endophthalmitis in humans and may select for more virulent microorganisms [19, 20]. Following injection or aspiration, the eye and vitreous body should be inspected for location of therapeutic (if injected) and if there are any adverse effects (e.g., hemorrhage), and these observations are recorded.

Porcine/Canine

The IVT injection or aspiration procedure in dogs and pigs is similar to that described in the rabbit. Pigs or dogs need to be anesthetized for IVT injection. Prior to injection, eyes are dilated with a combination of 2.5% phenylephrine HCL and 1% tropicamide HCL, followed by topical application of 0.5% proparacaine HCL. The eyes are irrigated with 5% betadine solution followed by sterile saline, as described previously for rabbits. After a sterile lid speculum is inserted, a 27- to 30-G needle is inserted though the conjunctiva and sclera 3 mm (pigs) to 5–6 mm (dogs) posterior to the superior limbus and angled posterior to avoid contact with the lens [22]. Injection volumes can be as high as 50–100 uL [22, 23]. For most animals, it is recommended to split doses of 100 uL into two separate injections, separated by 10 min. This time interval between injections is based on serial IOPs performed in NHPs, rabbits, and dogs following IVT dose with 50 uL or less. In NHPs, IOP has normalized by 10 min (personal communication, Dr. Seth Eaton). Alternatively, a 50 uL aqueous humor paracentesis may be performed prior to a 100 uL IVT injection to prevent elevation of IOP. Once the needle is removed, a cotton-tipped applicator or cellulose sponge is placed over the scleral hole to minimize reflux and vitreous incarceration [22]. Following injection or aspiration, the eye and vitreous body should be inspected for location of therapeutic (if injected) and if there are any adverse effects (e.g., hemorrhage), and these parameters are recorded. After surgery, animals are treated with atropine 1%, an antibiotic ointment, and pain medication as needed [22, 23].

Nonhuman Primates

Nonhuman primates have a lens-to-globe ratio similar to humans, which is smaller than the laboratory animal species described above. Therefore, needle insertion for IVT injection or aspiration may occur at an angle more perpendicular to the ocular surface with less risk of lens damage. A double-plane tunnel injection technique has also been recommended in humans to reduce injectate reflux through the sclera following needle disinsertion [24–26]. Following general anesthesia (see Table 2.1) and topical application of 1% tropicamide and 2.5% phenylephrine, the animal is placed in dorsal recumbency near the edge of the operating table. Proparacaine HCL 0.5% is applied topically, and the conjunctival and corneal surface is disinfected using 5% betadine solution and sterile saline irrigation, as described previously. It is preferable that the person performing the injection or aspiration uses magnification, such as an operating microscope or 3.5–5× magnifying loupes. After insertion of a lid speculum, a 27- to 31-G needle is inserted 2–3 mm posterior to the superotemporal or inferotemporal limbus into the sclera at 15–30° angle directed toward the posterior pole of the globe. The needle angle is then increased to 45–60° as it passes through the sclera and inserted 4–6 mm into the mid-vitreous. Following injection, the needle angle is then increased to near 90° prior to removal, and the injection site is compressed with a cotton-tipped applicator, cellulose sponge, or forceps to prevent reflux. A topical antibiotic is administered immediately after the completion of injection to minimize endophthalmitis.

Subconjunctival Injection

Subconjunctival (SC) injections are performed to administer topical therapeutic agents such as antibiotics or corticosteroids to the ocular surface and anterior segment following ocular surgery. This route, however, is also commonly investigated as a site for the injection of sustained-release drug formulations or implants to prolong the effect of and enhance the efficacy of drugs to the ocular surface and anterior segment [27–29]. Complications of SC injections are rare but may include SC hemorrhage or inadvertent penetration of the sclera at the injection site. Due to their small globe size and thin conjunctival membranes, SC injections are not commonly performed in mice and rats.

The procedure for SC injection is similar in most laboratory species including rabbits, dogs, pigs, and NHPs. Prior to injection, animals should be anesthetized (see Table 2.1). A topical anesthetic such as 0.5% proparacaine HCL is applied to the ocular surface. Additional local conjunctival analgesia can be achieved by applying topical 2% lidocaine viscous gel to the intended site of injection using a cotton-tipped applicator for 1–2 min, followed by a thorough rinsing of the site with sterile saline or BSS. A full aseptic ocular surface preparation should be performed using 5% betadine solution. Rabbits, dogs, and pigs are commonly placed in lateral recumbency, and NHPs are commonly placed in dorsal recumbency. The injector's wrists should be stabilized on the table edge or with towels or sandbags on either side of the animal's head. It is preferred that the injector use magnification, either with an operating microscope or 3.5–5× magnifying loupes. After the animal is positioned, a sterile, fenestrated drape may be placed over the animal and the eye. Only sterile instruments should be used to perform the injection. A wire eyelid speculum (or other suitable self-retaining speculum) is placed to provide adequate exposure of the eye. The eye is irrigated with sterile saline or balanced salt solution (BSS). SC injections can be performed at any anatomical location around the globe, but the dorsal and lateral (temporal) regions are the easiest to access in most laboratory species as the presence of the nictitating membrane can complicate the injection procedure in rabbits, dogs, and pigs. Depending on the properties of the injectate, the largest gauge needle that should be used for SC injections is a 21-G needle, and the volume injected should not exceed 300 uL. Depending on the intended location and volume of injection, as well as the characteristics of the injectate, the injector may wish to use stay sutures or have a surgical assistant manipulate the globe's position to facilitate the injection procedure. Once the eye has been positioned and stabilized, the conjunctiva is gently grasped immediately adjacent to the intended site of needle entry. The needle is inserted through the conjunctiva adjacent to the point of fixation, at least 4–5 mm posterior to the limbus, with the bevel facing upward, in an orientation roughly parallel to the limbus. Care is taken to keep the needle orientation parallel to the underlying sclera to avoid inadvertent penetration of the sclera with the needle. The entire bevel of the needle must be in the SC space prior to injection. Once the test material is injected, the needle is slowly removed, and a cotton-tipped applicator or ophthalmic surgical sponge is used to compress the injection site.

Retrobulbar

Retrobulbar injections are commonly performed in both physician-based and veterinary ophthalmology to provide analgesia and/or akinesia of the eye and periocular region for ocular surgery [30–33]. While this route is less commonly employed for administration of therapeutic agents, it has been investigated as a possible route for administration of drugs to the optic nerve and posterior segment [34, 35], circumventing some of the anatomical and physiological barriers of the ocular surface and anterior segment [36–38]. Complications of retrobulbar injection are uncommon but may include retrobulbar hemorrhage, penetration/laceration of the globe and optic nerve, postinjection cellulitis or abscess, direct intravascular injection, intrathecal injection, and elicitation of the oculocardiac reflex. Due to their comparatively smaller orbital volume in relation to globe size, retrobulbar injections are not typically performed in mice and rats. Furthermore, rodent species and rabbits possess a vascular retrobulbar sinus that must be avoided to prevent severe retrobulbar hemorrhage [39]. In addition, the presence of this retrobulbar sinus may markedly influence pharmacokinetic results and lack translatability to larger laboratory species or human patients.

The procedure for retrobulbar injection can be performed similarly in most laboratory species including dogs, pigs, and NHPs. Prior to injection, animals should be anesthetized (see Table 2.1). A full aseptic ocular surface preparation should be performed using 5% betadine solution. Dogs and pigs are commonly placed in lateral recumbency, and NHPs are commonly placed in dorsal recumbency. The injector's wrists should be stabilized on the table edge or with towels or sandbags on either side of the animal's head. After the animal is positioned, a sterile, fenestrated drape may be placed over the animal and the eye, ensuring adequate exposure of the periocular region circumferentially. Only sterile instruments should be used to perform a retrobulbar injection. The eye is irrigated with sterile saline or balanced salt solution (BSS). In dogs and pigs, a sterile 1.5″ 22-G spinal needle is used, mechanically bent to create a slight (approximately 20°) angle halfway between the hub and tip. The needle is inserted through the inferior-lateral (temporal) bulbar conjunctiva, corresponding to a point on the adjacent inferior eyelid, approximately 1/3 of the distance from the lateral canthus to the medial canthus. The needle is advanced until a "popping" sensation is felt indicating penetration of the fascia of the orbital septum. Thereafter, it is directed slightly dorsally and medially (nasally) to point toward the orbital apex. After the needle is advanced 1–2 cm, the injection is performed slowly. The needle is left in place for 30–60 s and then slowly withdrawn along the same path that it was introduced. The volume administered in a single injection should not exceed 2 mL.

Subretinal Injections

Subretinal (SR) injections are often required for delivery of drug, gene, or cell therapy products, targeted to treat outer retinal conditions of RPE or photoreceptor dysfunction or loss. The SR injection procedure is technically challenging, particularly in animal models of retinal degeneration, where the structural integrity of the retina may be compromised. Protocols for SR injection may vary based on the location of the targeted retinal cell population, the properties of the injectate used, and species selected for the investigation.

Rodents

There are many published protocols describing various techniques for SR injection in both rats and mice [40–44]. Injections can be performed in both neonates and adults, with injection volumes ranging from 0.5 uL in mice up to 10 uL in rats. The primary risk of SR injection in rodents is dependent upon the approach, with anterior approaches having the highest potential for lens damage and posterior approaches risking choroidal hemorrhage. These procedures can be performed with or without direct visualization of the injection, although regardless of the technique used, an operating or dissection microscope is required for the approach. Following general anesthesia (1–2% isoflurane or other suitable inhalant or injectable anesthetic) (see Table 2.1) and dilation of pupils with 0.5–1% tropicamide and 2.5% phenylephrine, the animal is placed under an operating microscope on a heating pad at 37–40 °C, and the eyes moistened with artificial tears [14]. The globe can be manually proptosed in mice to aid in visualization; however rats often require a speculum or suture placed behind the globe equator. A microscope coverslip can be placed on the cornea to improve the visibility of the fundus if direct visualization is utilized. Corneal approaches do not require any dissection, while limbal or posterior approaches may require dissection of conjunctiva and Tenon's capsule. A beveled needle as large as 27 G may be used to create the initial sclerotomy or corneal puncture, while a smaller approximately 33-G needle or a pulled glass pipette is used for the injection. The injection needle is placed either through the retina from an anterior approach or through the sclera, choroid, and retinal pigment epithelium from a posterior approach, and the injectate is delivered into the SR space slowly to induce a retinal detachment. Up to 100% of the retina can be detached, depending on volume of injectate used. If direct visualization is not utilized for the injection procedure, it is important to examine the eye using indirect ophthalmoscopy, fundus photography, or advanced imaging such as OCT to ensure delivery of injectate into the SR space and evaluate for damage to the lens, retina, or choroid.

Large Animals

Placement of a SR injection often has to be carefully considered in large animal models, as the goal is to deposit the injectate within a retinal region containing sufficient densities of the targeted cell population. This is a critical aspect of the injection procedure, since the injectate does not typically exhibit significant lateral spread beyond the margins of the induced retinal detachment [45]. Another factor that must be considered for SR injection is anatomical differences in location of the pars plana and the lens-to-globe ratio between large animal species. As stated previously, rabbits have a large lens-to-globe ratio and an anteriorly placed pars plana, making surgical approach to the entire retina from one scleral port extremely difficult. On the other end of the spectrum, nonhuman primates have a smaller lens-to-globe ratio and a more posterior pars plana, making surgical access to the retina very straightforward. Other than these considerations, the procedure for SR injection is similar across large animal species, and a standard protocol commonly involves the following: animals should be placed under general anesthesia. The eye to be injected is positioned facing upward and thoroughly irrigated with 5% betadine solution and immediately irrigated with sterile 0.9% saline. The pupils are dilated with 1.0% tropicamide and 10% phenylephrine, followed by application of a topical anesthetic, such as 0.5% proparacaine HCL. After positioning and antiseptic preparation of the eye, a sterile drape with a 2 cm diameter circular hole may be placed over the eye. Sterile instruments, an operating microscope with sterile handles, and a vitrectomy lens must be used. A wire lid speculum is placed to ensure adequate exposure of the eye, and a lateral canthotomy is often necessary to facilitate exposure of the superior and temporal pars plana and placement of transscleral cannula ports. These ports range in size from 20 to 27 G; valved cannulas abrogate the need for placement and removal of cannula plugs. For larger cannulas, a conjunctival peritomy is necessary to expose the sclera where cannula placement will occur, while smaller G cannulas can be placed in a sutureless manner through the intact conjunctiva. After measuring from the limbus to mark the pars plana, bipolar cautery may be used over the sites of scleral cannula placement to decrease intraocular hemorrhage. The temporal or superior quadrants of the eye are most commonly used for placement of the transscleral cannulas, which are inserted using a microvitreoretinal blade trocar angled toward the posterior pole of the globe to avoid lens damage. In dogs, which possess a tapetum, SR injections may be accomplished using only one transscleral cannula for the injection device and the surgical microscope as a light source. Atapetal species require the placement of a second cannula for insertion of a handheld light source into the globe. If vitrectomy is required prior to SR injection, a third cannula is placed, with a pre-placed 7-0 or 8-0 Vicryl suture, to facilitate irrigation of the posterior segment during the procedure and maintain intraocular pressure. Vitrectomy is frequently used to create space for the SR bleb to form during injection, although an aqueous humor paracentesis can also be performed for this purpose. Following completion of vitrectomy or aqueous paracentesis, a SR injection device is inserted through one of the transscleral cannulas. Many options exist for SR injection devices; most consist of a rigid outer cannula that matches the transscleral cannula size, with an extendable or fixed 38-41SC inner flexible injection cannula [46, 47]. This cannula is extended until the tip makes contact with the inner retinal surface. Proximity of the tip to the retinal surface is gauged by the relationship of the shadow cast by the injection cannula and the visualized cannula tip, coming closer together as the tip approaches the retinal surface. The tip should be placed on the retinal surface in a manner that occludes the bore of the cannula, so the resulting injection of fluid creates a retinotomy. In the author's experience, it is beneficial to place the cannula tip adjacent to, but not directly over, a retinal vessel to stabilize the tip during initiation of the injection. The injectate is then very slowly pushed through the cannula by a surgical assistant or automated injector controlled by the surgeon. As the SR bleb forms, the injection cannula should be carefully retracted but maintained within the retinotomy site during the entirety of the injection to prevent reflux of injectate. Once the entire dose volume is administered, the injection device is removed, and each transscleral cannula may be removed and sutured with 7-0 or 8-0 Vicryl, if required, and the infusion port is removed last with immediate tightening of the pre-placed suture. If conjunctival peritomy and lateral canthotomy were performed, these are then sutured closed. Postoperative treatment should include a combination of local and systemic anti-inflammatory and antibiotic therapy.

Rabbit

The rabbit is not a common model used for SR injection studies, in part due to their having a thinner retina than dogs or nonhuman primates, as well as a report of outer retinal degeneration following a 50 uL injection of phosphate-buffered saline [48]. Specific considerations when performing rabbit SR injections include an anteriorly positioned pars plana, requiring transscleral cannula placement only 1–2 mm posterior to the limbus [48, 49]. This, along with their large lens-to-globe ratio, makes the approach for SR injection challenging. In the authors' experience, it is much easier to initiate a SR injection in rabbits by placing the injection cannula immediately inferior to the optic nerve and myelinated vascular arcades, as these regions of the retina are thicker and tend to be more stable during SR bleb formation (J. Bartoe, personal communication).

Porcine/Canine

Both pigs and dogs are more commonly utilized for SR injection studies than rabbits. Pigs have large globes and a cone-rich retina, making them suitable models for many gene and cell therapy studies [50–52]. Dogs are a valuable gene therapy model due to a large number of naturally occurring heritable retinal degenerations that mimic the phenotype and genotype of human retinal dystrophies [53, 54]. The SR injection procedures in both species are straightforward as described above, with placement of transscleral ports 3–3.5 mm posterior to the limbus in pigs and 5–6 mm posterior to the limbus in the temporal and superior quadrants of dogs [50, 51].

Nonhuman Primate

The nonhuman primate has a nearly identical retinal anatomy to humans, most notably presence of a macula containing a central fovea made up exclusively of cone photoreceptors. Because of this, NHPs are regularly used for definitive safety studies during preclinical drug development. SR injection procedures in NHP can be performed as described above; however there are often modifications made based on the test material properties and targeted cell population. Reliable SR injection within the macular region is more difficult than peripheral injections, with risk of creating a macular hole at the site of the fovea during injection [47, 55]. When performed carefully, SR injections in NHPs have little effect on long-term functional or anatomical outcomes [56, 57]. Transscleral cannulas may be placed 2–3 mm posterior to the limbus during the surgical approach in cynomolgus macaques, the most common NHP species used for biomedical research [56–58].

Globe/Tissue Dissection for Ocular Drug Analysis and Pharmacokinetics

Proper sample collection is critical for ocular bioanalytical studies. Improper sample collection procedures can result in cross-contamination of tissues or fluids which will compromise the value of even the best bioanalytical techniques [59].

The biological ocular barriers that stop foreign substances including drugs from penetrating eyes or traveling across various tissues within the eye are destroyed immediately upon euthanasia of the animal, allowing drugs to equilibrate across tissues within the eye. To prevent this equilibration, eyes need to be enucleated immediately upon euthanasia and flash frozen in liquid nitrogen or in a dry ice/alcohol bath as soon as possible. The eyes must be maintained in a frozen state during dissection to prevent or minimize drug diffusion to adjacent tissues.

As mentioned previously, ocular tissues contain several drug-metabolizing enzymes. These may provide a challenge for the bioanalyst in that they must be prevented from acting on prodrug or active drug after the sample is collected. Therefore, before undertaking a study, it is important to determine how to stabilize prodrugs or metabolically unstable drugs and metabolites in collected samples. It may be necessary to add a known amount of modifier (antioxidant, protease inhibitor, or esterase inhibitor as the case may be) to the vials prior to dissection and sample collection.

During eye dissection, cross-contamination of ocular tissues must be avoided. Taking certain precautions during sample collection will help in this regard. If the samples are being collected after systemic exposure, the animals may need to be perfused with chilled saline solution before necropsy to avoid contamination from blood since some eye tissues (choroid, conjunctiva) are highly vascularized structures. If the samples are being collected after topical administration, the enucleated eye ball can be rinsed in cold buffer such as phosphate-buffered saline (PBS) followed by flash freezing of the eye. If several groups of animals are to be euthanized in a day, the placebo group should always be the first one to be euthanized and/or dissected followed by the low-dose group with the longest time point ahead of shorter time points, followed by the higher-dosed groups in a similar fashion. It is also essential to keep instruments clean during dissection to avoid cross-contamination of the various eye tissues.

The technique for eye dissection should be practiced using cadaver eyes from rabbit or another model animal before dissecting ocular tissues from actual study samples. The procedure and sequence for ocular tissue collection in rabbits is briefly described in this section. All equipment required during surgery, dry ice/alcohol bath, and pre-labeled/pre-weighed vials need to be arranged prior to euthanasia. Eyes are enucleated as soon as possible following euthanasia, and the eyeball should be quickly rinsed in cold buffer, blotted dry, and immediately flash frozen. If needed, eyelids, conjunctiva, and lacrimal glands are then collected and frozen at −80 °C. Dissection of the frozen eye can be performed immediately or on the day of collection or at a later date as long as the eye remains frozen at −80 °C. The frozen eye is placed on a cooled ceramic tile to avoid thawing of the eye during dissection. In order to prevent cross-contamination of ocular tissues, instruments should be thoroughly rinsed with PBS followed by methanol followed by PBS and blotted dry (beakers of PBS and methanol need to be placed adjacent to dissection area for rinsing of instruments). The eyeball is separated in half using a long razor blade (a new blade is to be used for each eye), typically into a dorsal and ventral half. The frozen aqueous humor is removed first and is placed into its labeled vial. The cornea sections are removed next, followed by lens and vitreous humor. The iris and ciliary body are usually removed together followed by the retina and choroid. The remaining sclera fragments are then placed in a vial. Since collected ocular tissue samples are very small in weight/volume, the entire sample is usually processed for drug quantification. It is therefore highly recommended that at the in-life facility, samples are collected in pre-weighed, pre-labeled vials and weighed again prior to storage under frozen conditions. The balance used for weighing samples needs to be calibrated prior to its use and must be able to weigh ocular tissues accurately in the mg range. The weight data need to be provided to the bioanalytical laboratory along with the samples as the analytical laboratory will rely on the information provided by the in-life facility to calculate concentrations (ng/g) in various ocular tissues. All samples are stored frozen (−80 °C) until analysis. If the bioanalytical laboratory is at a different location, samples need to be shipped frozen over dry ice using an overnight courier. The shipment should be made only Monday through Wednesday so as to avoid thawing of samples if held over the weekend.

Conclusions

The goal of this chapter was to establish guidelines and provide a basis for researchers, contract research laboratories, or other investigators to develop harmonized protocols for commonly performed ophthalmic procedures in laboratory animals. This chapter can be used as the basis for developing institutional standard operating procedure (SOP) documentation. Having similar protocols and SOPs among researchers and institutions will allow better comparison of studies and more efficient use of animals in research and overall enhance ocular research.

Acknowledgments The authors thank Justin Prater and David Culp of Powered Research for their assistance.

References

1. Urtti A. Challenges and obstacles of ocular pharmacokinetics and drug delivery. Adv Drug Deliv Rev. 2006;58(11):1131–5. https://doi.org/10.1016/j.addr.2006.07.027.
2. Walters TR, Lee SS, Goodkin ML, Whitcup SM, Robinson MR. Bimatoprost sustained-release implants for glaucoma therapy: 6-month results from a phase I/II clinical trial. Am J Ophthalmol. 2017;175:137–47. https://doi.org/10.1016/j.ajo.2016.11.020.
3. Aref AA. Sustained drug delivery for glaucoma: current data and future trends. Curr Opin Ophthalmol. 2016;25(2):112–7. https://doi.org/10.1097/ICU.0000000000000334.
4. Bawa G, Tkatchenko TV, Avrutsky I, Tkatchenko AV. Variational analysis of the mouse and rat eye optical parameters. Biomed Opt Express. 2013;4(11):2585–95. https://doi.org/10.1364/BOE.4.002585.
5. Thomasy SM, Raghunathan VK, Winkler M, et al. Elastic modulus and collagen organization of the rabbit cornea: epithelium to endothelium. Acta Biomater. 2014;10(2):785–91. https://doi.org/10.1016/j.actbio.2013.09.025.
6. Kulkarni PS. The role of endogenous eicosanoids in rabbit-intraocular inflammation. J Ocul Pharmacol. 1991;7(3):227–41.
7. Jampel HD, Brown A, Roberts A, Koya P, Quigley H. Effect of paracentesis upon the blood-aqueous barrier of cynomolgus monkeys. Investig Ophthalmol Vis Sci. 1992;33:165–71.
8. Allbaugh RA, Roush JK, Rankin AJ, Davidson HJ. Fluorophotometric and tonometric evaluation of ocular effects following aqueocentesis performed with needles of various sizes in dogs. Am J Vet Res. 2011;72(4):556–61. https://doi.org/10.2460/ajvr.72.4.556.

9. del Amo EM, Urtti A. Rabbit as an animal model for intravitreal pharmacokinetics: clinical predictability and quality of the published data. Exp Eye Res. 2015;137:111–24. https://doi.org/10.1016/j.exer.2015.05.003.
10. del Amo EM, Rimpelä A-K, Heikkinen E, et al. Pharmacokinetic aspects of retinal drug delivery. Prog Retin Eye Res. 2016;57:134–85. https://doi.org/10.1016/j.preteyeres.2016.12.001.
11. Del Amo EM, Vellonen KS, Kidron H, Urtti A. Intravitreal clearance and volume of distribution of compounds in rabbits: in silico prediction and pharmacokinetic simulations for drug development. Eur J Pharm Biopharm. 2015;95:215–26. https://doi.org/10.1016/j.ejpb.2015.01.003.
12. Peyman GA, Lad EM, Moshfeghi DM. Intravitreal injection of therapeutic agents. Retina. 2008;29(7):875–912. https://doi.org/10.1097/IAE.0b013e3181a94f01.
13. Falavarjani KG, Nguyen QD. Adverse events and complications associated with intravitreal injection of anti-VEGF agents: a review of literature. Eye. 2013;27(7):787–94. https://doi.org/10.1038/eye.2013.107.
14. Hombrebueno JR, Luo C, Guo L, Chen M, Xu H. Intravitreal injection of normal saline induces retinal degeneration in the C57BL/6J mouse. Transl Vis Sci Technol. 2014;3(2):3. https://doi.org/10.1167/tvst.3.2.3.
15. Da Costa R, Röger C, Segelken J, Barben M, Grimm C, Neidhardt J. A novel method combining vitreous aspiration and intravitreal AAV2/8 injection results in retina-wide transduction in adult mice. Investig Ophthalmol Vis Sci. 2016;57(13):5326–34. https://doi.org/10.1167/iovs.16-19701.
16. Gal-Or O, Dotan A, Dachbash M, et al. Bevacizumab clearance through the iridocorneal angle following intravitreal injection in a rat model. Exp Eye Res. 2016;145:412–6. https://doi.org/10.1016/j.exer.2016.02.006.
17. Dureau P, Bonnel S, Menasche M, Dufier JL, Abitbol M. Quantitative analysis of intravitreal injections in the rat. Curr Eye Res. 2001;22(1):74–7. https://doi.org/10.1076/ceyr.22.1.74.6974.
18. Xie Z, Chen F, Wu X, et al. Safety and efficacy of intravitreal injection of recombinant erythropoietin for protection of photoreceptor cells in a rat model of retinal detachment. Eye. 2012;26(1):144–52. https://doi.org/10.1038/eye.2011.254.
19. Merani R, Hunyor AP. Endophthalmitis following intravitreal anti-vascular endothelial growth factor (VEGF) injection: a comprehensive review. Int J Retina Vitreous. 2015;1(1):9. https://doi.org/10.1186/s40942-015-0010-y.
20. Avery RL, Bakri SJ, Blumenkranz MS, et al. Intravitreal injection technique and monitoring: updated guidelines of an expert panel. Retina. 2014;34(Suppl 1):S1–S18. https://doi.org/10.1097/IAE.0000000000000399.
21. Kowalski RP, Romanowski EG, Mah FS, Yates KA, Gordon YJ. Topical 0.5% moxifloxacin prevents endophthalmitis in an intravitreal injection rabbit model. J Ocul Pharmacol Ther. 2008;24(1):1–7. https://doi.org/10.1089/jop.2007.0071.
22. Olsen TW, Feng X, Wabner K, Csaky K, Pambuccian S, Cameron JD. Pharmacokinetics of pars plana intravitreal injections versus microcannula suprachoroidal injections of bevacizumab in a porcine model. Investig Ophthalmol Vis Sci. 2011;52(7):4749–56. https://doi.org/10.1167/iovs.10-6291.
23. Abarca EM, Salmon JH, Gilger BC. Effect of choroidal perfusion on ocular tissue distribution after intravitreal or suprachoroidal injection in an arterially perfused ex vivo pig eye model. J Ocul Pharmacol Ther. 2013;29(8):715–22. https://doi.org/10.1089/jop.2013.0063.
24. Ozkaya A, Alkin Z, Celik U, et al. Comparing the effects of three different intravitreal injection techniques on vitreous reflux and intraocular pressure. J Ocul Pharmacol Ther. 2013;29:325–9. https://doi.org/10.1089/jop.2012.0144.
25. Rodrigues EB, Grumann A, Penha FM, et al. Effect of needle type and injection technique on pain level and vitreal reflux in intravitreal injection. J Ocul Pharmacol Ther. 2011;27(2):197–203. https://doi.org/10.1089/jop.2010.0082.
26. De Stefano VS, Abechain JJ, de Almeida LF, et al. Experimental investigation of needles, syringes and techniques for intravitreal injections. Clin Exp Ophthalmol. 2011;39(3):236–42. https://doi.org/10.1111/j.1442-9071.2010.02447.x.

27. Tansey G, Yuan P, Bungay PM, Lutz RJ, Robinson MR, et al. Preclinical evaluation of a novel episcleral cyclosporine implant for ocular graft-versus-host disease. Investig Ophthalmol Vis Sci. 2005;46(2):655–62.
28. Jessen BA, MHI S, Kaur H, et al. Safety assessment of subconjunctivally implanted devices containing latanoprost in Dutch-belted rabbits. J Ocul Pharmacol Ther. 2013;29(6):574–85. https://doi.org/10.1089/jop.2012.0190.
29. Ang M, Ng X, Wong C, et al. Evaluation of a prednisolone acetate-loaded subconjunctival implant for the treatment of recurrent uveitis in a rabbit model. PLoS One. 2014;9(5):e97555. https://doi.org/10.1371/journal.pone.0097555.
30. Tejedor J. Anesthesia for small-incision cataract surgery. In: Manual small incision cataract surgery. Cham: Springer; 2016. p. 35–47.
31. Zundert VA, Kumar C, Jankovic D. Regional anesthesia in ophthalmology. In: Regional nerve blocks in anesthesia and pain therapy. Cham: Springer; 2015. p. 81–98.
32. Shilo-Benjamini Y, Pascoe PJ, Maggs DJ, Kass PH, Wisner ER. Retrobulbar and peribulbar regional techniques in cats: a preliminary study in cadavers. Vet Anaesth Analg. 2013;40(6):623–31. https://doi.org/10.1111/vaa.12060.
33. Accola PJ, Bentley E, Smith LJ, Forrest LJ, Baumel CA, Murphy CJ. Development of a retrobulbar injection technique for ocular surgery and analgesia in dogs. J Am Vet Med Assoc. 2006;229(2):220–5. https://doi.org/10.2460/javma.229.2.220.
34. Raghava S, Hammond M, Kompella UB. Periocular routes for retinal drug delivery. Expert Opin Drug Deliv. 2004;1(1):99–114. https://doi.org/10.1517/17425247.1.1.99.
35. Geroski DH, Edelhauser HF. Drug delivery for posterior segment eye disease. Investig Ophthalmol Vis Sci. 2000;41(5):961–4.
36. Okada AA, Wakabayashi T, Morimura Y, et al. Trans-Tenon's retrobulbar triamcinolone infusion for the treatment of uveitis. Br J Ophthalmol. 2003;87(8):968–71. https://doi.org/10.1136/bjo.87.8.968.
37. Sen HN, Vitale S, Gangaputra SS, et al. Periocular corticosteroid injections in uveitis: effects and complications. Ophthalmology. 2014;121(11):2275–86. https://doi.org/10.1016/j.ophtha.2014.05.021.
38. Waite D, Wang Y, Jones D, Stitt A, Raj Singh TR. Posterior drug delivery via periocular route: challenges and opportunities. Ther Deliv. 2017;8(8):685–99. https://doi.org/10.4155/tde-2017-0097.
39. Davis FA. The anatomy and histology of the eye and orbit of the rabbit. Trans Am Ophthalmol Soc. 1929;27:400.2–441.
40. Timmers AM, Zhang H, Squitieri A, Gonzalez-Pola C. Subretinal injections in rodent eyes: effects on electrophysiology and histology of rat retina. Mol Vis. 2001;7:131–7.
41. Qi Y, Dai X, Zhang H, et al. Trans-corneal subretinal injection in mice and its effect on the function and morphology of the retina. PLoS One. 2015;10(8):e0136523. https://doi.org/10.1371/journal.pone.0136523.
42. Wert KJ, Skeie JM, Davis RJ, Tsang SH, Mahajan VB. Subretinal injection of gene therapy vectors and stem cells in the perinatal mouse eye. J Vis Exp. 2012;(69):4286. https://doi.org/10.3791/4286.
43. Park SW, Kim JH, Park WJ, Kim JH. Limbal approach-subretinal injection of viral vectors for gene therapy in mice retinal pigment epithelium. J Vis Exp. 2015;(102):e53030. https://doi.org/10.3791/53030.
44. Westenskow PD, Kurihara T, Bravo S, et al. Performing subretinal injections in rodents to deliver retinal pigment epithelium cells in suspension. J Vis Exp. 2015;(95):52247. https://doi.org/10.3791/52247.
45. Bruewer AR, Mowat FM, Bartoe JT, Boye SL, Hauswirth WW, Petersen-Jones SM. Evaluation of lateral spread of transgene expression following subretinal AAV-mediated gene delivery in dogs. PLoS One. 2013;8(4):e60218. https://doi.org/10.1371/journal.pone.0060218.
46. Komáromy AM, Varner SE, De Juan E, Acland GM, Aguirre GD. Application of a new subretinal injection device in the dog. Cell Transplant. 2006;15(6):511–9. https://doi.org/10.3727/000000006783981701.

47. Xue K, Groppe M, Salvetti AP, MacLaren RE. Technique of retinal gene therapy: delivery of viral vector into the subretinal space. Eye. 2017;31(9):1308–16. https://doi.org/10.1038/eye.2017.158.
48. Bartuma H, Petrus-Reurer S, Aronsson M, Westman S, André H, Kvanta A. In vivo imaging of subretinal bleb-induced outer retinal degeneration in the rabbit. Investig Ophthalmol Vis Sci. 2015;56(4):2423–30. https://doi.org/10.1167/iovs.14-16208.
49. Hirata M, Yasukawa T, Wiedemann P, et al. Fundus autofluorescence and fate of glycoxidized particles injected into subretinal space in rabbit age-related macular degeneration model. Graefes Arch Clin Exp Ophthalmol. 2009;247(7):929–37. https://doi.org/10.1007/s00417-009-1070-1.
50. Monés J, Leiva M, Peña T, et al. A swine model of selective geographic atrophy of outer retinal layers mimicking atrophic AMD: a phase I escalating dose of subretinal sodium iodate. Investig Ophthalmol Vis Sci. 2016;57(10):3974–83. https://doi.org/10.1167/iovs.16-19355.
51. Mussolino C, della Corte M, Rossi S, et al. AAV-mediated photoreceptor transduction of the pig cone-enriched retina. Gene Ther. 2011;18(7):637–45. https://doi.org/10.1038/gt.2011.3.
52. Koss MJ, Falabella P, Stefanini FR, et al. Subretinal implantation of a monolayer of human embryonic stem cell-derived retinal pigment epithelium: a feasibility and safety study in Yucatán minipigs. Graefes Arch Clin Exp Ophthalmol. 2016;254(8):1553–65. https://doi.org/10.1007/s00417-016-3386-y.
53. Petersen-Jones SM, Komáromy AM. Dog models for blinding inherited retinal dystrophies. Hum Gene Ther Clin Dev. 2015;26(1):15–26. https://doi.org/10.1089/humc.2014.155.
54. Acland GM, Aguirre GD, Ray J, et al. Gene therapy restores vision in a canine model of childhood blindness. Nat Genet. 2001;28:92–5. https://doi.org/10.1038/ng0501-92.
55. Campochiaro PA, Lauer AK, Sohn EH, et al. Lentiviral vector gene transfer of endostatin/angiostatin for macular degeneration (GEM) study. Hum Gene Ther. 2017;28(1):99–111. https://doi.org/10.1089/hum.2016.117.
56. Ochakovski GA, Peters T, Michalakis S, et al. Subretinal injection for gene therapy does not cause clinically significant outer nuclear layer thinning in normal primate foveae. Investig Ophthalmol Vis Sci. 2017;58(10):4155–60. https://doi.org/10.1167/iovs.17-22402.
57. Nork TM. Functional and anatomic consequences of subretinal dosing in the cynomolgus macaque. Arch Ophthalmol. 2012;130(1):65. https://doi.org/10.1001/archophthalmol.2011.295.
58. Lai CM, Shen WY, Brankov M, et al. Long-term evaluation of AAV-mediated sFlt-1 gene therapy for ocular neovascularization in mice and monkeys. Mol Ther. 2005;12(4):659–68. https://doi.org/10.1016/j.ymthe.2005.04.022.
59. Gilger BC. Ocular pharmacology and toxicology. Arch Ophthalmol. 1967;78(4):534–62. https://doi.org/10.1001/archopht.1967.00980030536023.

Chapter 3
Harmonization of Lesion Nomenclature in Laboratory Animals

Joshua T. Bartoe, Cynthia S. Cook, Martin Bussieres, Robert J. Munger, and Michael H. Brown

Abstract The goal of this chapter is to provide consensus for the harmonization of preclinical terminology for ultimate adoption on studies submitted to US Food and Drug Administration (FDA) and other global regulatory agencies. Included is a list of descriptive-based terminology for anatomical subsections of the eye with associated definitions and synonyms. We are recommending use of this harmonized terminology for description of common lesions observed spontaneously or associated with test article-induced changes. The tables provided contain listings for all necessary base-root lesions, while recommended modifiers are addressed in the section text. Additionally, there are representative images for selected lesions to provide the reader specific examples of the ocular changes they may encounter on ophthalmology examinations.

Keywords Terminology · Ocular lesions · Laboratory animal · Ocular toxicology · Harmonization

---

Endorsed by the American College of Veterinary Ophthalmologists (ACVO).

J. T. Bartoe (✉)
MPI Research, Mattawan, MI, USA
e-mail: Joshua.Bartoe@mpiresearch.com

C. S. Cook
Veterinary Vision, Inc., San Carlos, CA, USA
e-mail: Cook1@VeterinaryVision.com

M. Bussieres
V&O Services Inc., Saint-Lazare, QC, Canada
e-mail: mb@eyelab.ca

R. J. Munger
Animal Ophthalmology Clinic, Dallas, TX, USA
e-mail: eyedvm@aol.com

M. H. Brown
Animal Eye Center of New Jersey, Little Falls, NJ, USA
e-mail: muro127@aol.com

B. C. Gilger et al. (eds.), *Standards for Ocular Toxicology and Inflammation*,
https://doi.org/10.1007/978-3-319-78364-2_3

Introduction

Scientists engaged in the choreographed process of preclinical drug development agree that a common "language" for effectively communicating study observations and data between investigators, both in the same as well as different fields, provides a powerful tool for the submission of data to the global regulatory bodies that make final approval decisions based on these data. In pursuit of this common "language," toxicological pathologists were the early trailblazers.

Separate initiatives were started in the late 1980s both in the United States by the STP (Society of Toxicologic Pathology) and in Europe by the RITA database group (*R*egistry of *I*ndustrial *T*oxicology *A*nimal-data) resulting in the internationally recognized publications *SSNDC Guides for Toxicologic Pathology* (STP) and *International Classification of Rodent Tumours Part 1, The Rat* and *International Classification of Rodent Tumors, The Mouse* (RITA). In the mid-1990s, it was determined an effort to eliminate discrepancies between the published nomenclature systems and to reach a common consensus would be of additive value. In 2005, the Strategic and Regulatory Policy Committee (SRPC) of STP started the initiative "Revision of Standardized Nomenclature for Lesions in the Rat and Mouse." RITA was asked by the STP for cooperation, and in November of 2005, RITA members compiled the so-called "INHAND" proposal (*In*ternational *Ha*rmonization of *N*omenclature and *D*iagnostic Criteria). In 2006 both the British and Japanese Societies of Toxicologic Pathology joined this initiative, at which point the project became truly a global effort. The *G*lobal *E*ditorial and *S*teering *C*ommittee (GESC) is guiding the activities of the *O*rgan System *W*orking *G*roups (OWG) which are responsible for generating preferred nomenclature and diagnostic criteria, which represent the consensus of the international collaborators and are made available through goRENI website portal.

In 2004, the US Food and Drug Administration (FDA) launched the Critical Path Initiative with the strategy to drive innovation in the scientific processes through which medical products are developed, evaluated, and manufactured. Through this initiative, the SEND standard was developed under the auspices of CDISC, a non-profit organization formed to establish standards supporting the acquisition, exchange, submission, and archive of nonclinical and clinical research data and metadata. On December 17, 2017, the latest FDA SEND Mandate for providing regulatory submissions in electronic format came into force. All organizations must now use the appropriate FDA-supported standards, formats, and terminologies specified in the FDA Data Standards Catalog for NDA, ANDA, IND, and certain BLA submissions.

CDISC quickly realized the value of the independent efforts already undertaken by the INHAND initiative toward adoption of a globally sanctioned "language" for discussion of pathologic lesions in numerous species relevant to toxicology studies. CDISC is currently working closely with the INHAND GESC to adopt INHAND terminology as the SEND mandated submission lexicon.

We, as representatives of the American College of Veterinary Ophthalmologists (ACVO) working on preclinical drug development, recognize the inherent weakness of historical use of a non-standardized set of diagnostic terminology which in many cases is individualized to specific contract research organizations (CROs) and even isolated testing facilities within a CROs network. As such we are in a key position to create and oversee a common standard lexicon for description of in-life ophthalmology observations and have had preliminary discussions with the SEND Controlled Terminology group concerning essential steps toward ultimate acceptance of our recommended terminology as ultimately mandated SEND lexicon. We recognize that each ACVO Diplomate has received unique training and likely has personal preference for how ocular findings are described. Therefore, no single list of finding descriptions is likely to be perfect, and updates in the future are expected especially as new compounds that produce their own unique collection of ocular changes are investigated. However, the power of a harmonized list of ocular findings lies in its widespread adoption and use by veterinary ophthalmologists and vision researchers around the globe. What follows in this chapter is an initial list of ACVO-endorsed terminology to describe common ocular findings observed on preclinical toxicology and medical device safety studies. The ultimate goal of this simple lexicon is to allow an observer to efficiently and effectively communicate essential information about location, size, and extent of ocular observations. The intent of this recommended terminology list is to describe the appearance and localization of ocular changes considered outside the range of normal variation thus allowing these changes to be localized by different observers in the in-life phase as well as by pathologists in the post-life study phases. We assume that the study anatomical pathologist would ultimately be responsible for determination of diagnostic microscopic characteristics and/or etiology of these ocular changes. We strongly urge the reader to adopt this preferred terminology.

Orbit and Globe

This section covers recommended terminology for the globe as a whole and the orbit. Terms are listed in the section where the primary abnormality exists. For example, although exophthalmos describes forward displacement of the globe, the abnormality that causes it is orbital. Proptosis is at the most severe spectrum of exophthalmos but carries a distinctly poor prognosis for vision and is thus listed separately. Terms are listed without specific regard to cause or whether congenital or acquired. For example, with a single clinical exam, it may be difficult to distinguish between microphthalmia and phthisis bulbi. Although causally different, both are listed as "globe, small." Other clinical findings would be expected, and histopathology may be needed to confirm the ultimate diagnosis.

Blood collection from the retrobulbar region of laboratory rodents can be the source of iatrogenic lesions including orbital hemorrhage resulting in exophthalmos. In extreme situations, trauma to the globe can result in a variety of lesions [1]. The orbital venous sinus in the hamster, gerbil, and mouse is comparably larger than the orbital venous plexus in the rat leading to a recommendation that the lateral tail vein be used in rats [2, 3].

Recommended modifier terminology to further describe specific location, size, and extent of orbit or globe lesions includes:

Location: superior, inferior, temporal, nasal (alternatively, quadrants may be used—superotemporal, inferotemporal, inferonasal, superonasal), anterior, posterior.

Size: millimeter/centimeter scale (depending on species) or relative to corneal diameter (for instance, "said lesion is approximately half of the corneal diameter").

Extent: minimal, mild, moderate, or severe.

Orbit		
Observation	Definition	Photo + legend
Enophthalmos	Posterior displacement of the globe within the orbit	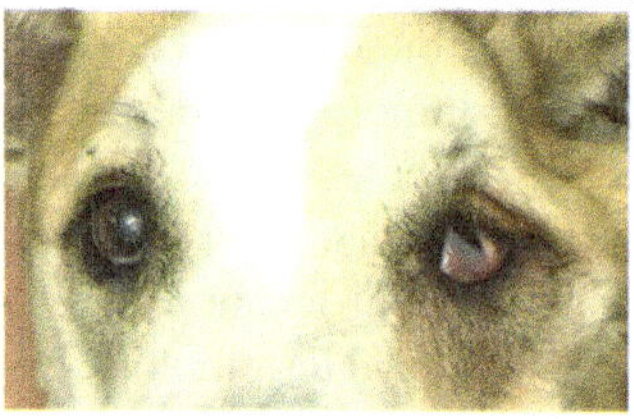 Dog. Neurogenic muscle atrophy resulting in enophthalmos and protrusion of the third eyelid
Exophthalmos	Anterior displacement of the globe relative to the orbit Includes cyst, neoplasia, inflammation, and congenital choristoma consisting of encapsulated dermal structures Synonyms: Proptosis, exorbitism	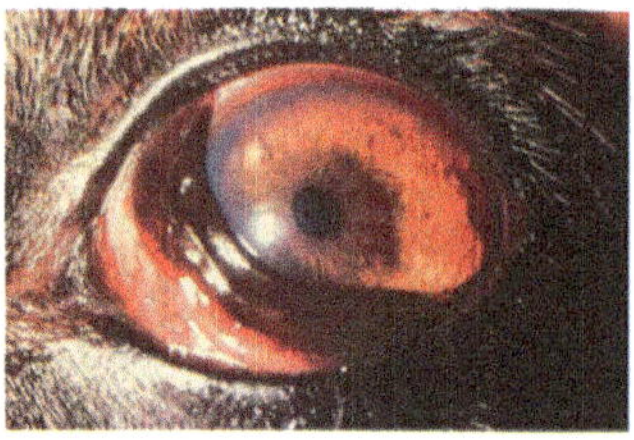 Dog. Note also protrusion of the third eyelid, miosis
		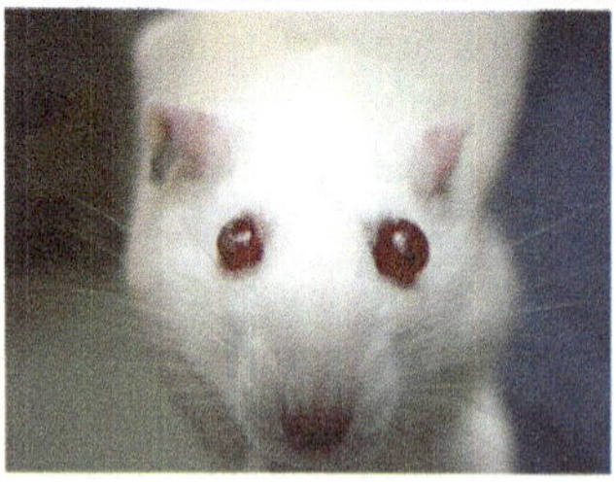 Sprague Dawley rat (photo courtesy of David Wilkie)
Hemorrhage	Extravascular blood within the orbit. Most often traumatic	See photo below under Proptosis

(continued)

Orbit		
Observation	Definition	Photo + legend
Proptosis	Severe anterior displacement of the globe relative to the orbit, often associated with blindness due to globe and/or optic nerve damage. In laboratory rodents may be seen as a complication of blood sampling Synonym: Exophthalmos, exorbitism	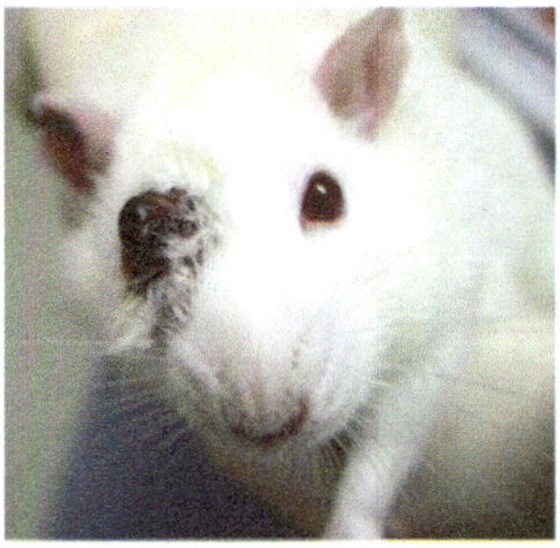 Sprague Dawley rat. Proptosis caused by severe orbital hemorrhage following blood sampling (photo courtesy of David Wilkie)
		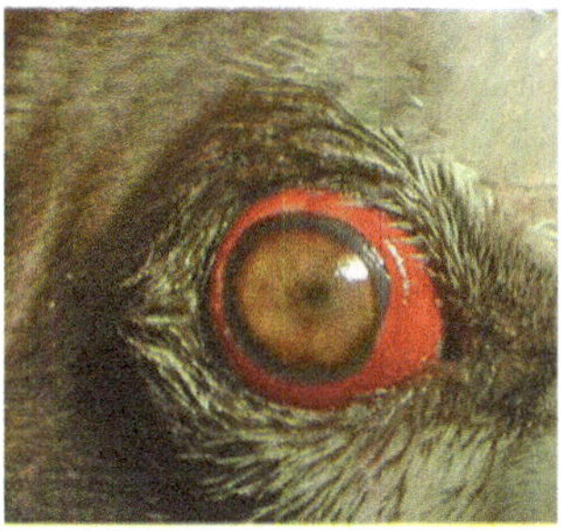 Dog

Globe		
Observation	Definition	Photo + legend
Deviated	Visual axis deviated (direction should be noted: Superior, inferior, nasal, temporal) Synonym: Exotropia, esotropia, cyclotropia, hypertropia, hypotropia, strabismus	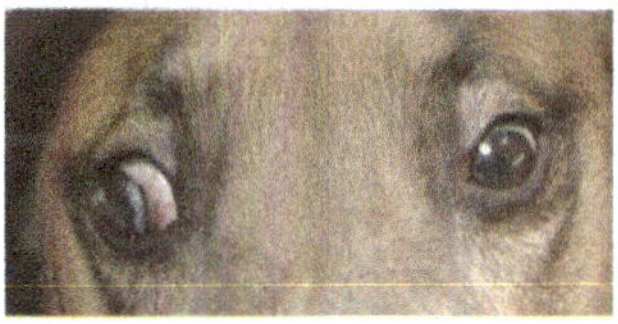 Dog. Right eye exotropia with associated peripheral corneal opacity (degeneration)
Globe enlarged	Globe enlargement, usually acquired due to elevated IOP (glaucoma) or intraocular mass Synonym: Buphthalmos, megophthalmos, megaloglobus, macrophthalmos	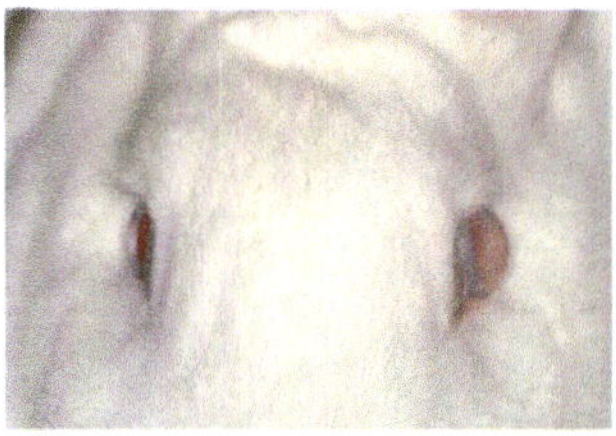 New Zealand white rabbit

(continued)

Globe		
Observation	Definition	Photo + legend
		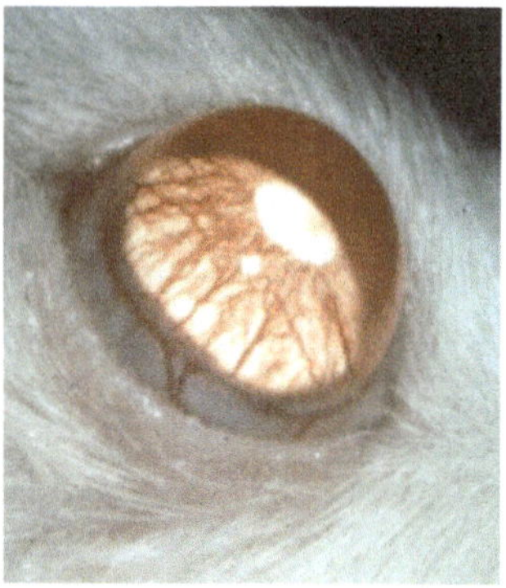 Sprague Dawley rat (photo courtesy of David Wilkie)
Globe not visible	Congenital absence of the globe. Globe may appear to be absent in severe microphthalmia Synonym: Anophthalmia	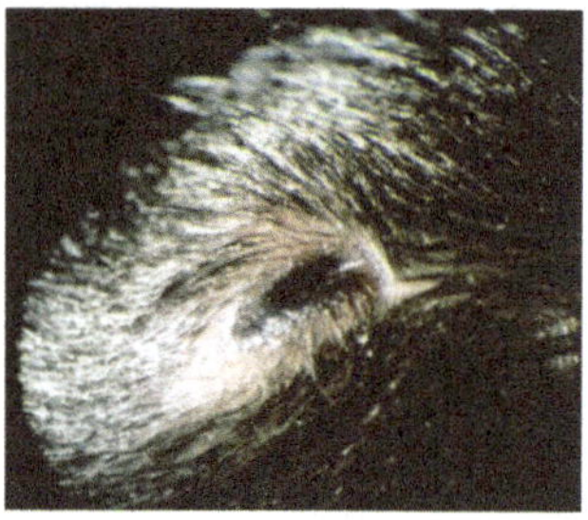 C57Bl/6J mouse
Globe small	May be congenital due to developmental hypoplasia or acquired due to shrinkage of the globe Synonym: Microphthalmia (congenital), phthisis bulbi (acquired)	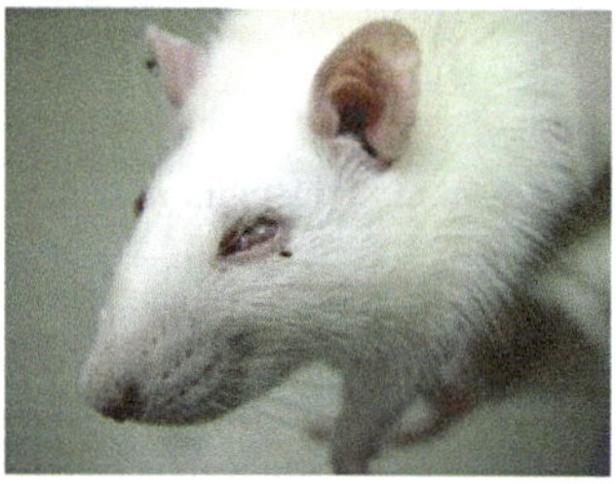 Rat (photo courtesy of David Wilkie)

(continued)

Globe		
Observation	Definition	Photo + legend
		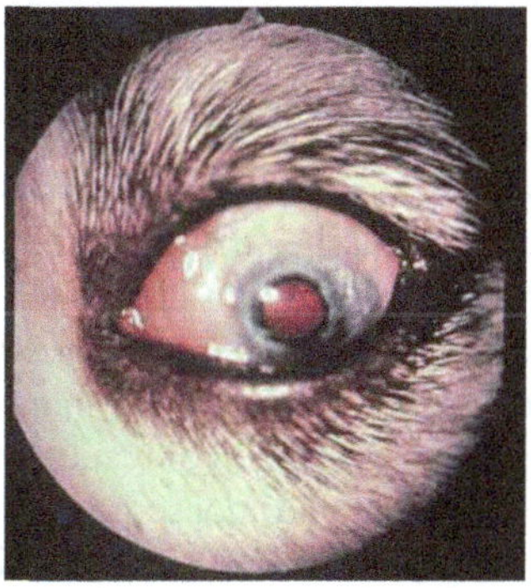 Dog. Note the globe is proportionally smaller than the palpebral fissure. More commonly, both the globe and fissure are similarly reduced in size
Neoplasia	Space-occupying proliferation of neoplastic cells. May originate within any ocular tissue. May be primary or secondary by extension or metastasis	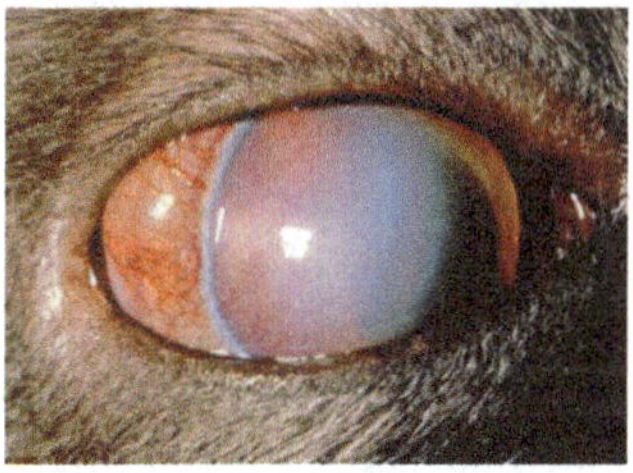 Dog. Intraocular neoplasia with thickening under the sclera and corneal opacity
Rupture/ laceration	Full thickness defect in the cornea or sclera. Most commonly traumatic. May result in phthisis bulbi (see above under "globe small")	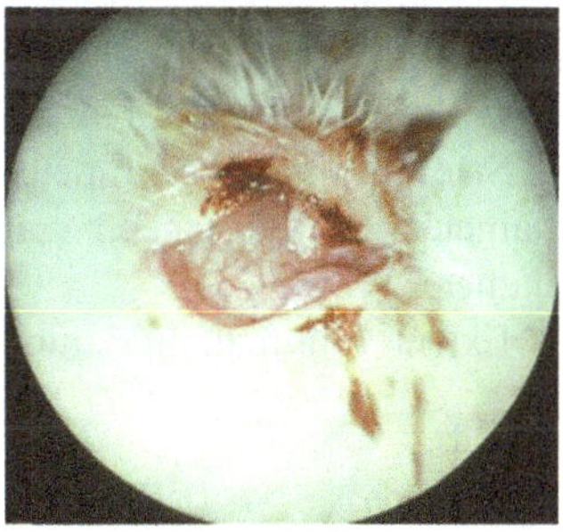 Sprague Dawley rat
Synoph-thalmia	Failure of separation of the ocular anlage, resulting in a single midline globe Synonym: Cyclopia	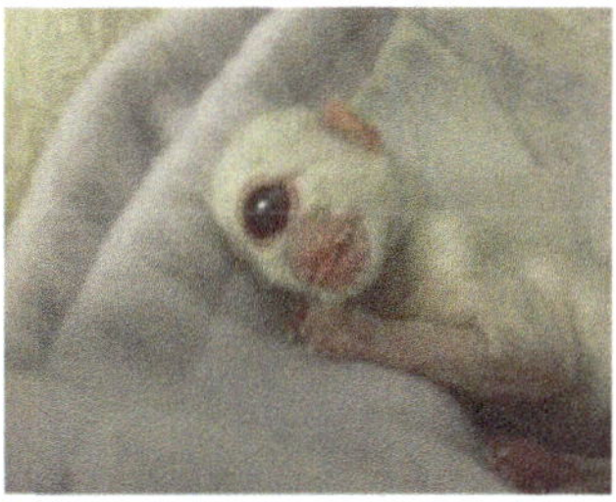 Newborn kitten

Eyelids, Adnexa, and Conjunctiva

This section describes recommended terminology for the eyelids, adnexa, lacrimal glands, and nasolacrimal drainage system. There are wide anatomical variations in these structures between species, most notably, the presence of a third eyelid and associated gland in nonhuman primate (NHP) laboratory species. However, these are also tissues that have responses to inflammation that are species-specific with variations between pigmented and nonpigmented strains of the same species. For example, in rabbits, minimal manipulation of the eyes, even during examination, can result in transient conjunctival hyperemia. The examiner needs to be familiar with interpretation of results within the context of background biological behavior.

The rat and mouse have both intra-orbital and extra-orbital lacrimal glands as well as a Harderian gland that is associated with the third eyelid but is distinct from the third eyelid (nictitans). The guinea pig has a large intra-orbital lacrimal gland. The Mongolian gerbil has both nictitans and Harderian glands [4, 5].

Rabbits have a prominent Harderian gland that is absent in NHP and dog. The high lipid concentration in this gland allows rabbits to have a very slow blink cycle. In addition, rabbits also have a lacrimal and nictitans gland. Swelling of these glands can result in visible protrusion within the medial canthal region.

Chromodacryorrhea in laboratory rodents refers to red discoloration of the tears resulting in periocular staining. This can be seen associated with ocular inflammation, as a test article effect, but is also seen incidentally associated with generalized stress and with infections such as sialodacryoadenitis virus (SDA) [6–10].

The nasolacrimal drainage system is likewise a species variable. The rabbit lacks a lacrimal sac and has a single outflow punctum [11].

Recommended modifier terminology to further describe specific location, size, and extent of eyelid, adnexal, or conjunctival lesions includes:

Location: superior, inferior, temporal, nasal (alternatively quadrants may be used—superotemporal, inferotemporal, inferonasal, superonasal), proximal, distal, marginal, palpebral, or bulbar.

Size: millimeter/centimeter scale (depending on species) or relative to corneal diameter (for instance, “said lesion is approximately half of the corneal diameter”).

Extent: minimal, mild, moderate, or severe.

Eyelids		
Observation	Definition	Photo + legend
Alopecia	Loss of eyelid hair	See photo below for eyelid swelling
Blepharophimosis	Congenitally narrow palpebral fissure Synonyms: Blepharostenosis	
Blepharospasm	Spasm of the eyelid resulting in physiologic narrowing of the palpebral fissure, most commonly due to pain	

(continued)

Eyelids		
Observation	Definition	Photo + legend
Chalazion/ hordeolum	Swelling caused by impaction (chalazion) or infection (hordeolum) of the meibomian gland(s). Synonym: Meibomian cyst, stye	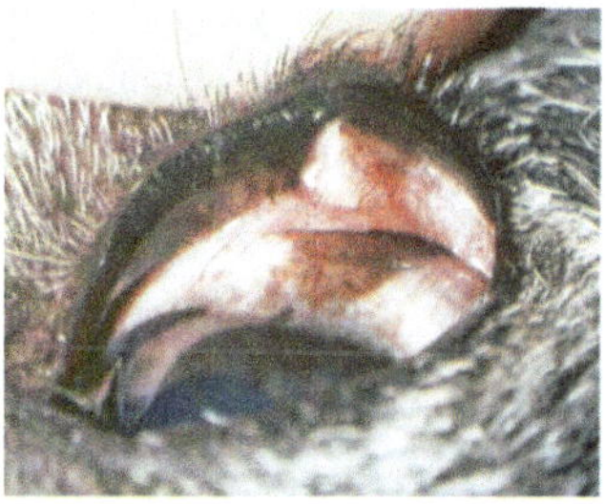 Dog
Coloboma	Congenital defect of the eyelid margin	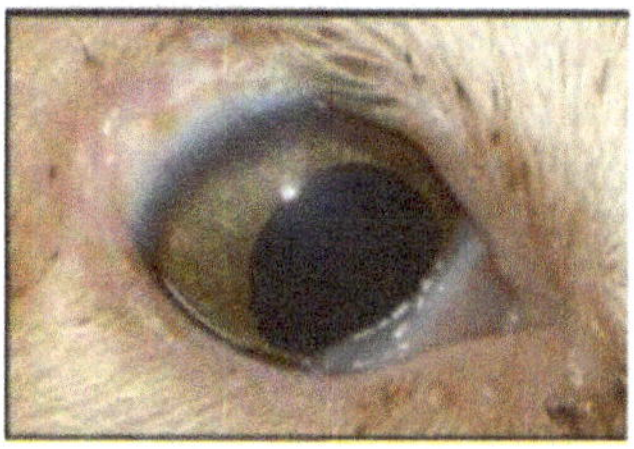 Cat
Depigmentation	Loss of eyelid pigment Synonym: Vitiligo	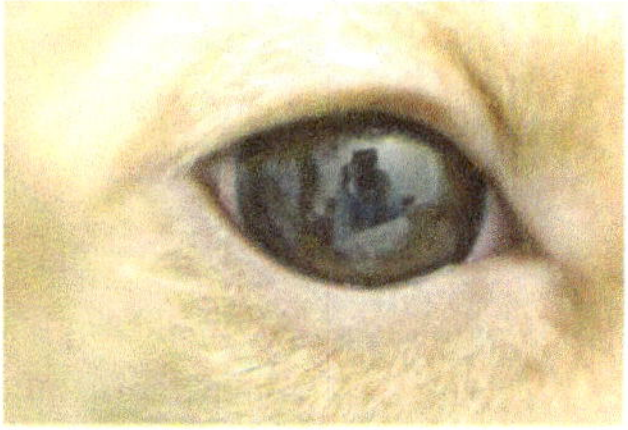 Dog
Distichiasis/ectopic cilia	Aberrant cilia	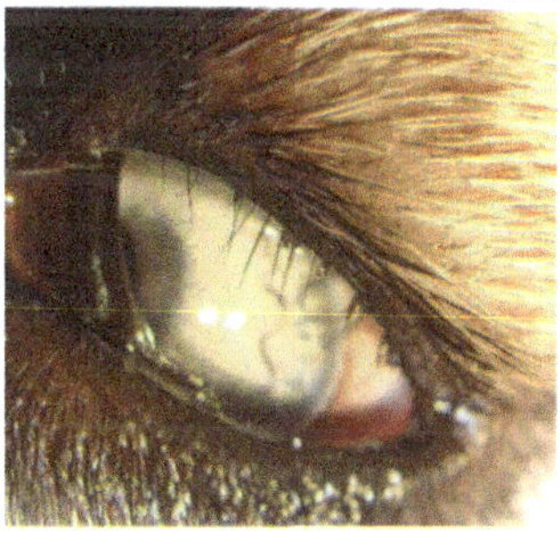 Dog

(continued)

Eyelids		
Observation	Definition	Photo + legend
Ectropion	Outward rolling of the eyelid margin, or other eyelid laxity that results in failure of contact of the eyelid margin with the cornea	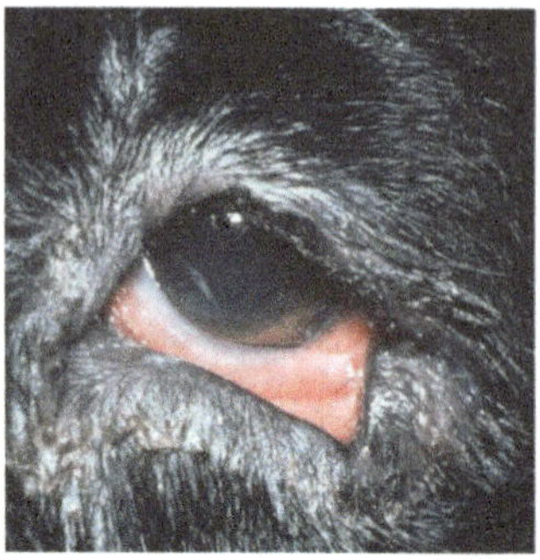 Dog
Entropion	Inward rolling of the eyelid margin	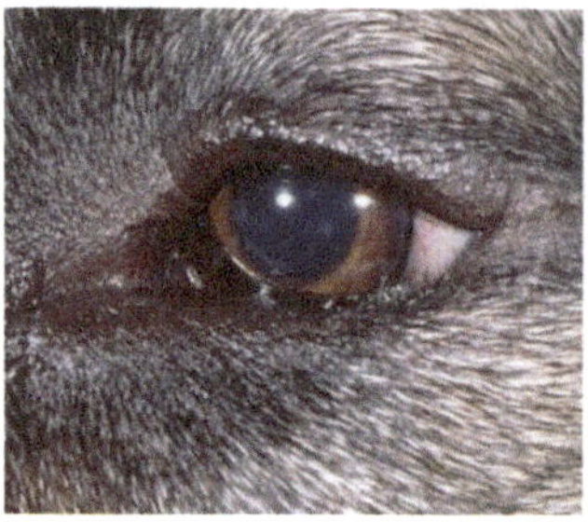 Dog. Lower eyelid is affected
Erythema	Hyperemia of eyelid skin	See photo below for eyelid swelling
Hyperpigmentation	Increased pigment (most commonly melanin, other pigments possible). May occur as a normal variation	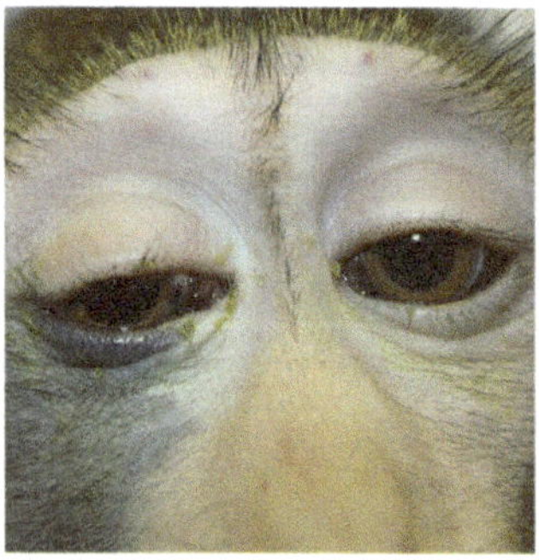 Cynomolgus macaque. Regional dermal hyperpigmentation involving the face and lower lid. Normal variation

(continued)

Eyelids		
Observation	Definition	Photo + legend
Laceration	Traumatic injury involving the eyelid margin	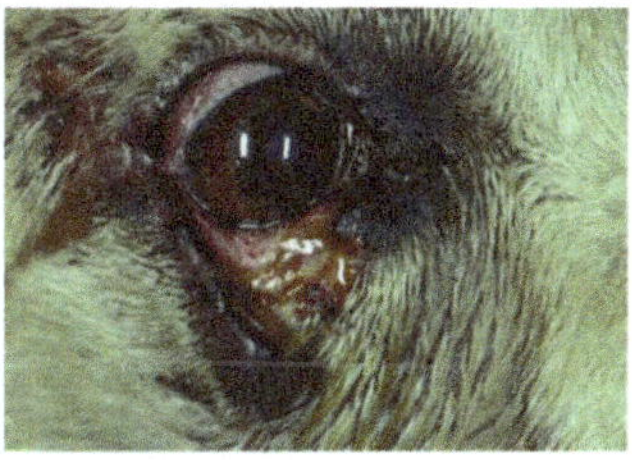 Dog
Lagophthalmos	Failure of complete closure of the palpebral fissure, often associated with secondary corneal pathology	
Mass	Space-occupying lesion to include dermoid, neoplasm, cyst, inflammatory nodule, granuloma	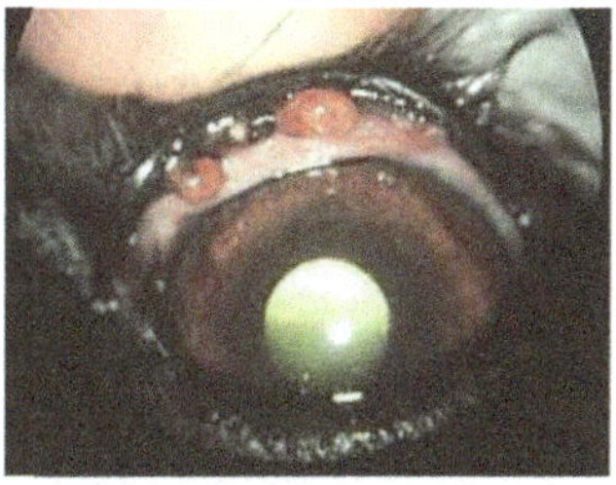 Dog. Multiple eyelid cysts
Ptosis	Congenital or acquired condition that causes drooping of the upper eyelid. May be congenital or acquired. Most commonly associated with Horner's syndrome	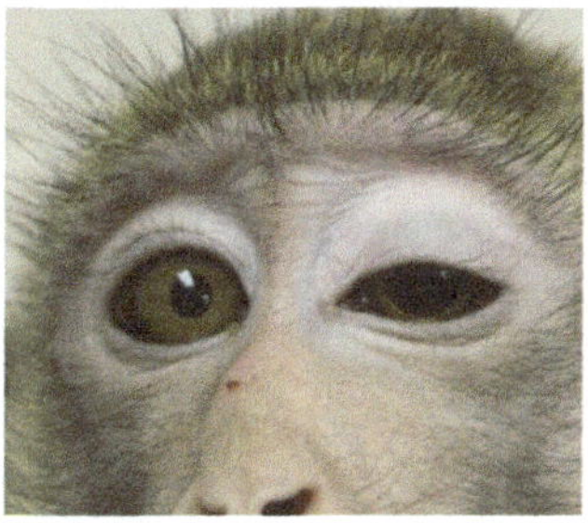 Primate. Left ptosis
		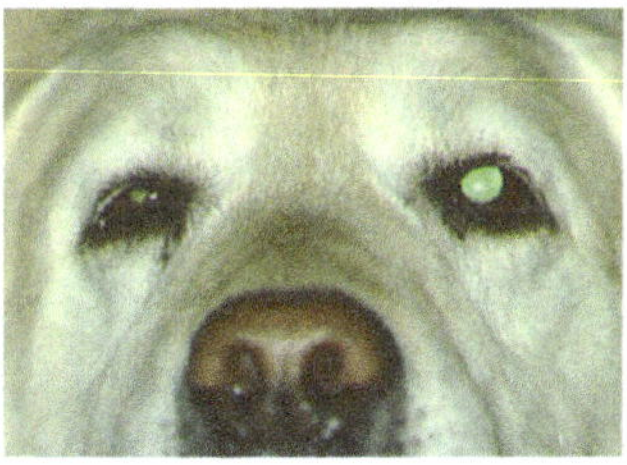 Dog. Right ptosis associated with Horner's syndrome. Note the typical accompanying miosis when compared with the left eye

(continued)

Eyelids		
Observation	Definition	Photo + legend
Scar	Acquired contraction of eyelid, usually following trauma	
Swelling/edema	Increase in extracellular fluid Synonyms: Blepharitis, blepharedema	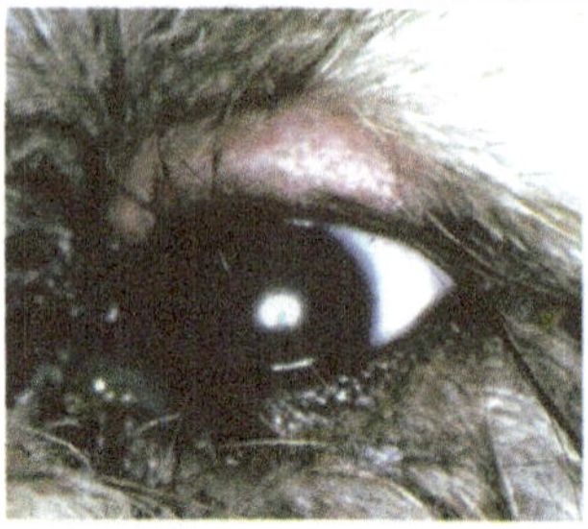 Dog
		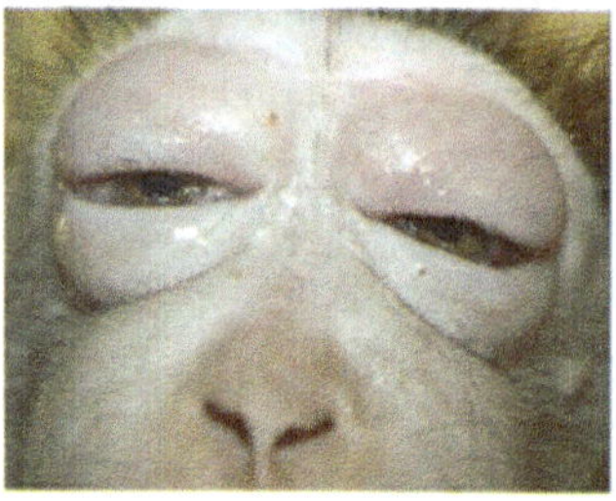 Primate

Conjunctiva		
Observation	Definition	Photo + legend
Conjunctival proliferation	Proliferation of the conjunctiva to overlie the cornea. Usually post-inflammatory and most common in rabbits Synonyms: Pseudopterygium, conjunctival overgrowth	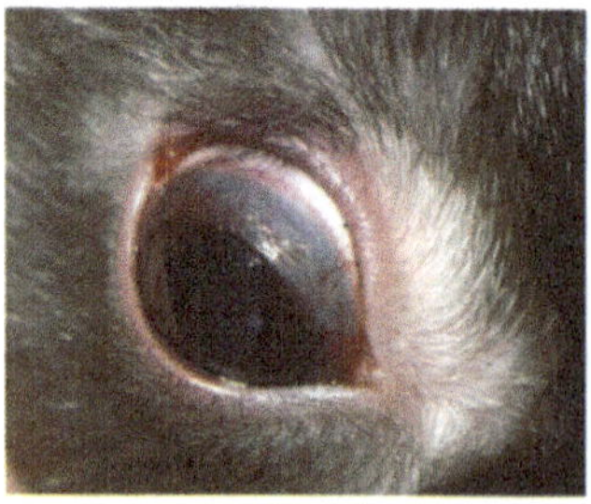 Dutch belted rabbit (photo courtesy of David Wilkie)
Dermoid	Congenital choristoma consisting of dermal elements within the conjunctiva and cornea	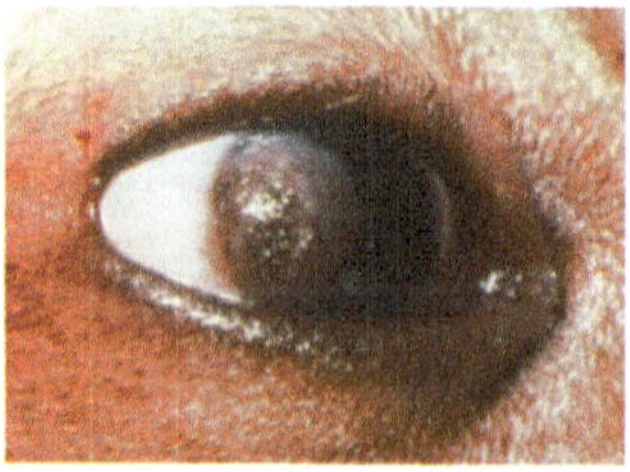 Dog

(continued)

Conjunctiva		
Observation	Definition	Photo + legend
Discharge	Ocular discharge that may originate from secretions of the lacrimal gland(s), meibomian glands, conjunctival goblet cells. May or may not be inflammatory. Identification should include color and consistency (serous, mucoid, purulent, hemorrhagic) (see Chap. 5 for scoring)	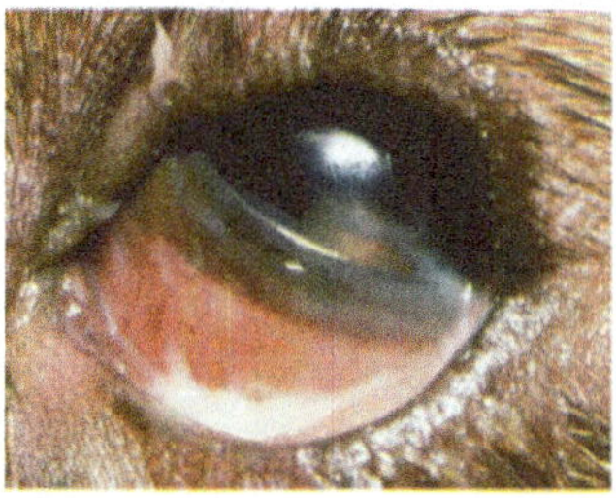 Dog. Mucoid discharge
		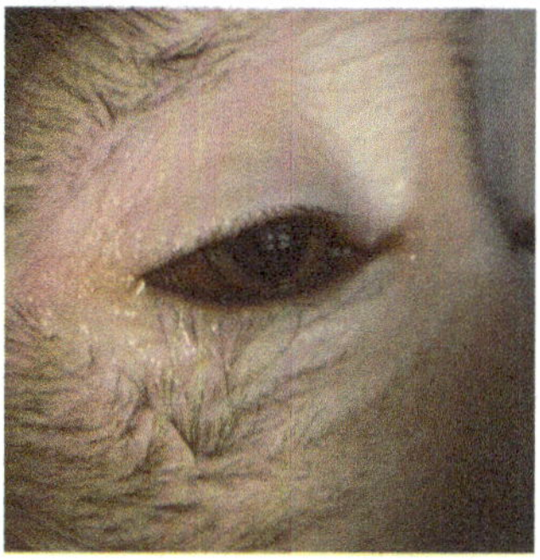 Primate. Serous discharge
Hemorrhage	Extravascular accumulation of red blood cells	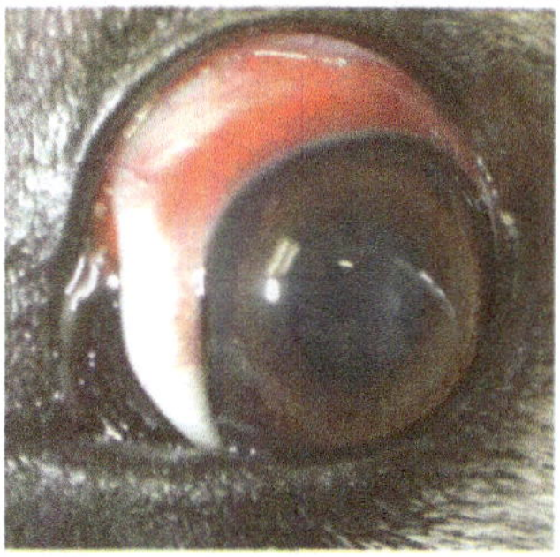 Dog
		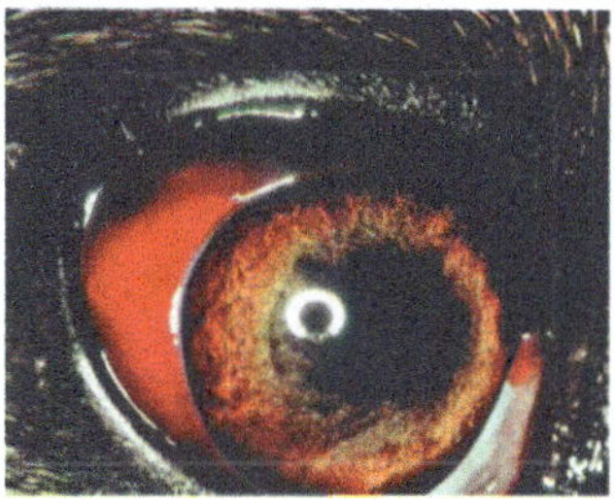 Dog

(continued)

Conjunctiva		
Observation	Definition	Photo + legend
Hyperemia	Vascular engorgement of the conjunctiva Synonyms: Vascular injection, redness, injection, congestion (see Chap. 5 for scoring)	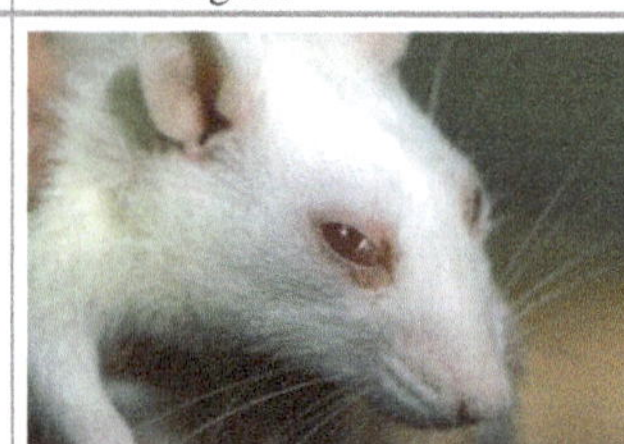 Rat (photo courtesy of David Wilkie)
		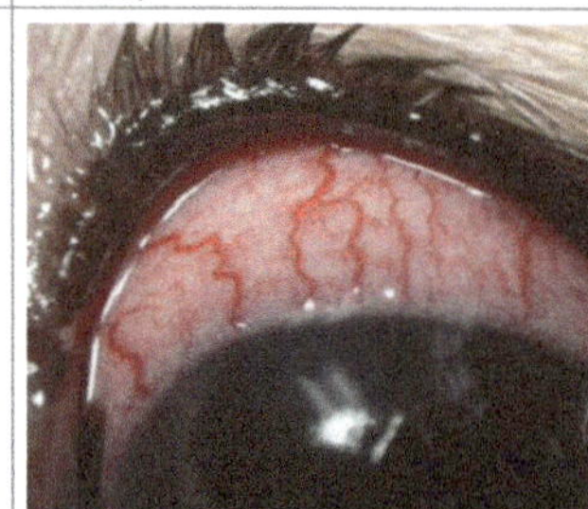 Dog
Hyperpigmentation	Increased pigment (most commonly melanin, other pigments possible)	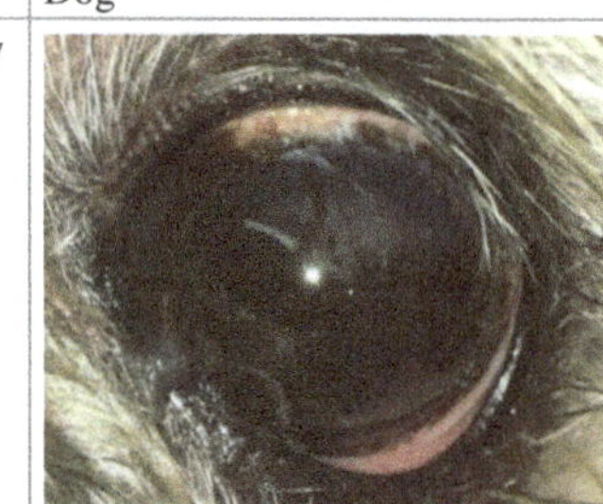 Dog. Corneal and conjunctival pigment
		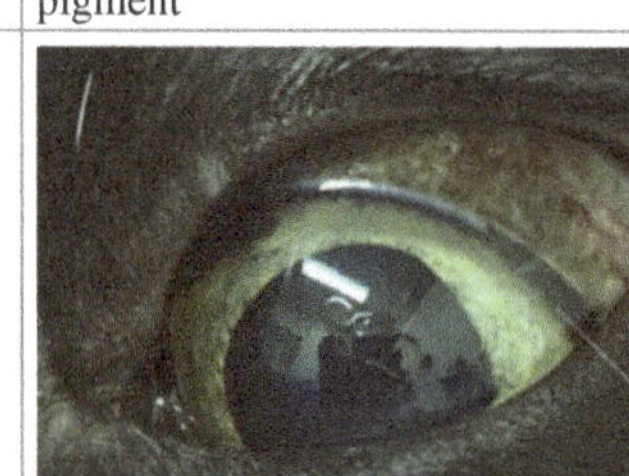 Cat. Dog. Conjunctival pigment

(continued)

Conjunctiva		
Observation	Definition	Photo + legend
Mass	Space-occupying lesion (includes cyst, neoplasia, inflammation)	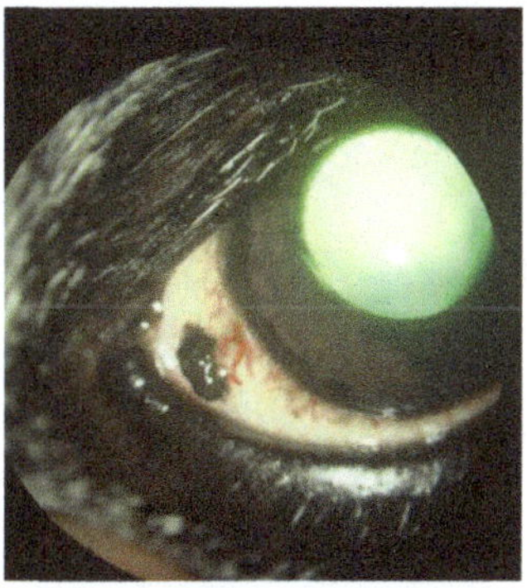 Dog. Conjunctival melanoma
Swelling	Increase in extracellular fluid Synonyms: Chemosis (see Chap. 5 for scoring)	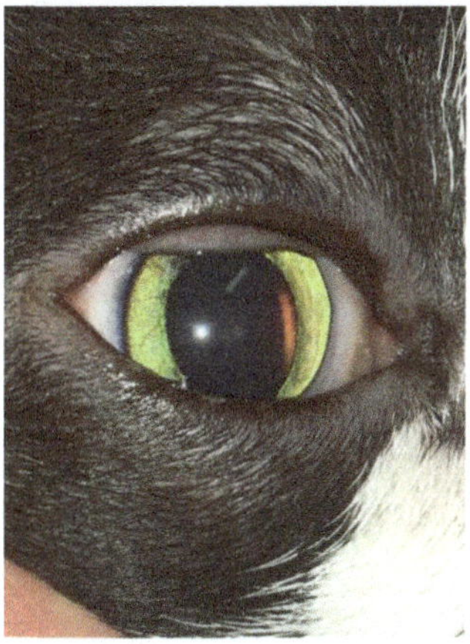 Cat. Mild chemosis
		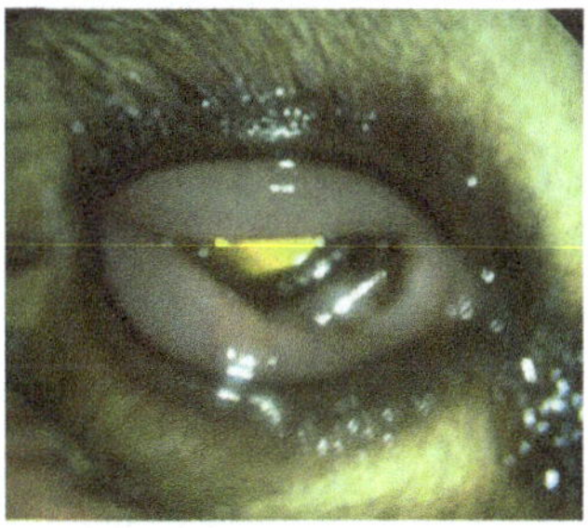 Cat. Severe chemosis

(continued)

Conjunctiva		
Observation	Definition	Photo + legend
Symblepharon	Acquired conjunctival fibrosis resulting in adhesions between the bulbar and palpebral conjunctiva and/or cornea, often with reduced size of the palpebral fissure Synonyms: Ankyloblepharon, blepharosynechia	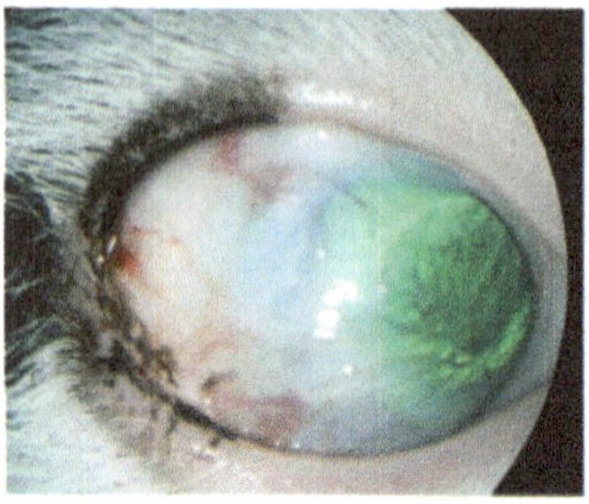 Cat. Note the conjunctival proliferation over the corneal surface

Third eyelid (in nonprimate species)		
Observation	Definition	Photo + legend
Cartilage anomaly	Congenital malformation of the cartilage of the third eyelid	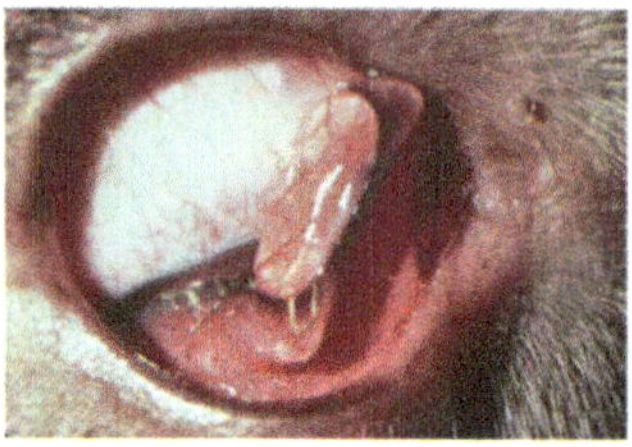 Dog
Depigmentation	Reduced pigment	
Gland prolapse	Prolapse of the gland of the third eyelid	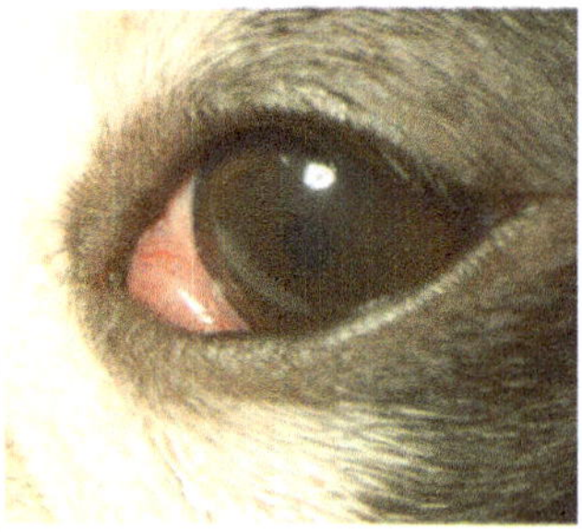 Dog
Hyperemia	Vascular engorgement of the conjunctiva of the third eyelid Synonyms: Vascular injection, redness, injection, congestion (see Chap. 5 for scoring)	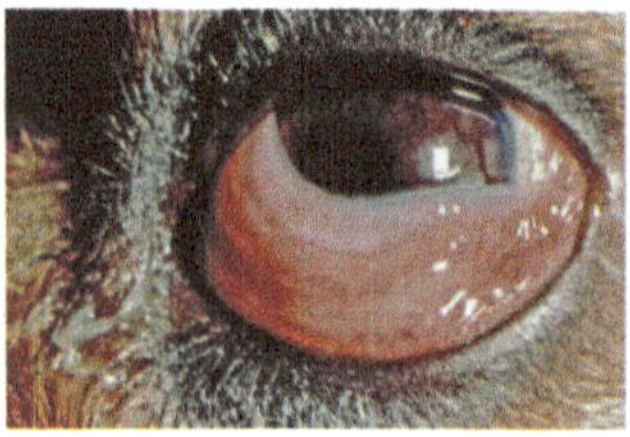 Dog

(continued)

Third eyelid (in nonprimate species)		
Observation	Definition	Photo + legend
Laceration	Traumatic injury to the third eyelid. May involve conjunctiva and the supportive cartilage, gland, or a combination	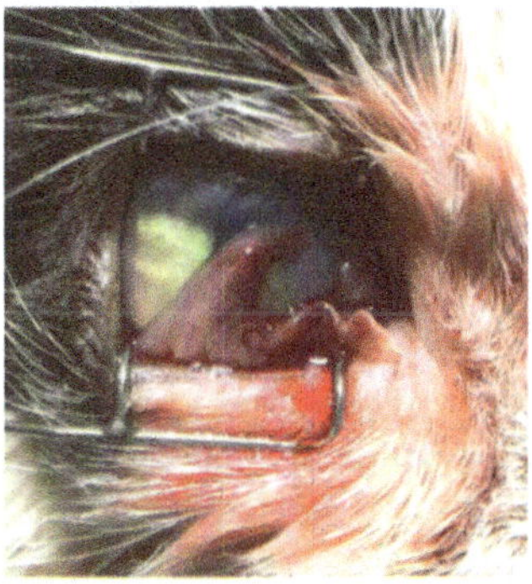 Cat
Lymphoid follicles	Nodular thickening, usually on the posterior surface, consisting of accumulation of lymphocytes	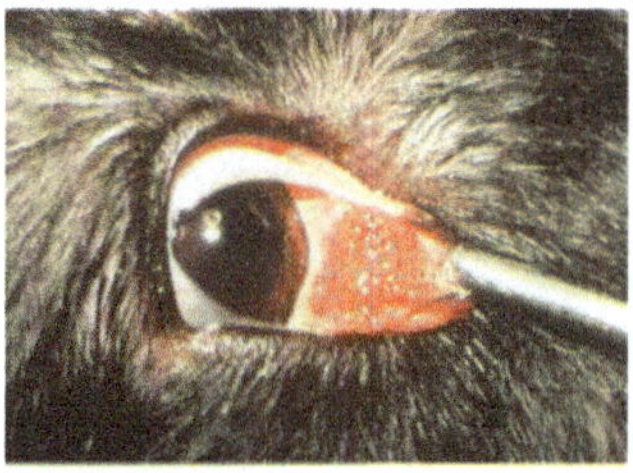 Dog
Mass	Space-occupying lesion (includes cyst, neoplasia, inflammation)	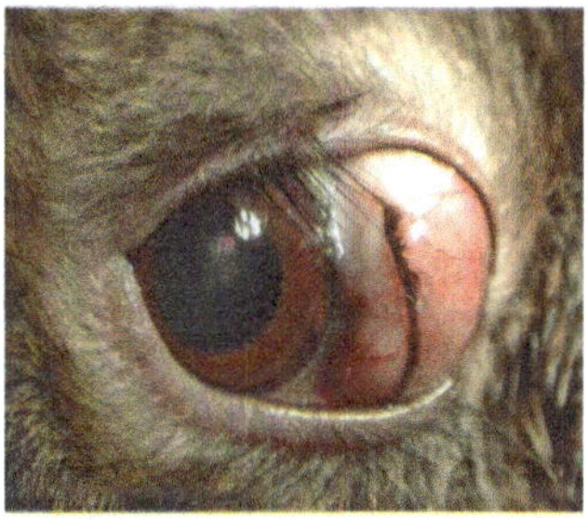 Rabbit: Third eyelid mass

Nasolacrimal		
Observation	Definition	Photo + legend
Chromodacryorrhea	Epiphora associated with red-colored (suspected porphyrin laden) secretions	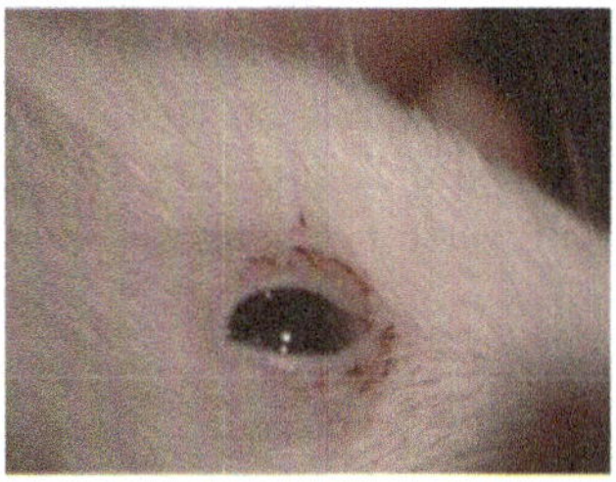 Rat. Mild example

(continued)

Nasolacrimal		
Observation	Definition	Photo + legend
Cyst/mass	Space-occupying lesion within the nasolacrimal duct	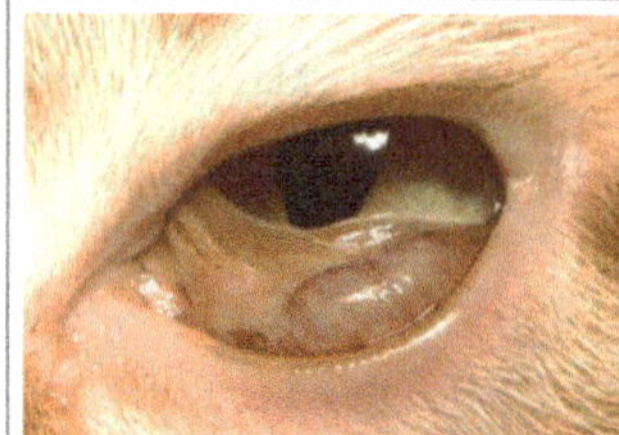 Cat. Lacrimal cyst
Dacryocystitis	Inflammation of the nasolacrimal duct. May be associated with obstruction	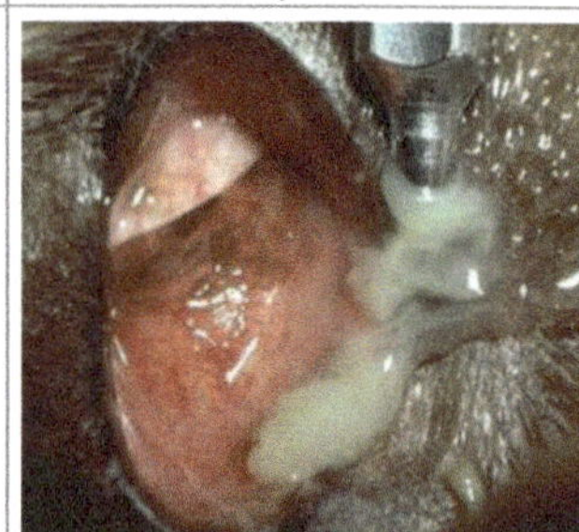 Dog. Purulent exudate being flushed from the inferior nasolacrimal punctum

Cornea and Sclera

The recommended terminology described in this section covers evaluation of the external tunics of the eye: cornea and sclera. In addition to providing protection for the internal structures of the globe through structural rigidity, a primary function of the cornea is refraction of light from the surroundings onto a focused path for photon detection by the neurosensory retina. Both the corneal epithelium and more importantly the corneal endothelium play an active role in maintenance of corneal transparency. Topically applied, intraocularly injected, or systemically delivered compounds can potentially affect function of these cell populations, with a common adverse toxicologic finding being loss of corneal transparency. While a population of limbal-based stem cells provides constant renewal of corneal epithelial cells, allowing a chance for recovery after toxicologic insult, regeneration of corneal endothelial cells in common mammalian laboratory species is extremely limited with significant toxicity to corneal endothelial cell populations frequently resulting in irreversible change.

Many of the corneal terminology recommended in this section can be used to describe observations that periodically arise in all commonly utilized species for toxicology and medical device safety and efficacy studies. In some cases terminology is included that has a strong preponderance in specific species and/or strains of that species, perhaps the most notable of these being “crystalline deposits” which is intended to supersede the historical terminology "corneal dystrophy," "corneal crystals," or other related variations for the frequently bilateral, multifocal, superficial epithelial/stromal; white to gray deposits observed with high prevalence in certain strains of rats (including: Sprague-Dawley, Wistar, Fischer, etc.); and oval to ring-shaped deposits in the axial/paraxial epithelium/stroma observed occasionally in Beagle dogs or more rarely in various alternate locations of other species.

Recommended modifier terminology to further describe specific location, size, and extent of corneal of scleral lesions includes:

Location: superior, inferior, temporal, nasal (alternatively quadrants may be used—superotemporal, inferotemporal, inferonasal, superonasal), epithelial, superficial stromal, mid-stromal, deep stromal, or endothelial.

Size: millimeter/centimeter scale (depending on species) or relative to corneal diameter (for instance, "said lesion is approximately half of the corneal diameter").

Extent: minimal, mild, moderate, or severe.

Cornea		
Observation	Definition	Photo + legend
Cellular infiltrate	Migration into and accumulation of cells within the corneal stroma Modifiers of location, extent, and depth should be included	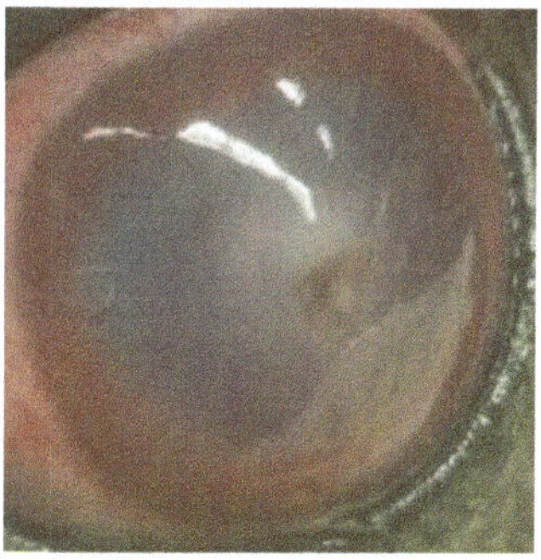 Dog. Corneal vascularization, corneal edema, and conjunctival injection also present
Crystalline deposits	Abnormal deposition of extracellular material (lipid, mineral, other) along the epithelial basement membrane or within the superficial layers of the stroma Synonyms: Corneal dystrophy, corneal crystals, mineralization	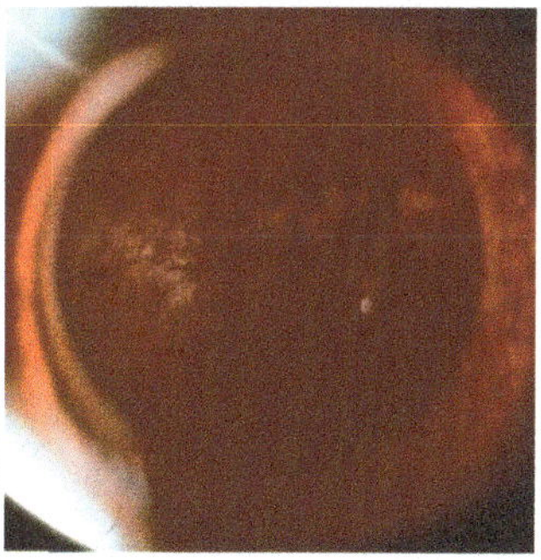 Rat. Crystalline deposits

(continued)

Cornea		
Observation	Definition	Photo + legend
		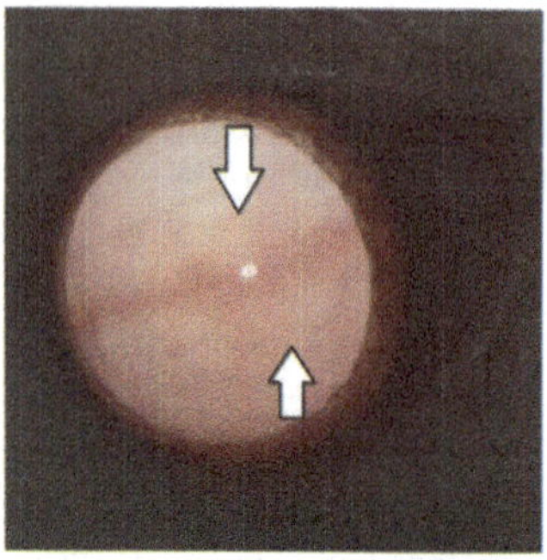 Rat
		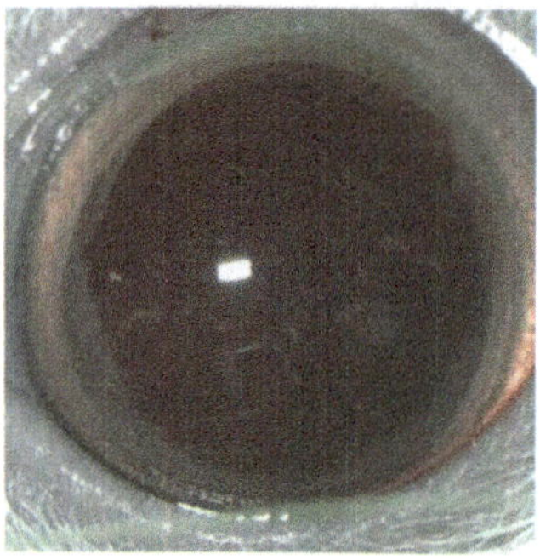 Rat
		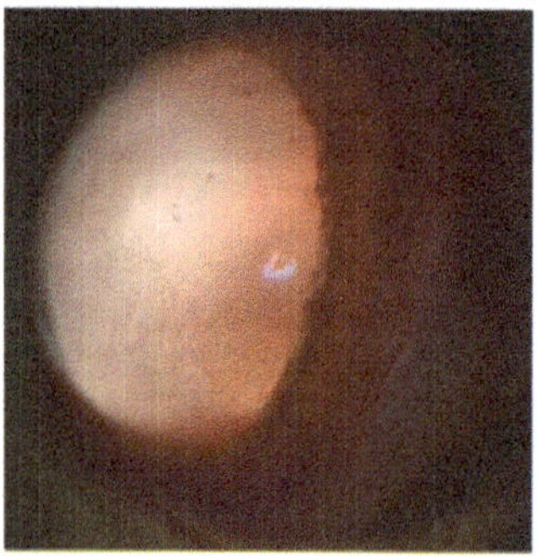 Rat

(continued)

Cornea		
Observation	Definition	Photo + legend
Cyst	Cells or fluid entrapped within a stroma pocket/s Synonyms: Epithelial inclusion, stromal bulla Modifiers of color, location, extent, and depth should be included	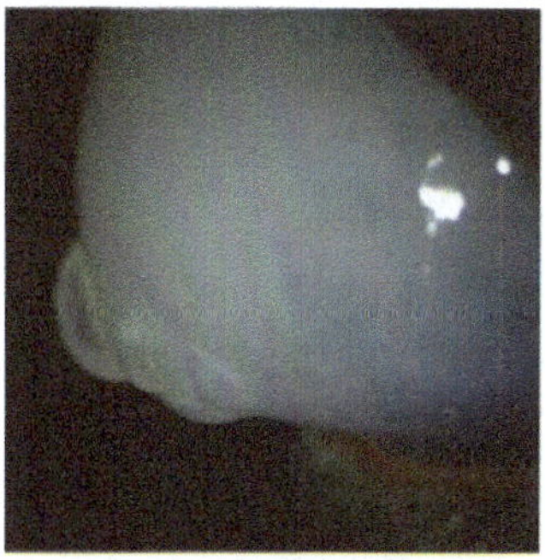 Rabbit. Corneal edema also present
		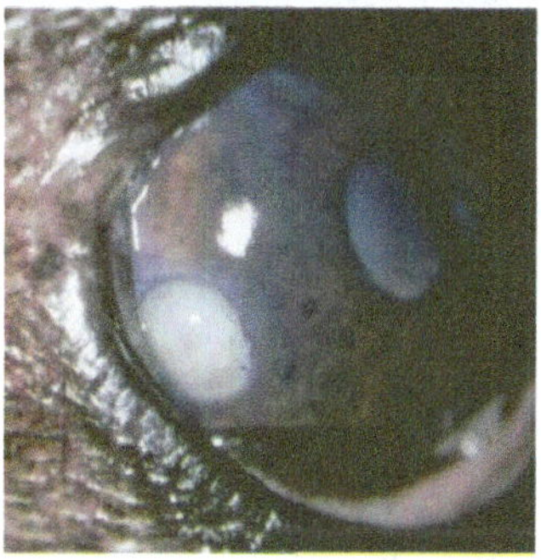 Dog. Perilimbal epithelial inclusion cyst
Edema	Fluid accumulating between and expanding the lamellar collagen structure of the corneal stroma Modifiers of location, extent, and depth should be included	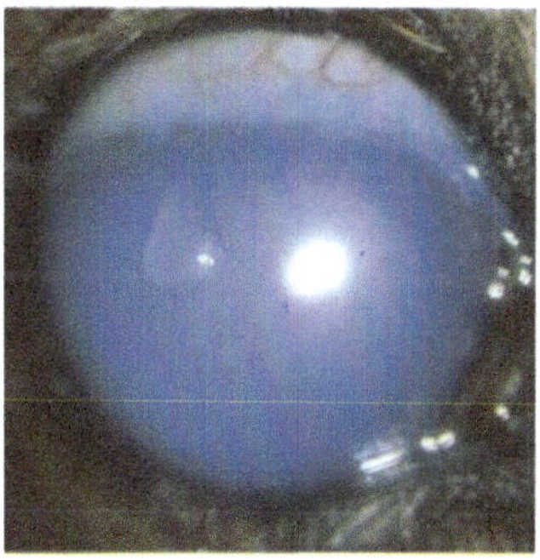 Dog

(continued)

Cornea		
Observation	Definition	Photo + legend
Epithelial and basement opacity	Spontaneous or acquired opacities in the superficial cornea, usually bilateral Synonym: Corneal dystrophy	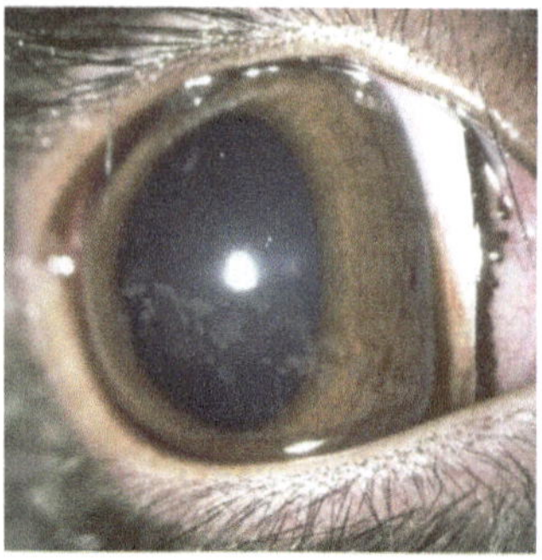 Rabbit. Corneal epithelial opacities
Facet	Re-epithelialized, partial-thickness corneal stromal defect	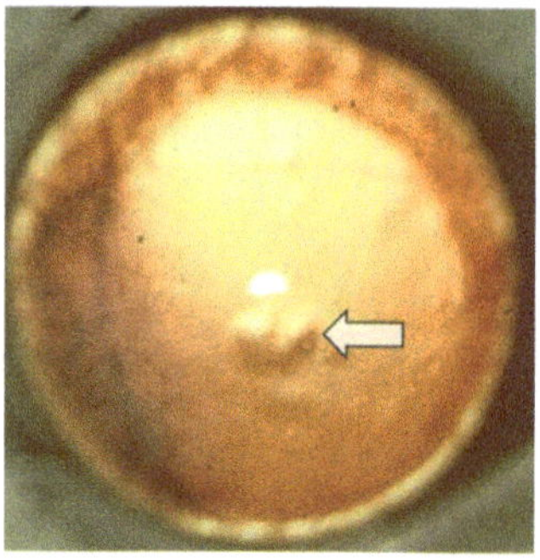 Rat
Hemorrhage	Free red blood cells within the corneal stroma Modifiers of location, extent, and depth should be included	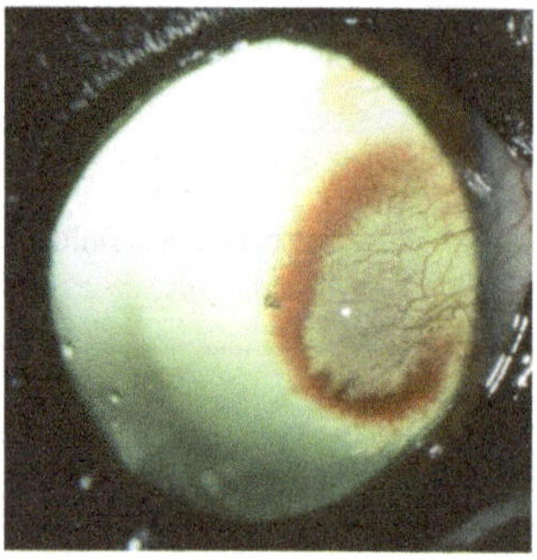 Dog. Corneal vascularization also present

(continued)

Cornea		
Observation	Definition	Photo + legend
Keratoconus	Progressive defect resulting in thinning and bulging of the corneal stroma. May occur as a congenital abnormality or through acquired progressive loss of corneal integrity If lined by uveal tissue, this is a staphyloma	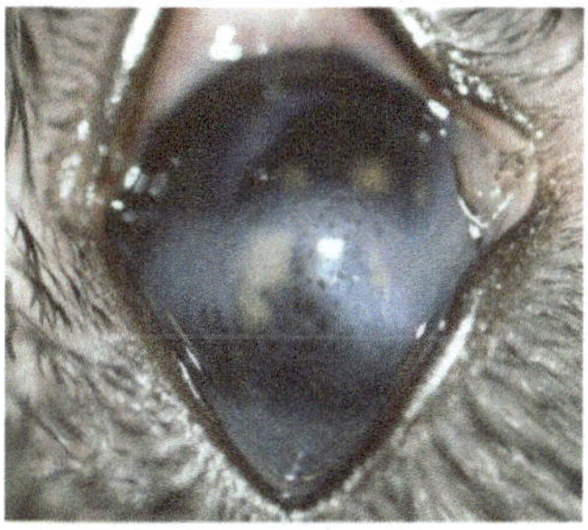 Chinchilla
Keratomalacia	Liquefaction of corneal stromal collagen due to presence of degradative enzymes secreted from infecting bacteria or invading neutrophils	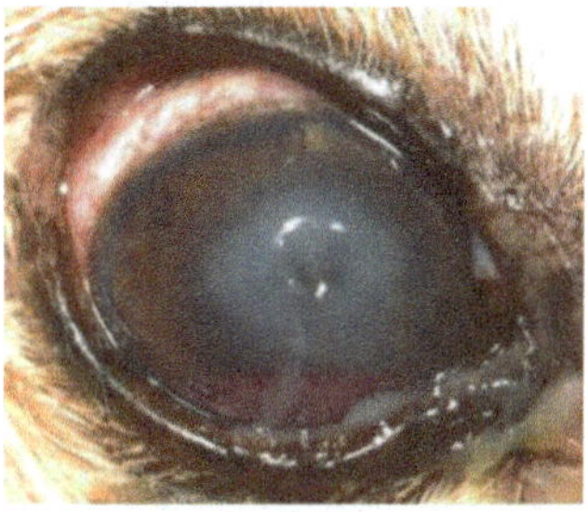 Dog. Axial lesion
Lipidosis	Foci of lipid within the stroma or deep layers of the corneal epithelium Synonyms: Arcus lipoides, corneal arcus Modifiers of location, extent, and depth should be included	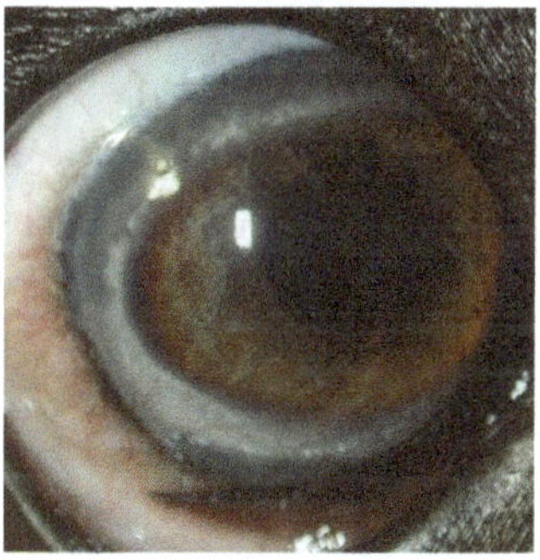 Dog. Perilimbal lipid infiltrate
Mass	Space-occupying corneal lesion Synonyms: Neoplasia, choristoma	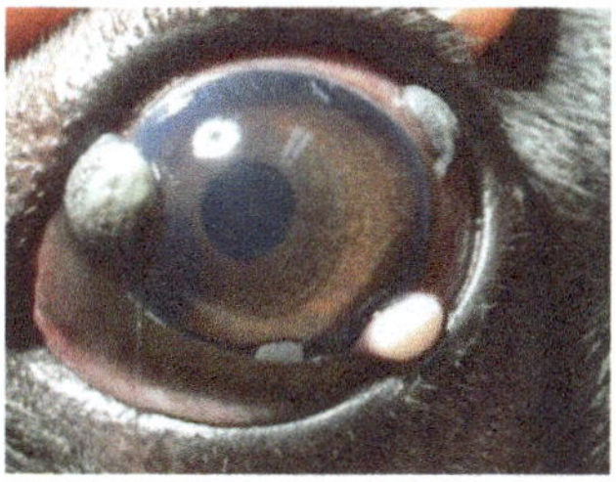 Dog. Corneal and conjunctival masses (papillomas)

(continued)

Cornea		
Observation	Definition	Photo + legend
		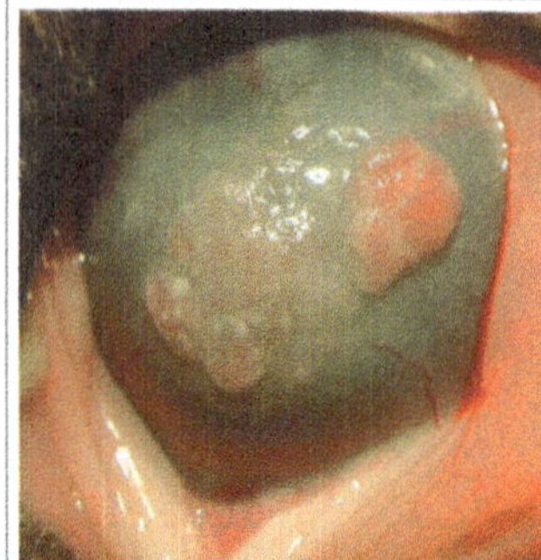 Dog. (corneal squamous cell carcinoma)
Opacity, other	Modifiers of location, extent, and depth should be included	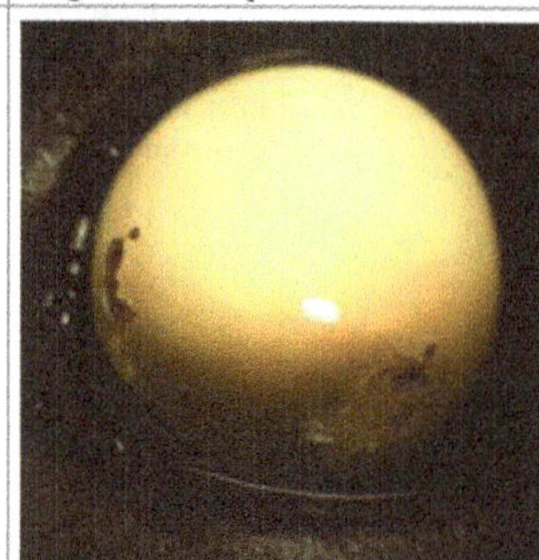 Dog. Endothelial
Pigmentation	Pigment (most commonly melanin, other pigments possible) present within the corneal epithelium or stroma Modifiers of location, extent, and depth should be included	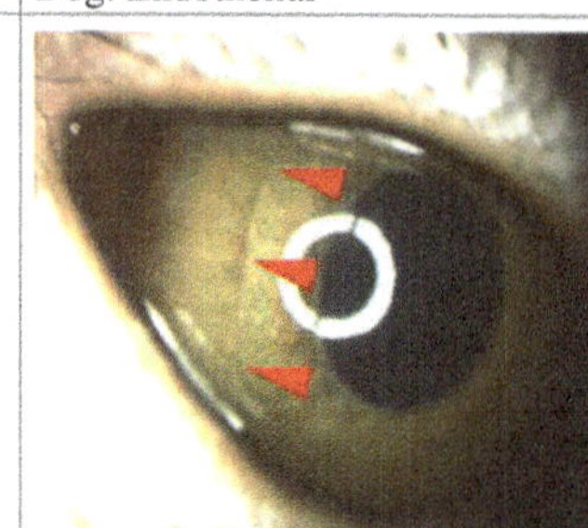 Primate
		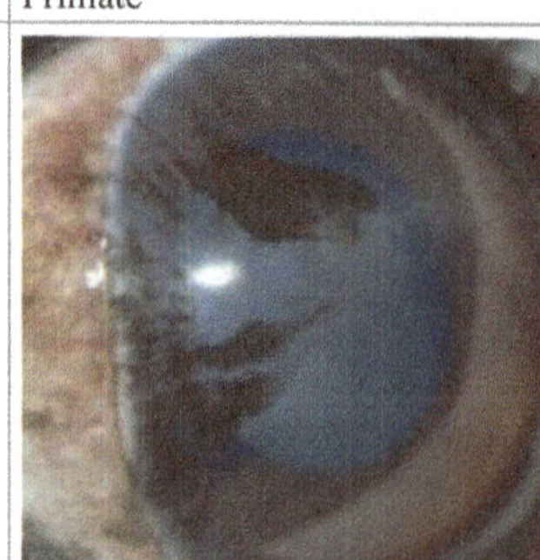 Dog

(continued)

Cornea		
Observation	**Definition**	**Photo + legend**
Scar	Opacity representing area of presumed fibrosis, usually well-defined	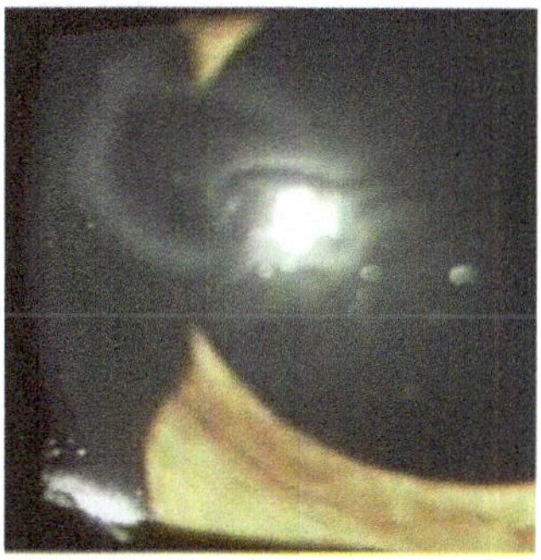 Primate. Focal lesion
		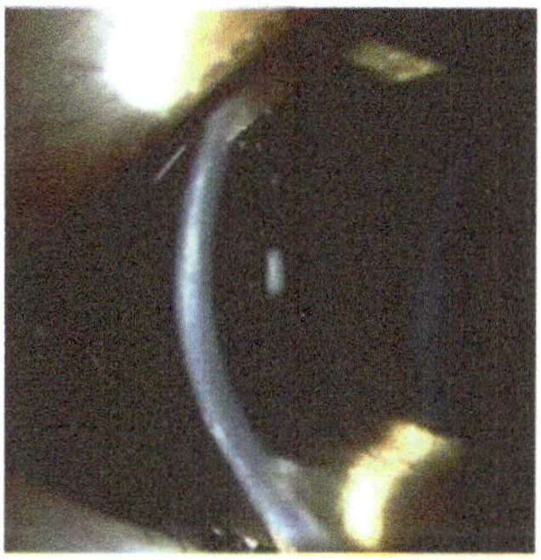 Primate (slit-lamp corneal section)
		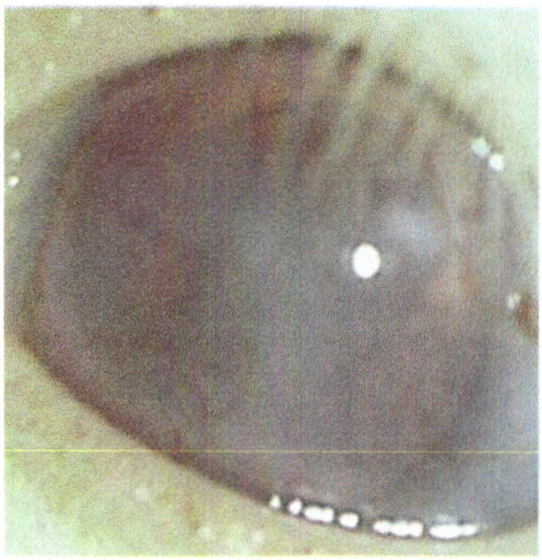 Rat. Diffuse

(continued)

Cornea		
Observation	Definition	Photo + legend
Tear film defect	Inadequate production or spreading of the precorneal tear film Synonyms: Dry eye, corneal desiccation, keratoconjunctivitis sicca	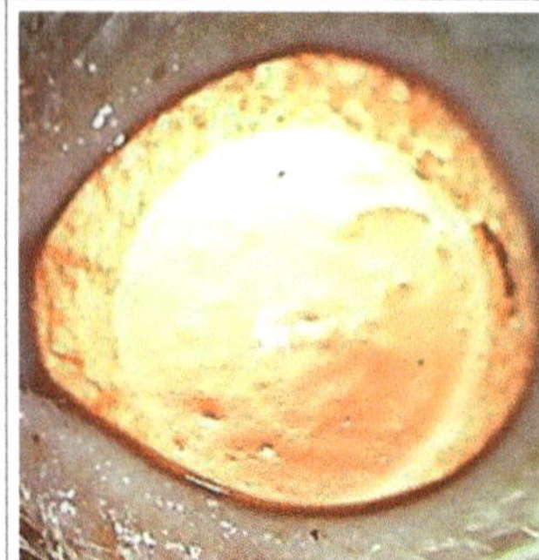 Rat
		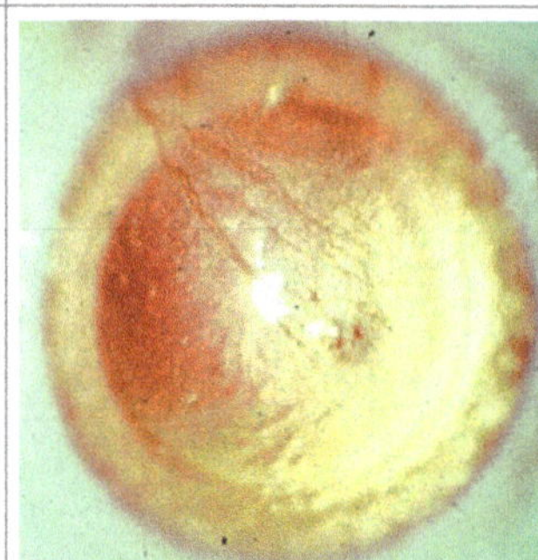 Rat. Note also corneal vascularization
Ulcer	Full-thickness loss of corneal epithelium with or without concurrent loss of underlying corneal stroma. Epithelial defect commonly identified by fluorescein uptake by corneal stroma Modifiers of location, extent, and depth should be included See Chap. 5 for scoring of fluorescein staining	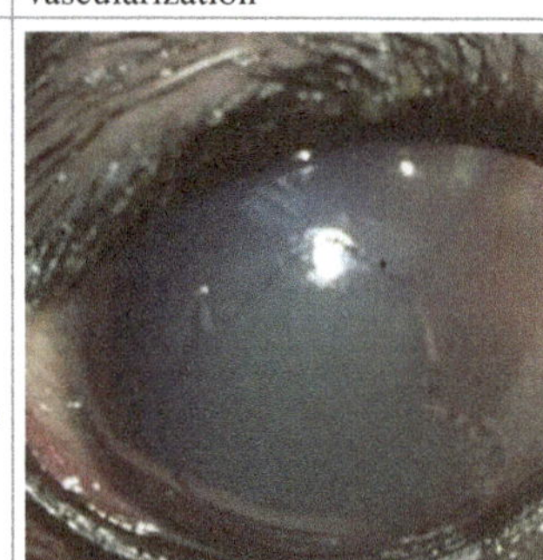 Dog

(continued)

Cornea		
Observation	Definition	Photo + legend
		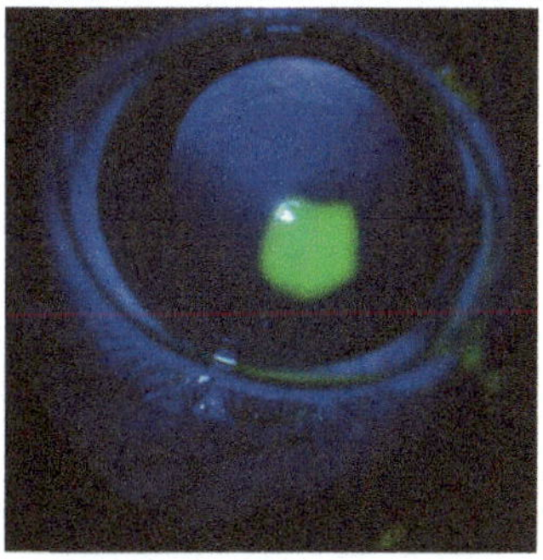 Rabbit. Ulcer delineated with fluorescein stain
Vascularization	Patent blood vessels abnormally present within the corneal stroma Synonyms: Pannus Modifiers of location, extent, and depth should be included See Chap. 5 for scoring	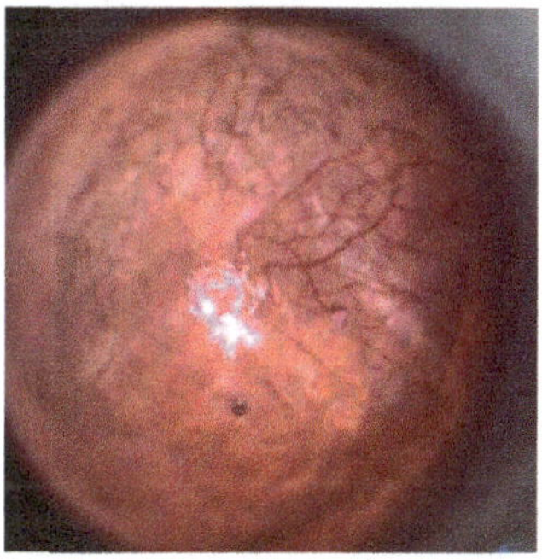 Rat
		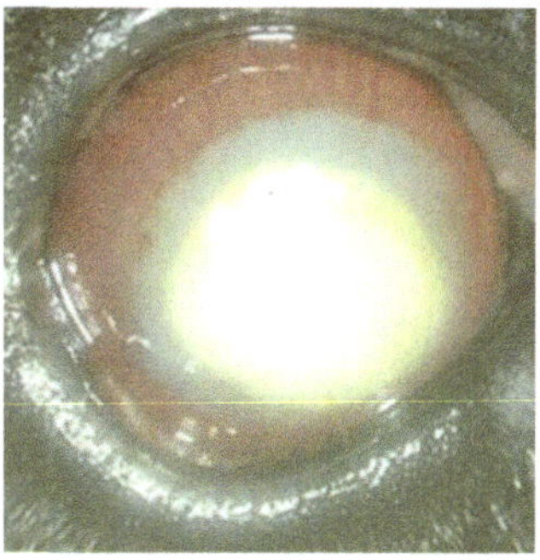 Guinea pig. Axial cellular infiltrate also present

(continued)

Sclera		
Observation	Definition	Photo + legend
Hyperpigmentation	Pigment (most commonly melanin, other pigments possible) present within the sclera (location, depth, and color indicated)	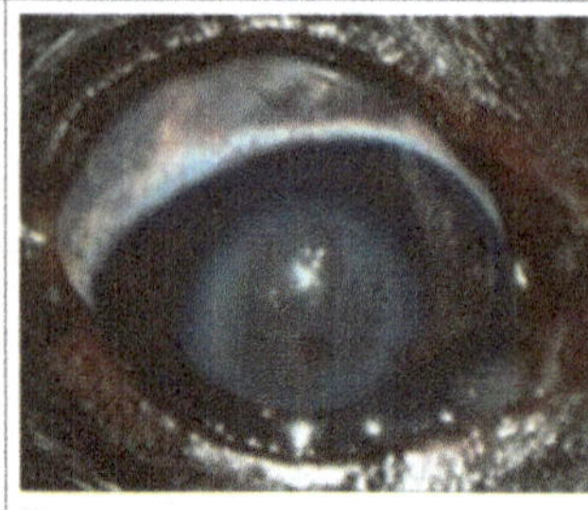 Dog
Mass	Space-occupying scleral lesion	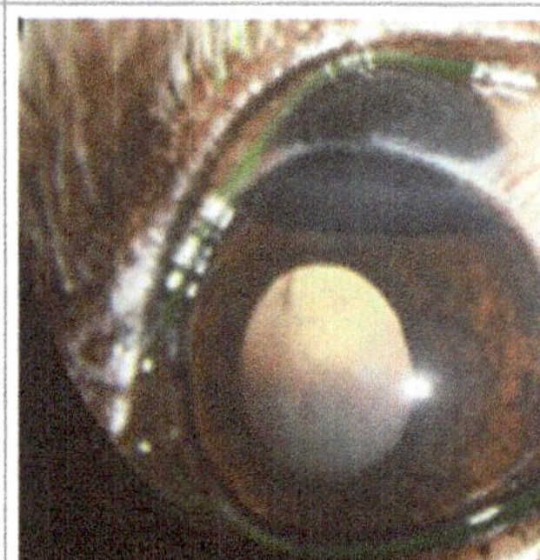 Dog. Mass, pigmented
		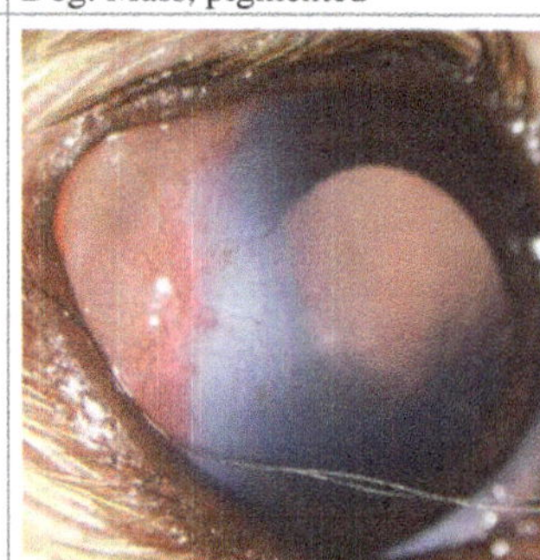 Dog. Inflammatory proliferation. Note dilated vasculature
Vascular injection	Dilation of episcleral vasculature	See above accompanying a proliferative inflammatory lesion

Aqueous/Anterior Chamber

Aqueous humor is the normally transparent fluid produced by the ciliary body epithelium that fills the anterior chamber, pupil, and posterior chamber. Aqueous humor exits the eye through the iridocorneal angle via the corneoscleral trabecular and uveoscleral outflow pathways; the balance of production and outflow maintains normal intraocular pressure. Aqueous humor provides oxygen, nutrition, and waste removal for the avascular lens and cornea. Breakdown of the blood ocular barrier produces alterations of aqueous humor components, as materials from the blood plasma are leached into the eye, ultimately affecting its transparency. Such alterations may include increased proteins, cells, and fibrin (see Chap. 5 for methods of describing and scoring such alterations). Inflammation reduces aqueous humor production resulting in decreased intraocular pressure (ocular hypotony), while obstruction of the outflow will result in increased intraocular pressure (ocular hypertension).

Recommended modifier terminology to further describe specific location, size, and extent of aqueous humor and anterior chamber lesions includes:

Location: superior, inferior, temporal, nasal (alternatively quadrants may be used—superotemporal, inferotemporal, inferonasal, superonasal), anterior, posterior, or equatorial.

Size: millimeter/centimeter scale (depending on species) or relative to corneal diameter (for instance, "said lesion is approximately half of the corneal diameter").

Extent: minimal, mild, moderate, or severe.

Observation	Definition	Photo + legend
Anterior chamber, deep	Increased space between cornea and iris/lens. Causes include posterior displacement of lens and decreased volume of the lens as may occur in hypermature cataract	See examples above under "globe, enlarged" for rat and rabbit
Anterior chamber, shallow	The space between the iris/lens and the cornea is shallower than normal. Causes include anterior displacement of the iris/lens, intumescent cataract, iris bombé, swelling of the iris	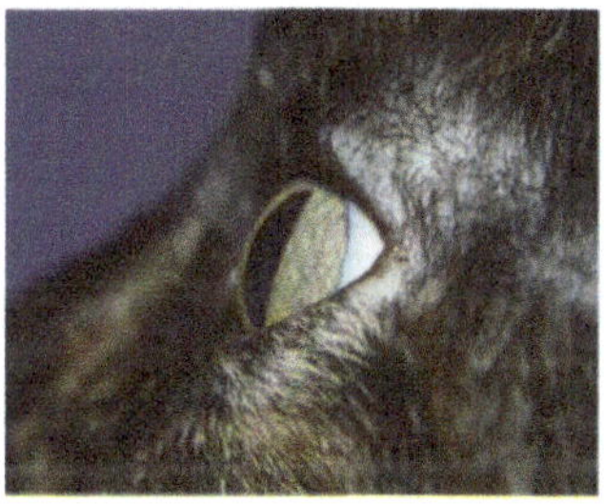 Cat. Forward displacement of the vitreous, lens, iris so that the iris is nearly contacting the inner cornea
		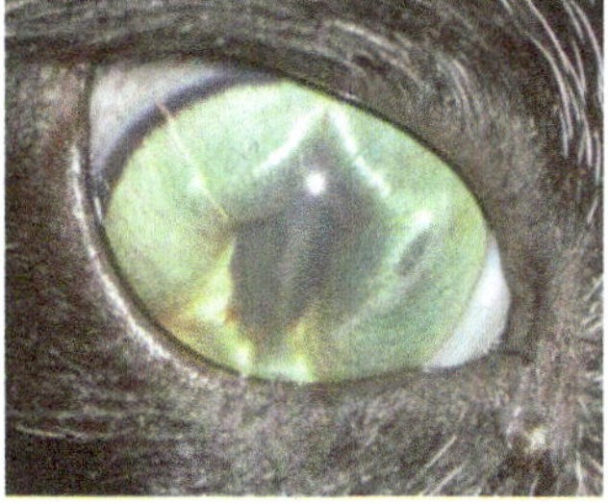 Cat. Posterior synechia with secondary iris bombé

(continued)

Observation	Definition	Photo + legend
Cells	Cells are visible as particles in the aqueous when illuminated by a beam of light passing through the anterior chamber Modifiers of color and extent should be included See Chap. 5 for scoring	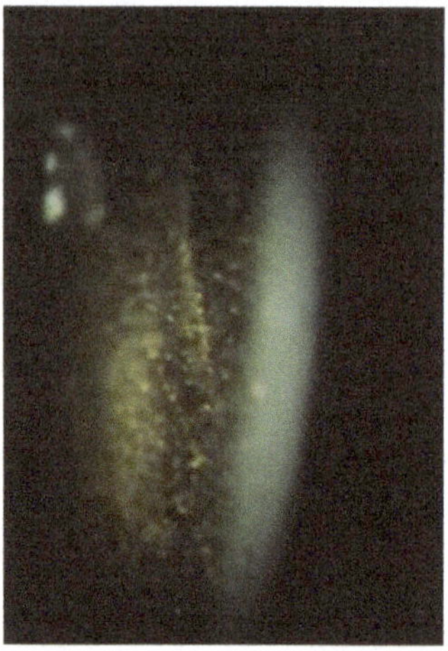 Dutch-belted rabbit
Flare	Tyndall phenomenon whereby protein in the aqueous humor is visible when a beam of light is passed through the anterior chamber See Chap. 5 for scoring	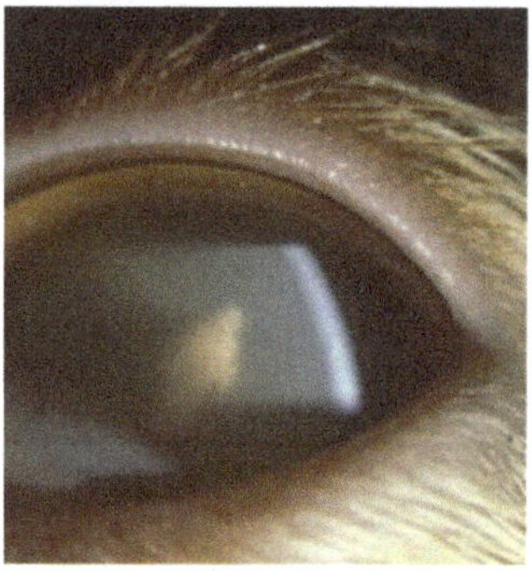
Hyphema	Blood in the anterior chamber	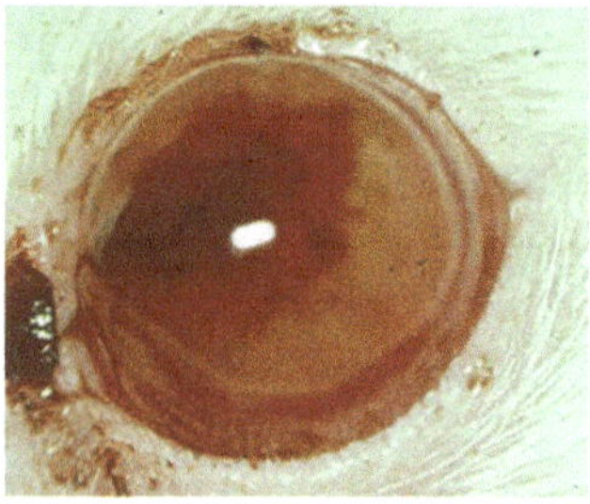 Rat

(continued)

Observation	Definition	Photo + legend
Hypopyon	Inflammatory cells in the anterior chamber. See Chap. 5 for further description of intraocular inflammation	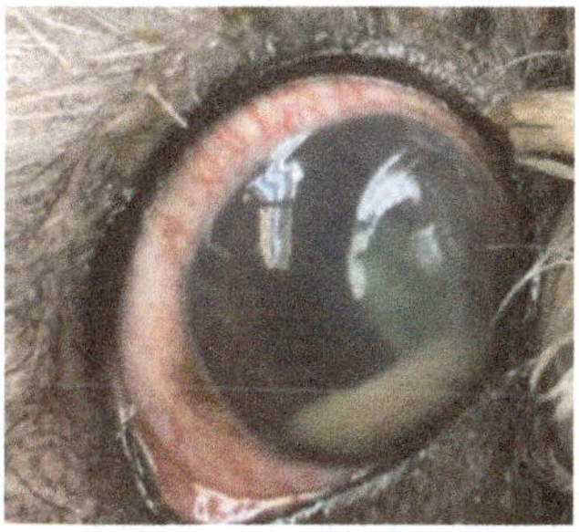 Dog
		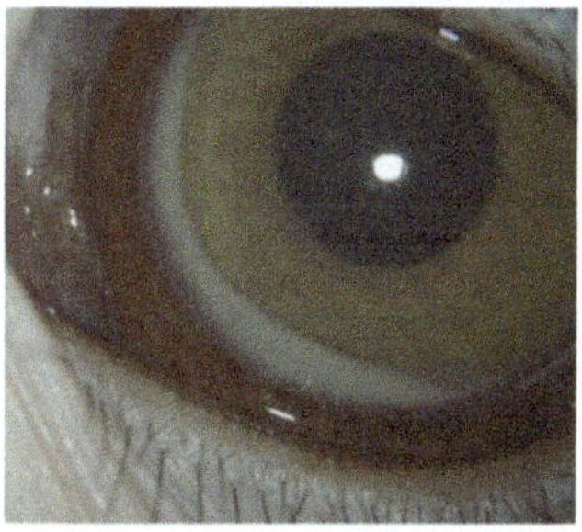 Primate
Keratic precipitates	Accumulations of inflammatory cells, fibrin, and pigment on the inferior corneal endothelium Modifiers of color and extent should be included See Chap. 5 for further description of intraocular inflammation	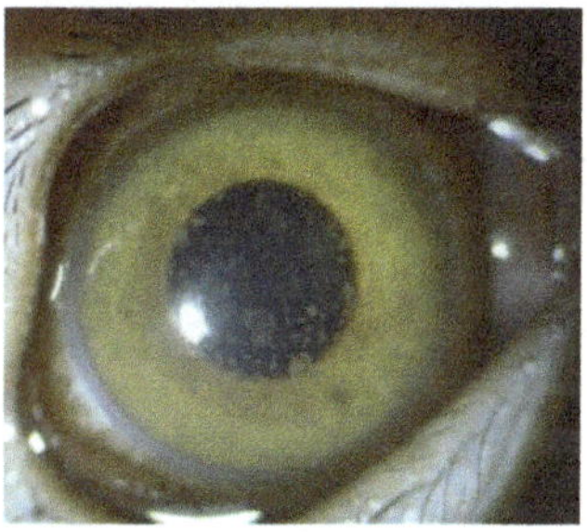 Primate
		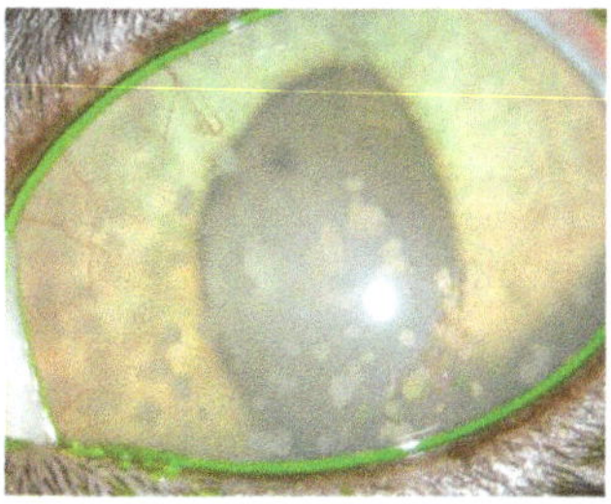 Cat

(continued)

Observation	Definition	Photo + legend
Lipemic aqueous	Lipid accumulation within the aqueous. Synonym: lipemic aqueous	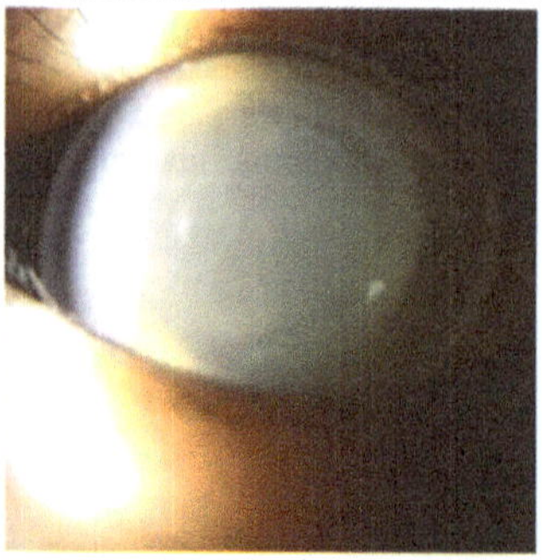 Primate
		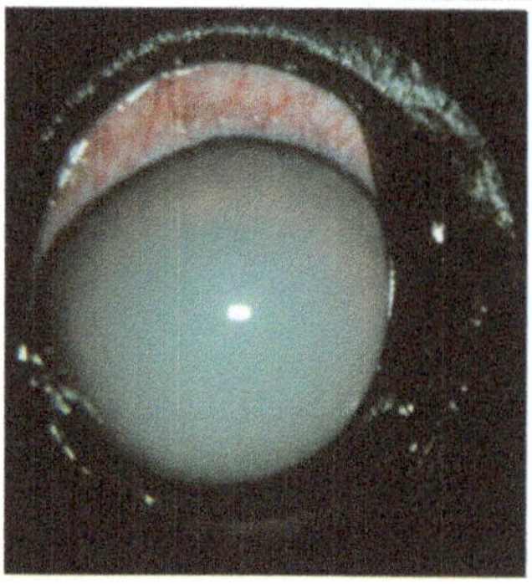 Dog
Plasmoid	Proteins and fibrin in aqueous occurring as a result of marked compromise of the blood-aqueous barrier	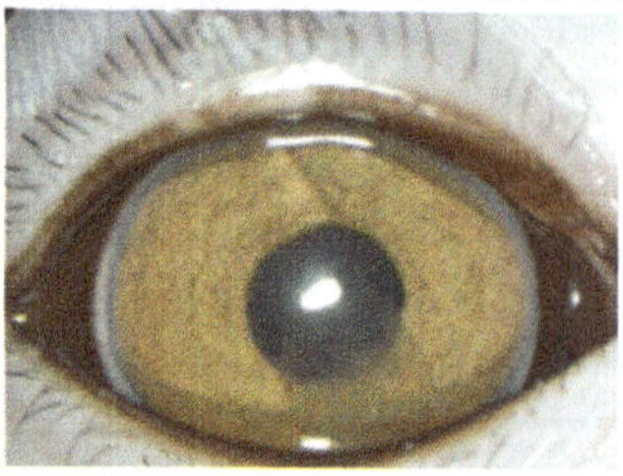 Primate
		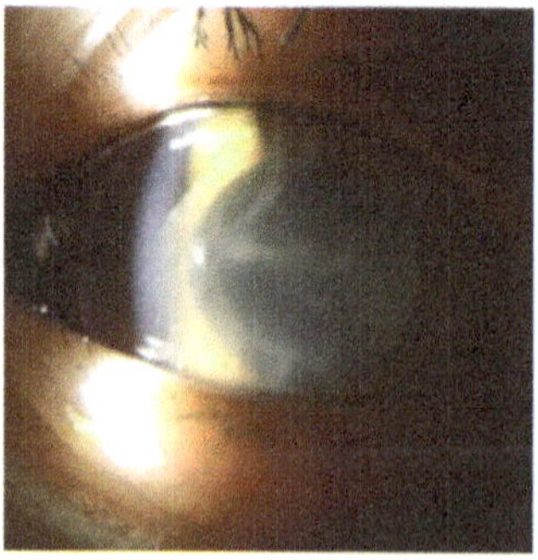 Primate

(continued)

Observation	Definition	Photo + legend
Vitreous strands	Clear strands of vitreous are visible in the anterior chamber. Differentiate from PPMs as the strands arise from behind the iris and enter the AC through the pupil	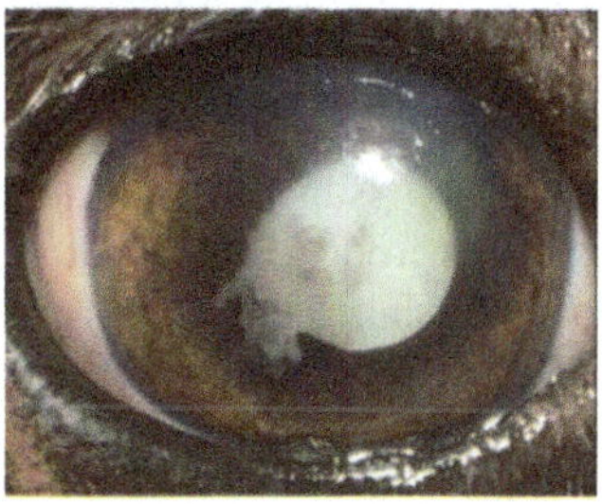 Dog. Cataract also present

Iris and Ciliary Body

The uvea is the inner vascular coat of the eye and consists of three distinct parts: iris/pupil, ciliary body/ciliary processes, and choroid. The iris and pupil regulate quantity of light passing through the lens and vitreous to the retina. One simple but critical means of assessing retinal function is the observation of an appropriate pupillary light reflex (PLR). Functions of the ciliary body and the ciliary processes include production of the aqueous humor and lenticular accommodation, respectively. The third component of the uvea is the choroid; which provides circulation, nutrition, and waste removal for the outer retina. Uveitis is inflammation of the uvea as a whole and may be divided into subsets that involve just the iris (iritis), the ciliary body (cyclitis), and choroid (choroiditis) or combinations of the above, e.g., iridocyclitis (iris and ciliary body), or the entire uvea, i.e., panuveitis. Uveitis may be infectious (bacterial, fungal, or viral), and the immune system plays an important role in responding to infection or as idiopathic immune-mediated or even autoimmune processes. Aggregations of lymphocytes may be resident in the uvea and participate in immune responses. Adhesions (synechiae) that form between the iris and lens or cornea or both may impede aqueous outflow resulting in secondary glaucoma. In addition, scarring over time can further interfere with function. Atrophy of the ciliary processes can result in ocular hypotony and atrophy of the eye in severe cases.

The recommended terminology described in this section covers the evaluation of the iris and ciliary body. Examination requires that the examiner have good knowledge and understanding of the variations that occur in different species as well as familiarity with variations in pigmentation of these structures. Every examination should begin with evaluation of the overall iris and pupil as well as the response of the pupil to direct and consensual light stimulation. The examiner must be familiar with normal vascular integrity and the appearance of congestion especially in pigmented versus nonpigmented eyes. Examinations must include evaluations before and after dilation of the pupils with attention to variations in pupil response and shape that may occur due to the administration of a test article or a procedural intervention. Findings should be correlated with histopathological findings.

Recommended modifier terminology to further describe specific location, size, and extent of iris and ciliary body lesions includes:

Location: superior, inferior, temporal, nasal (alternatively quadrants may be used—superotemporal, inferotemporal, inferonasal, superonasal), anterior, posterior, proximal, distal, or marginal.

Size: millimeter/centimeter scale (depending on species) or relative to corneal diameter (for instance, "said lesion is approximately half of the corneal diameter").

Extent: minimal, mild, moderate, or severe.

Iris and Ciliary Body		
Observation	Definition	Photo + legend
Atrophy	Spontaneous progressive thinning of the iris stroma	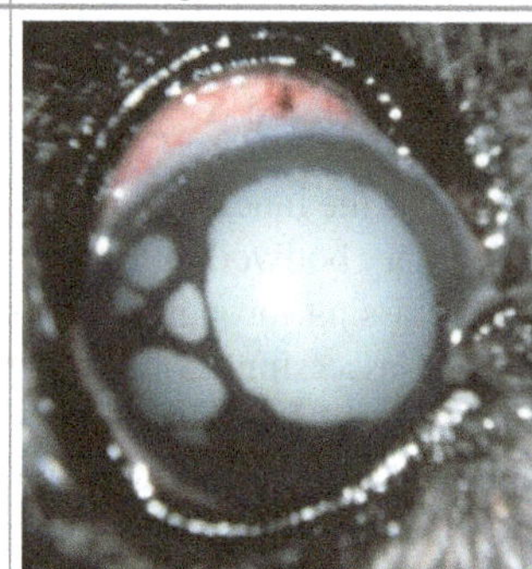 Dog. Also note complete cataract and conjunctival hyperemia. Corectopia present
Coloboma/ hypoplasia	A congenital partial or full-thickness defect in the iris	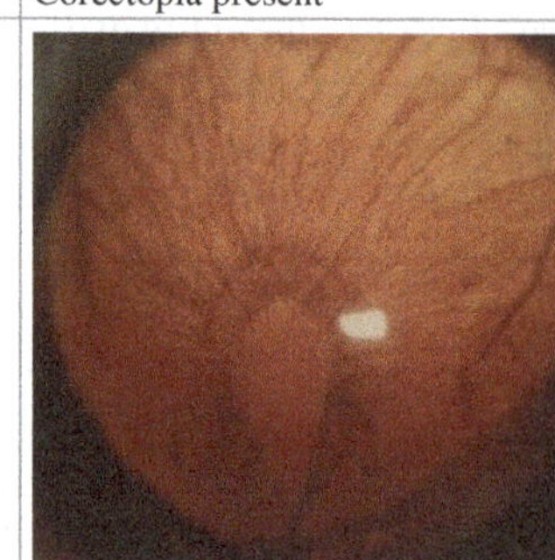 Rat. "Typical" 6 o'clock location. Corectopia present

(continued)

Iris and Ciliary Body		
Observation	Definition	Photo + legend
		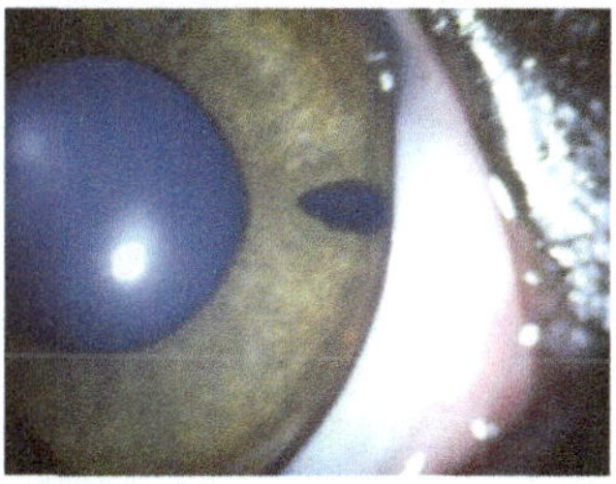 Primate. Atypical location
		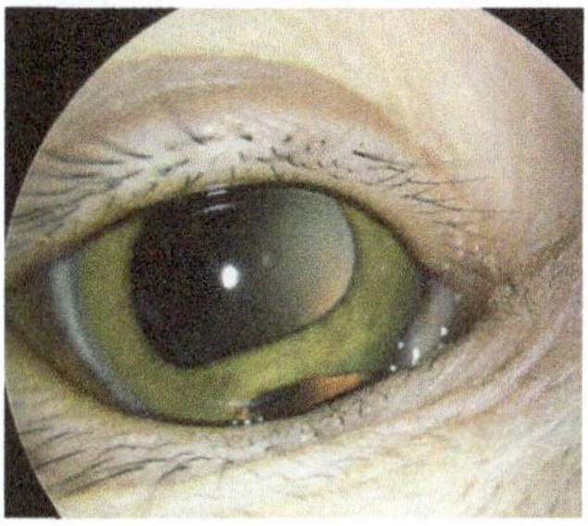 Primate
Congestion	Vascular injection of the iridal vessels Synonyms: Hyperemia, iris involvement See Chap. 5 for scoring	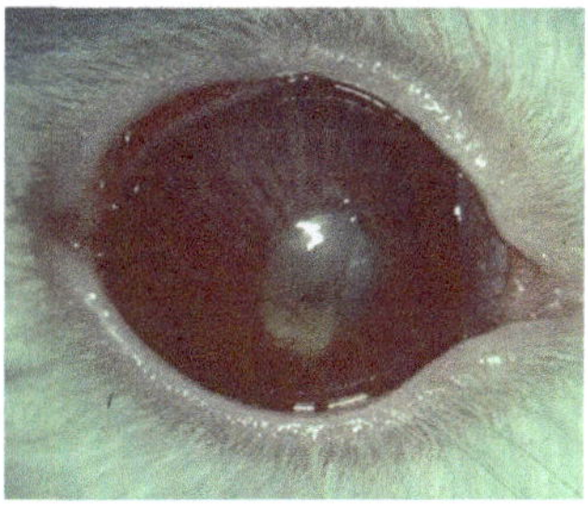 Rat
Corectopia/polycoria	Anomalous position of the pupil (corectopia). Multiple pupils (polycoria)	See examples above under iris atrophy and coloboma
Cyst	A cyst arising from the iris or ciliary body. May be pigmented or nonpigmented	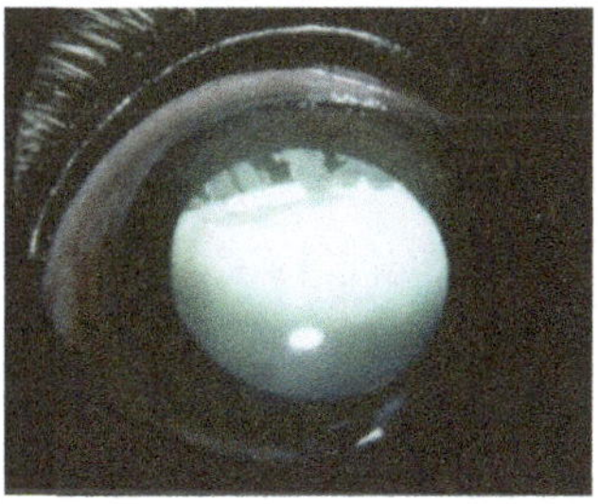 Dog. Lens coloboma and ciliary body cysts

(continued)

Iris and Ciliary Body		
Observation	Definition	Photo + legend
		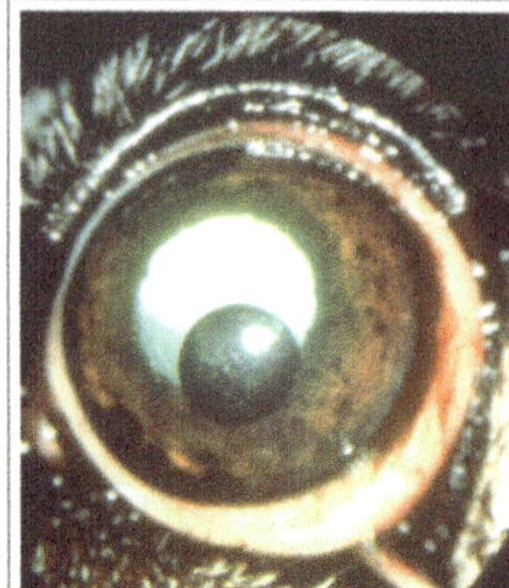 Dog
Depigmentation	Loss of iris pigment	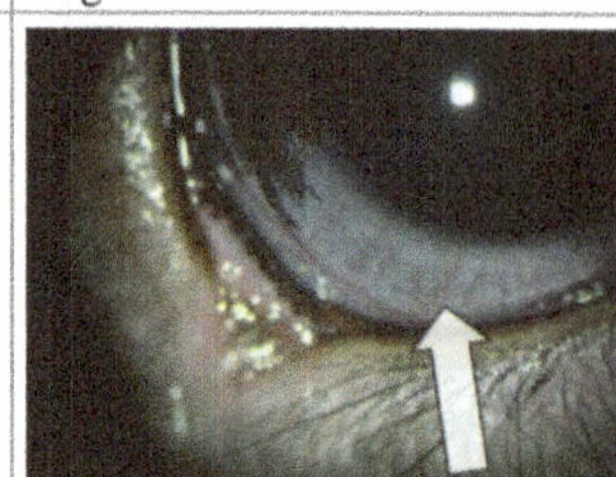 Dutch belted rabbit. Iris depigmentation
Dyscoria	An irregular or distorted shape to the pupil. Causes include atrophy of the iris, anterior or posterior synechiae, iris coloboma, traumatic injury to the iris	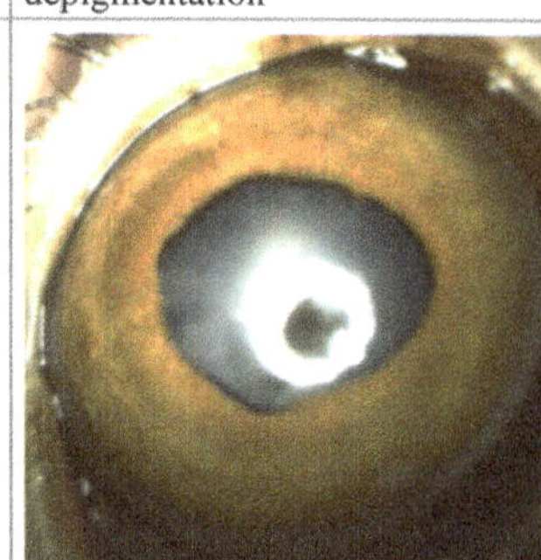 Primate. Note also cortical cataract and iris hyperpigmentation

(continued)

Iris and Ciliary Body		
Observation	Definition	Photo + legend
		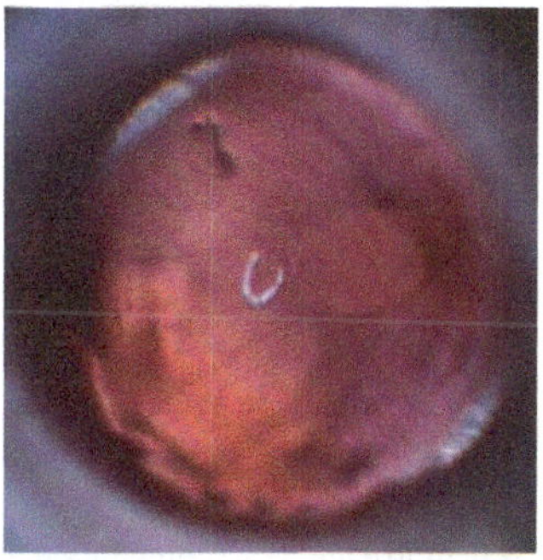 Mouse
		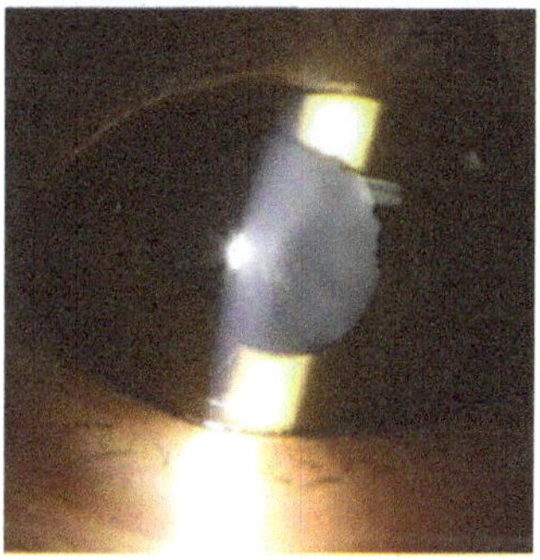 Primate. Lens cortical opacity also present
Hyperpigmentation	Increased pigmentation of the iris. May be localized or diffuse. When localized, may be an incidental finding	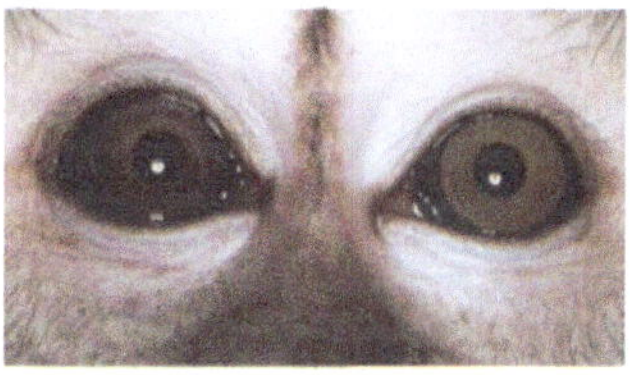 Primate
		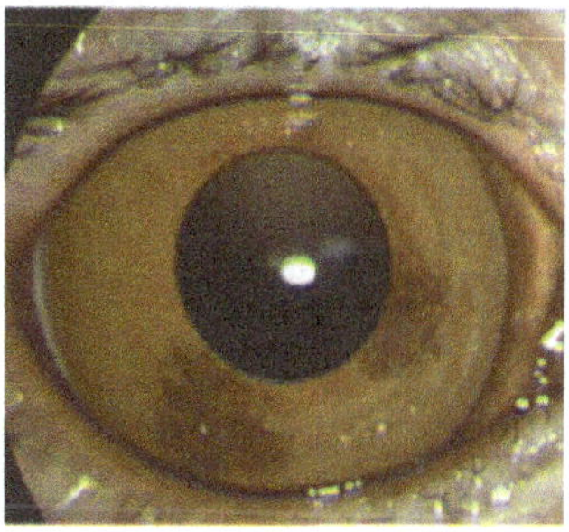 Primate

(continued)

Iris and Ciliary Body		
Observation	Definition	Photo + legend
		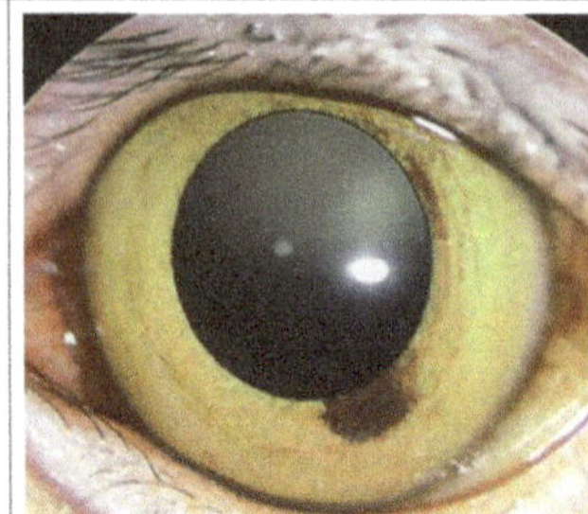 Primate
Iris hemorrhage	Free blood within iris stroma. May be transient in juvenile animals	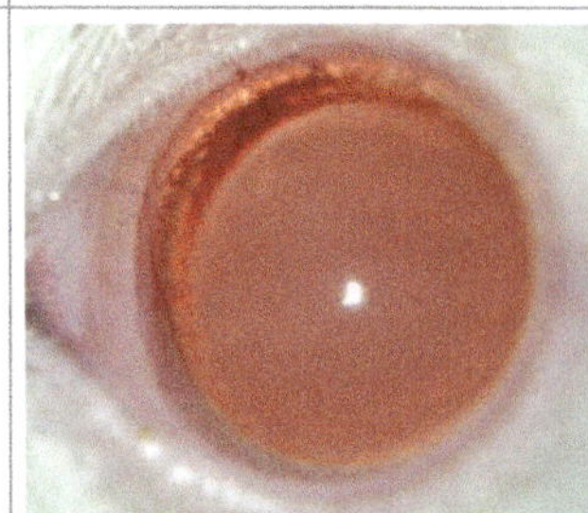 Rat. There is also fibrin in the anterior chamber
		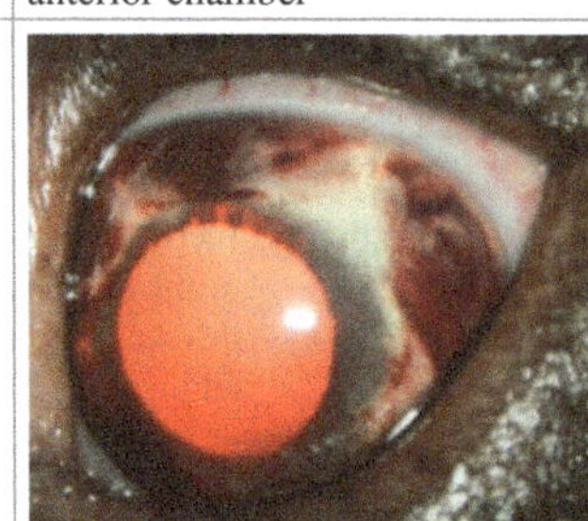 Dog. Iris hemorrhage within a subalbinotic (blue/gray) iris
Limited view	Inability to visualize iris detail due opacity of cornea and/or anterior chamber	

(continued)

Iris and Ciliary Body		
Observation	Definition	Photo + legend
Mass		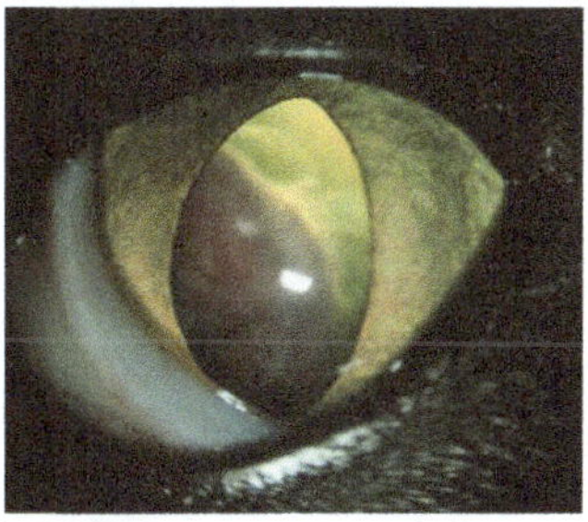 Cat. Ciliary body mass visible within the pupil
		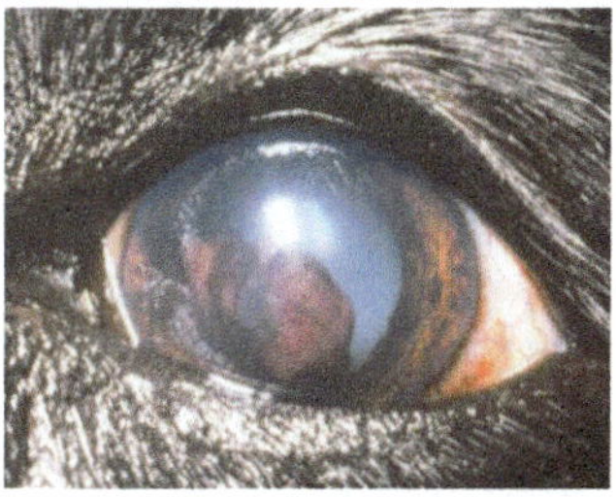 Dog
		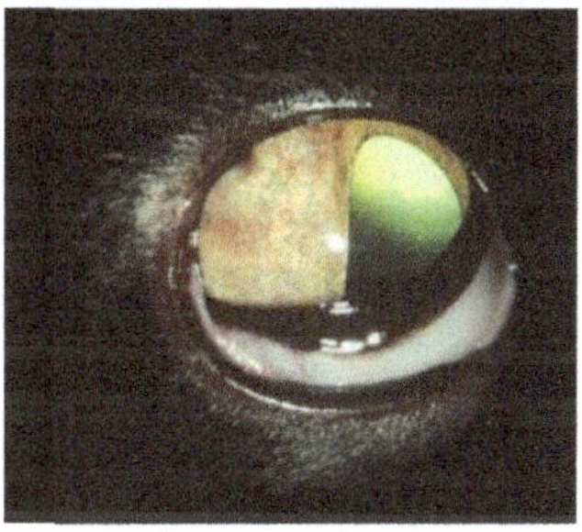 Cat
Persistent pupillary membranes (PPM)	Incomplete resorption of embryonal vasculature and mesenchymal tissues resulting in retained iris strands that attach at the collarette region of the iris and extend to another part of the iris surface, the lens, or the cornea	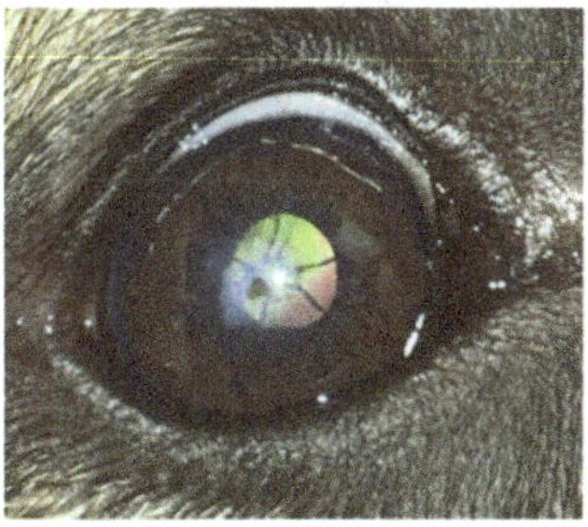 Dog. PPM attached to the cornea and anterior lens with associated opacities in each area

(continued)

Iris and Ciliary Body		
Observation	Definition	Photo + legend
		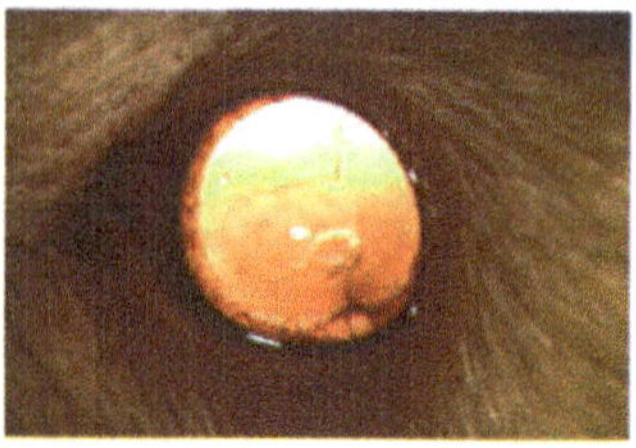 Rat
		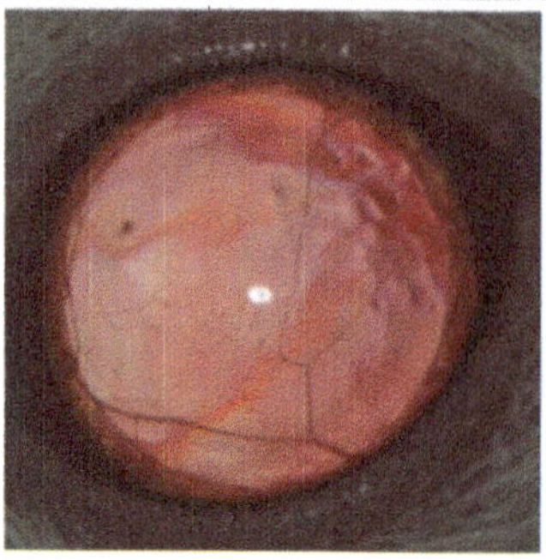 Rat
Synechia, anterior	Post-inflammatory adhesion of the iris to the cornea	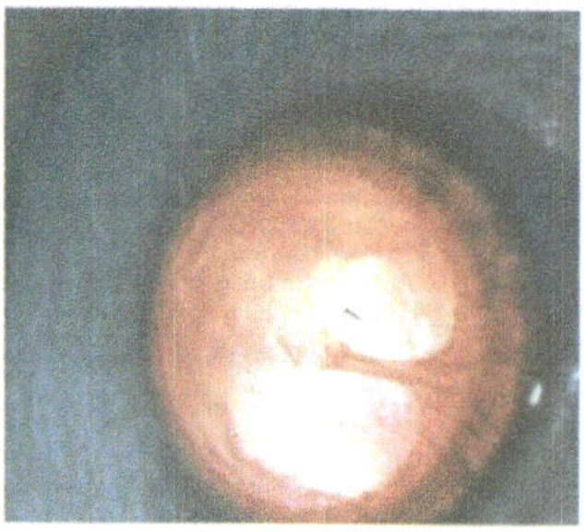 Rat (photo courtesy of David Wilkie)
		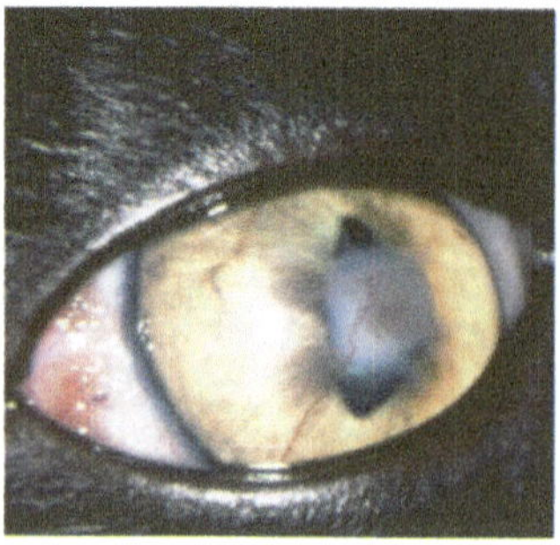 Cat

(continued)

Iris and Ciliary Body		
Observation	Definition	Photo + legend
Synechia, posterior	Post-inflammatory adhesion of the iris to the lens	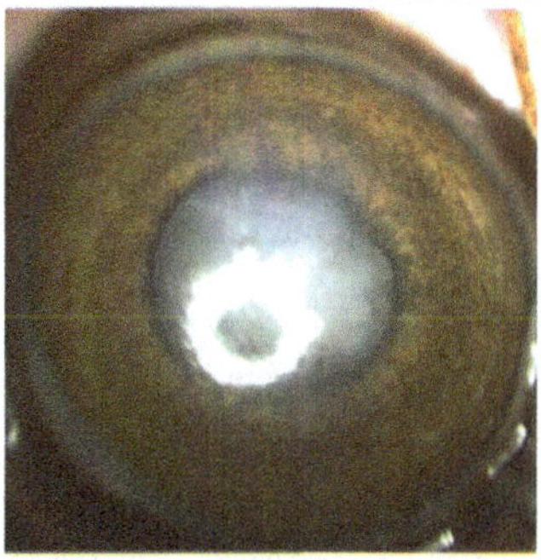 Primate. Entropion uveae, pigment on anterior lens capsule, iridal stromal hyperpigmentation, and cortical lens opacity also present
		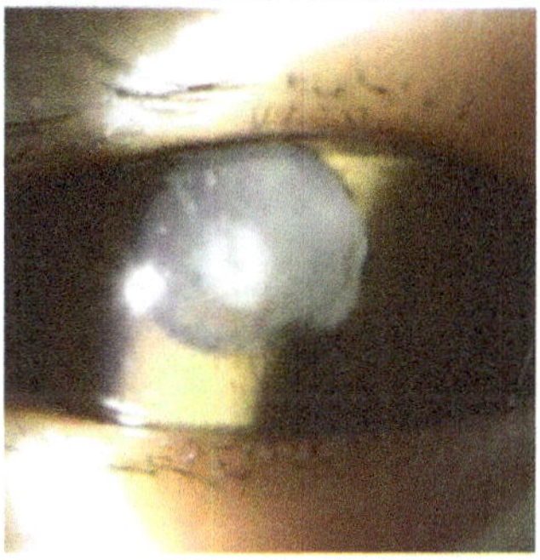 Primate. Cortical cataract also present

Lens

The lens is the metabolically active structure of the eye that focuses light on the retina. Technically a cataract is defined as any opacity of the lens that may vary from punctate, multifocal, intermediate, to diffuse. Evaluation of the lens requires slit-lamp biomicroscopy. Regions of the lens that are observed with biomicroscopy are capsular (involving the lens capsule that encloses the lens fibers), cortical (including sub-capsular areas), nuclear (the center of the lens), and equatorial (the area where lenticular zonules insert and lens epithelial cells differentiate and elongate). The lens epithelial cells continue to produce new lens fibers throughout life resulting in the nuclear region representing the oldest portion of the lens and the differentiating lens fibers comprising the layers of the lens cortex. These metabolically active lens epithelial cells are a common site for toxicological effects from compounds entering the eye, with a common ultimate endpoint of developing lens opacity (clinically referred to as cataract).

Location: superior, inferior, temporal, nasal (alternatively quadrants may be used—superotemporal, inferotemporal, inferonasal, superonasal), anterior, posterior, capsular, subcapsular, cortical, perinuclear, nuclear, and equatorial.

Size: punctate, intermediate, diffuse, and multifocal.

Lens		
Observation	Definition	Photo + legend
Aphakia	Lens not observed	
Capsule rupture	Rupture of the anterior or posterior lens capsule with release of lens material. Often associated with secondary inflammation	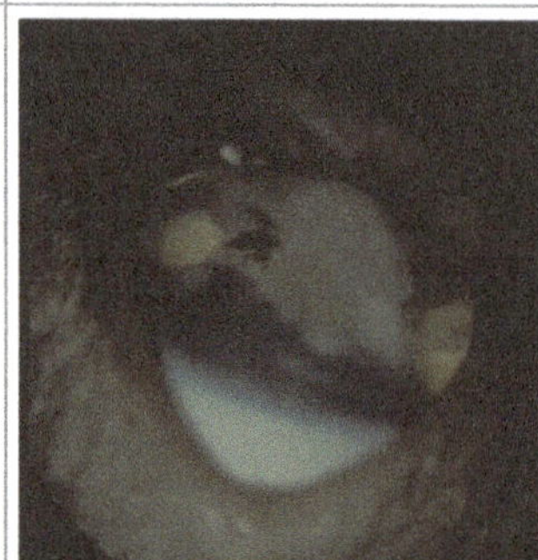 Rabbit
		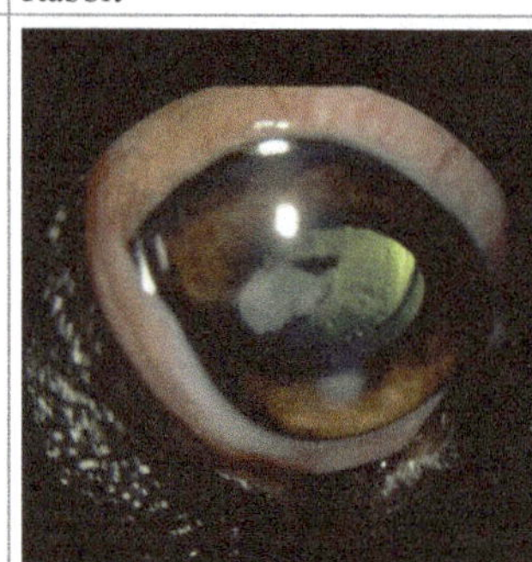 Rabbit. Lens cortex is protruding into the anterior chamber. Note also the pigment on the anterior lens capsule
Cells, capsular	Inflammatory cells on the anterior or posterior capsule. The cells may be white to tan in color Modifiers of color and extent should be included See Chap. 5 for further description of intraocular inflammation	

(continued)

Lens		
Observation	Definition	Photo + legend
Cells, cortical	Inflammatory cells in the lens cortex. When observed, it is most commonly associated with *Encephalitozoon cuniculi* in rabbits	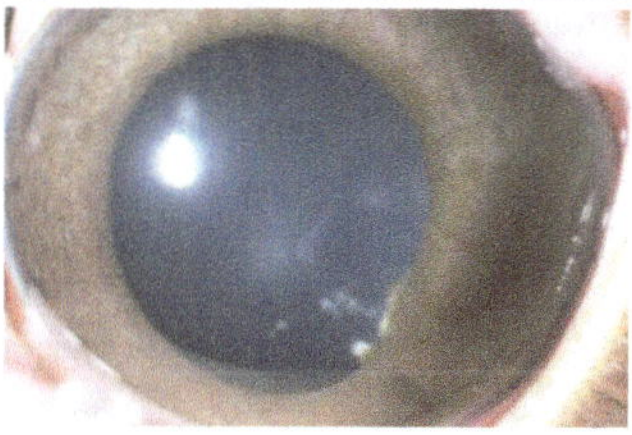 Rabbit. Posterior synechia and dyscoria also present
Coloboma	Developmental abnormality resulting in a segmental defect of the lens. The lens zonules are usually absent in the affected area	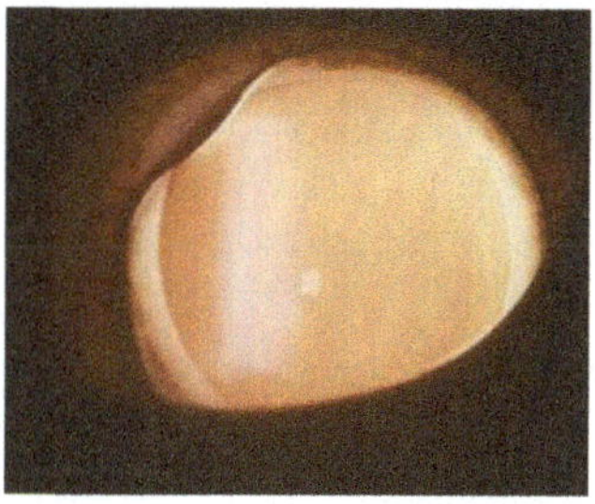 New Zealand white rabbit. Lens defect from 10–11 o'clock viewed with retroillumination
		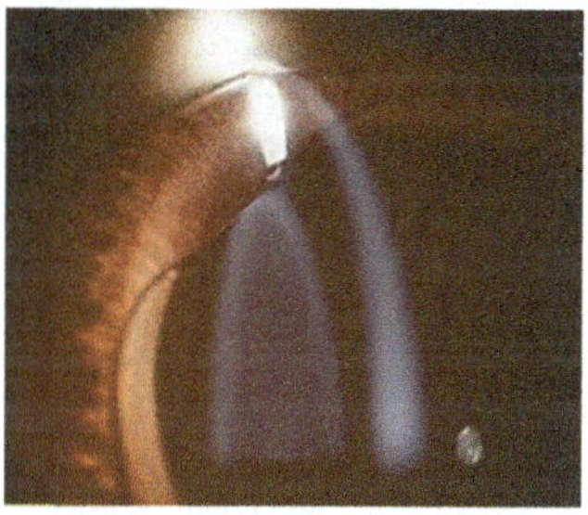 Same eye viewed with slit-lamp biomicroscopy
Lenticonus	Developmental abnormality resulting in anterior or posterior protrusion of the lens	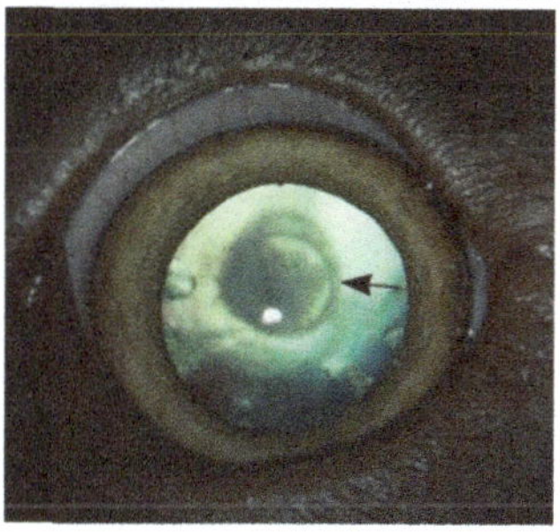 Dog. Posterior lenticonus

(continued)

Lens		
Observation	Definition	Photo + legend
Limited view	Visualized of lens detail prevented by opacification of the cornea and/or anterior chamber	
Luxation/ subluxation	Displacement of the lens caused by partial or complete breakdown of the zonule fibers. If complete, may be anterior or posterior	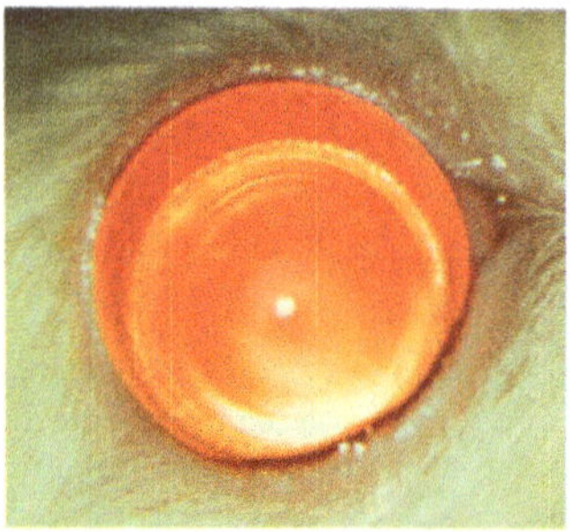 Rat
		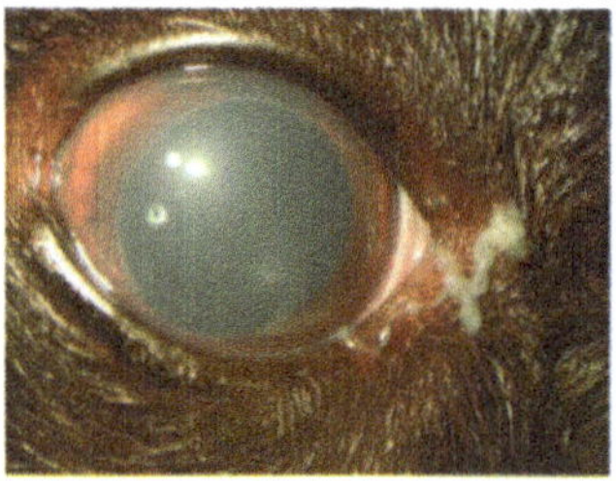 Dog. Anterior luxation
Microphakia	Abnormally small lens	
Opacity, capsular	Opacity limited to lens capsule (anterior, posterior, or equatorial) Modifiers of location (anterior, posterior, equatorial) and extent should be included Synonym: Cataract See Chap. 5 for further description of cataract assessment	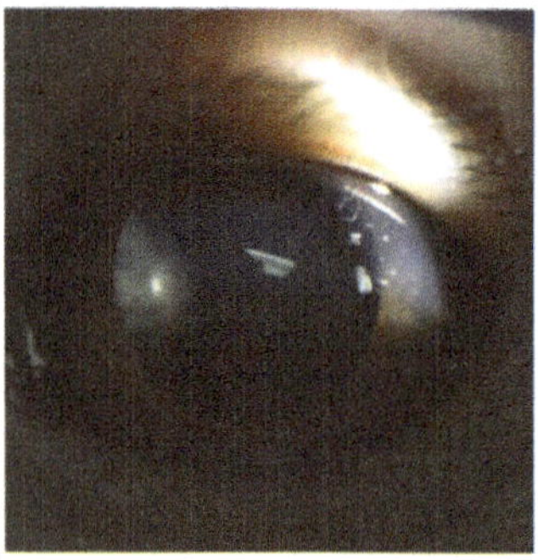 Primate. Posterior capsular opacity

(continued)

Lens		
Observation	Definition	Photo + legend
Opacity, complete	Opacity involving the entire lens Synonym: Cataract See Chap. 5 for further description of cataract assessment	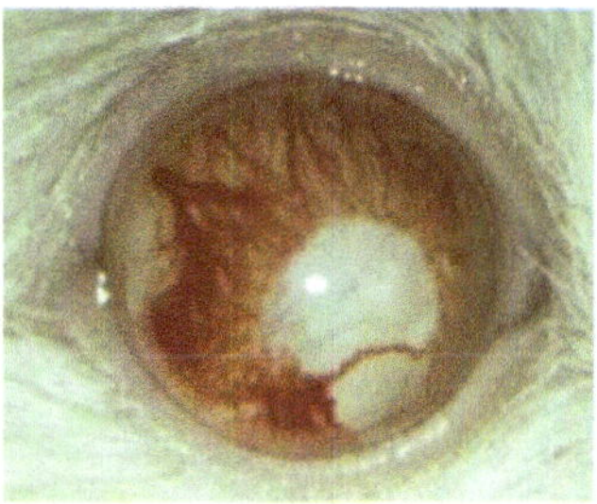 Rat. Note also iridal congestion and complete cataract
		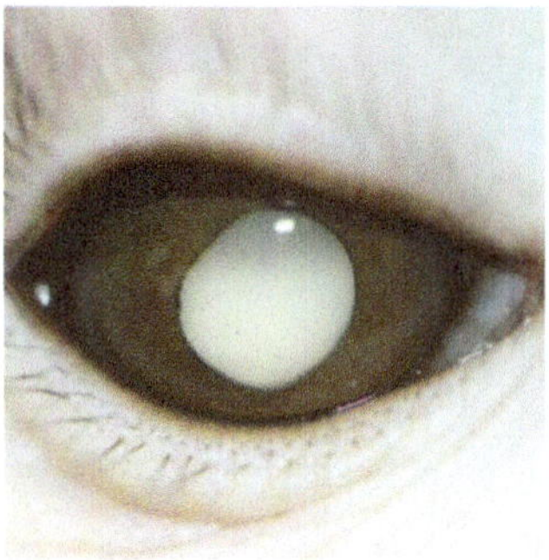 Primate. Note also iris hyperpigmentation, dyscoria. This cataract is liquefied and hypermature
Opacity, cortical	Opacity involving the lens cortex Modifiers of location (anterior, posterior, equatorial) and extent should be included Synonym: Cataract See Chap. 5 for further description of cataract assessment	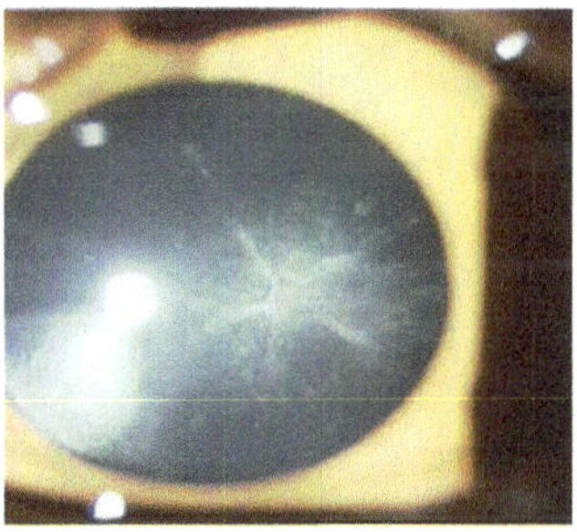 Primate. Posterior cortex affected

(continued)

Lens		
Observation	Definition	Photo + legend
		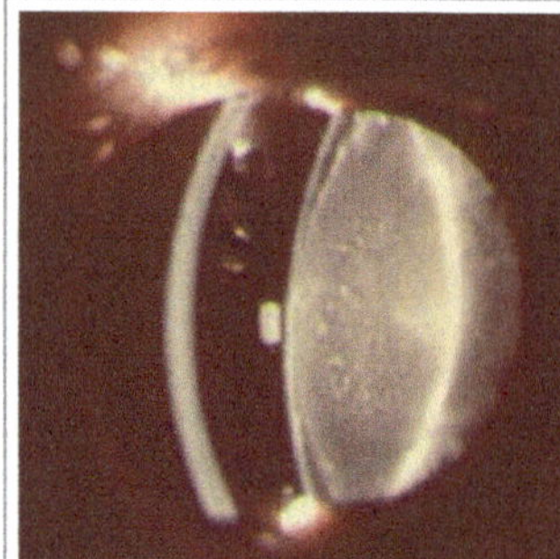 Primate. Diffuse anterior, posterior, and nuclear cortical opacity
		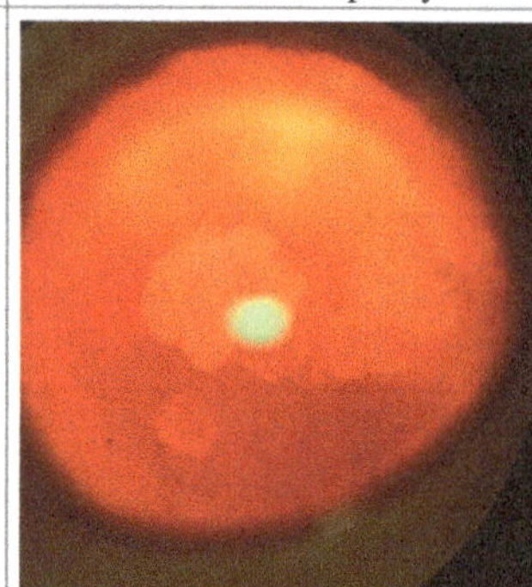 Rat. Posterior cortical opacity
		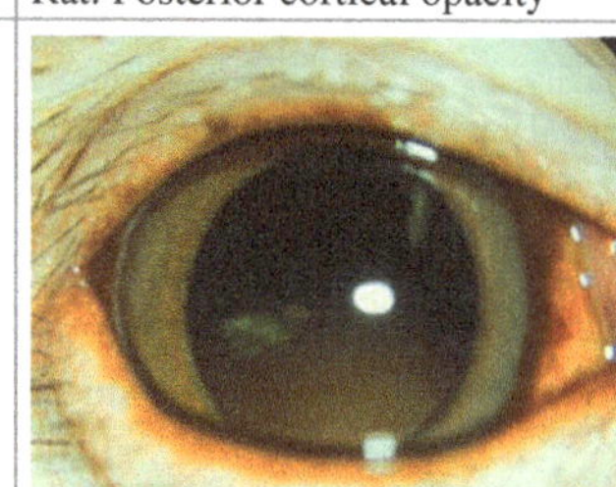 Primate. Multifocal linear posterior cortical opacities

(continued)

Lens		
Observation	Definition	Photo + legend
		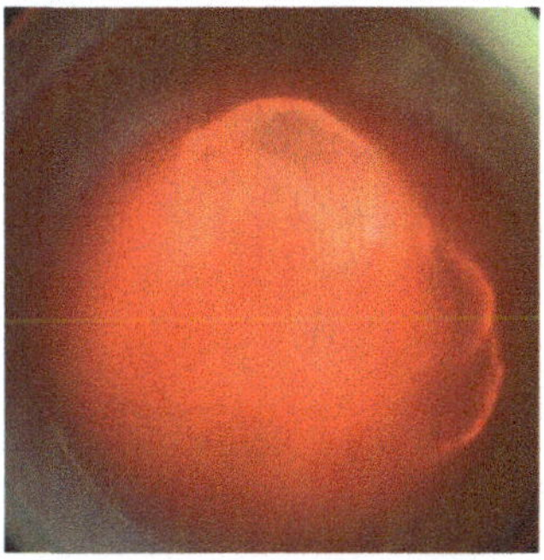 Mouse
		 Rat
		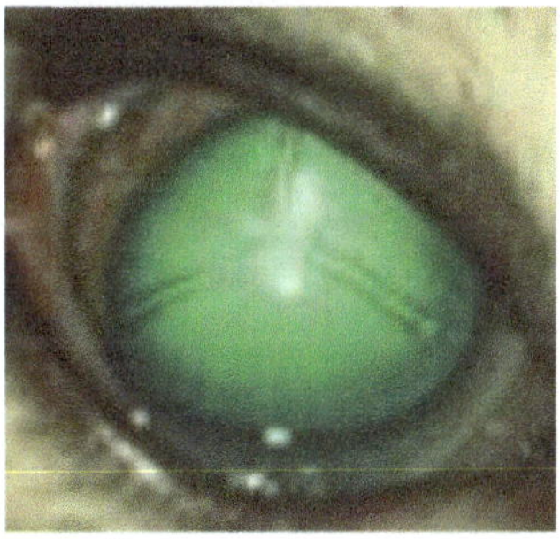 Cat

(continued)

Lens		
Observation	Definition	Photo + legend
Opacity, nuclear	Opacity involving the nuclear region of the lens See Chap. 5 for scoring	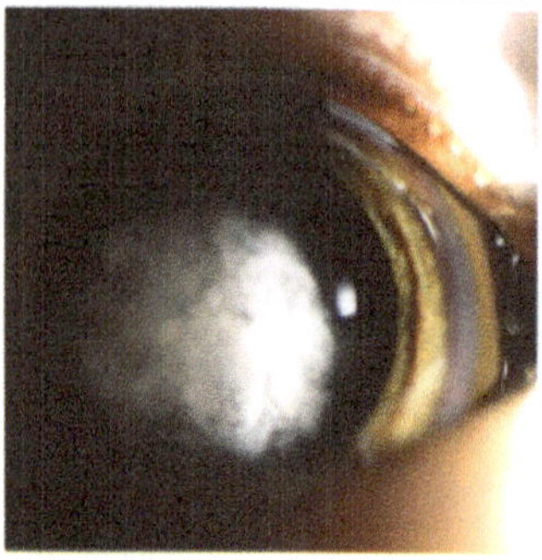 Primate
		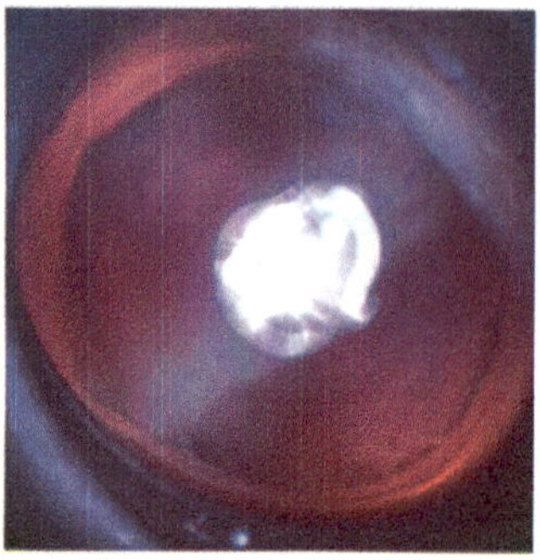 Guinea pig
Pigmentation	Pigment on the lens capsule. Can be seen as a consequence of inflammation or as an isolated inconsequential finding on pretest examination	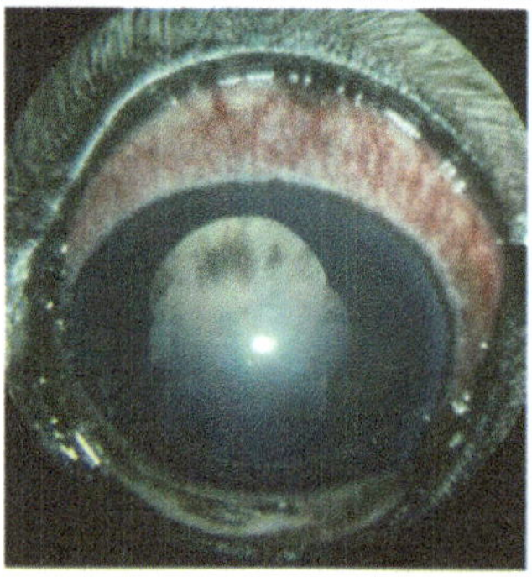 Dog. Note also dyscoria

(continued)

Lens		
Observation	Definition	Photo + legend
		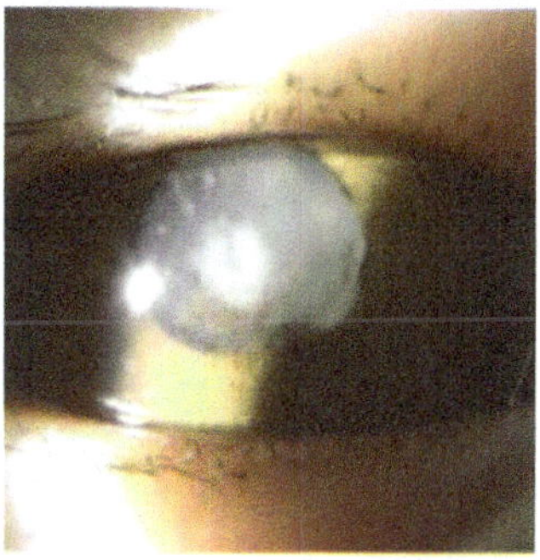 Primate. Pigment on anterior lens capsule (cortical opacity is also present)
		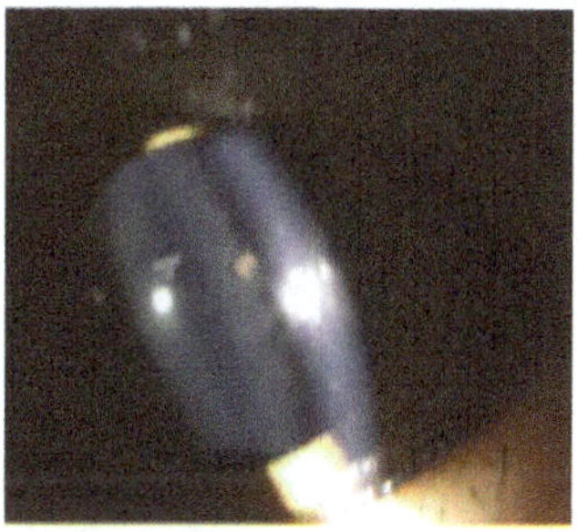 Primate. Multifocal pigment on anterior lens capsule
Prominent lens suture	Increased density of lens sutures. Considered anomalous variation	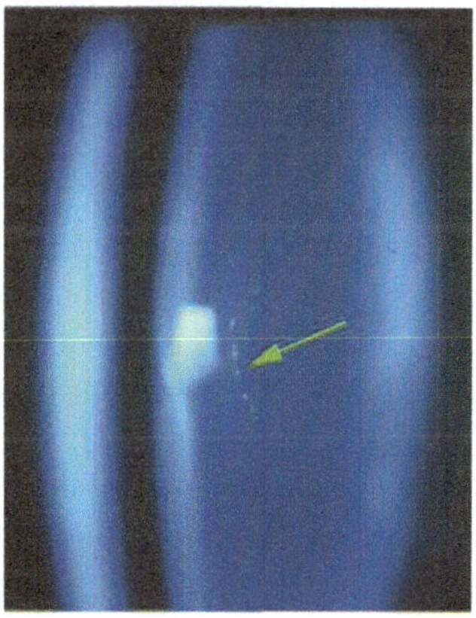 Pinpoint opacities along the anterior lens sutures

(continued)

Lens		
Observation	Definition	Photo + legend
Vacuoles	Circular translucencies in lens cortex	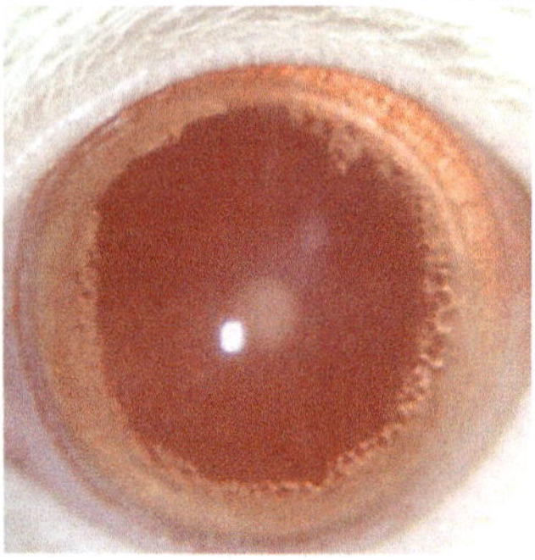 Rat. Equatorial lens vacuole (diabetic model)
		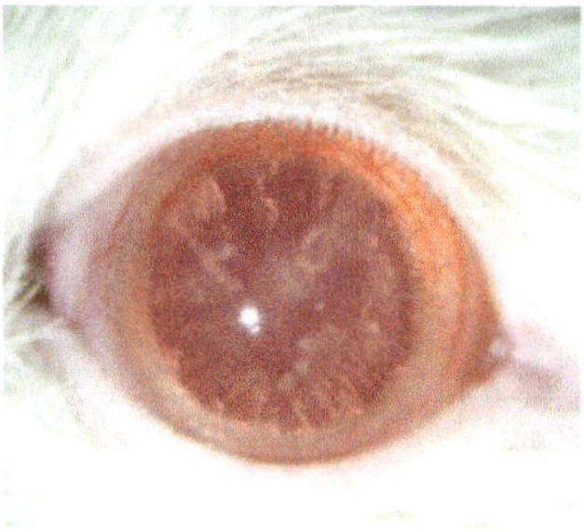 Rat (diabetic model)

Vitreous Humor

Terminology used to describe findings within the vitreous includes congenital malformations and acquired abnormalities which may be degenerative or inflammatory. Species born with fused eyelids have eyes that are developmentally immature compared with NHP. Transient persistence of embryonic structures including the primary vitreous is often seen in juvenile individuals. Strictly speaking, anything other than transparent vitreous in a mature animal is considered abnormal.

Location: superior, inferior, temporal, nasal (alternatively quadrants may be used—superotemporal, inferotemporal, inferonasal, superonasal), anterior, posterior, central, or peripheral.

Size: millimeter/centimeter scale (depending on species) or relative to optic nerve head (ONH) widths (for instance, "said lesion is approximately three ONH widths").

Extent: minimal, mild, moderate, or severe.

Vitreous		
Observation	Definition	Photo + legend
Cells	For complete description, refer to Chap. 5	
Degeneration	Liquefaction of the vitreous Synonym: Syneresis	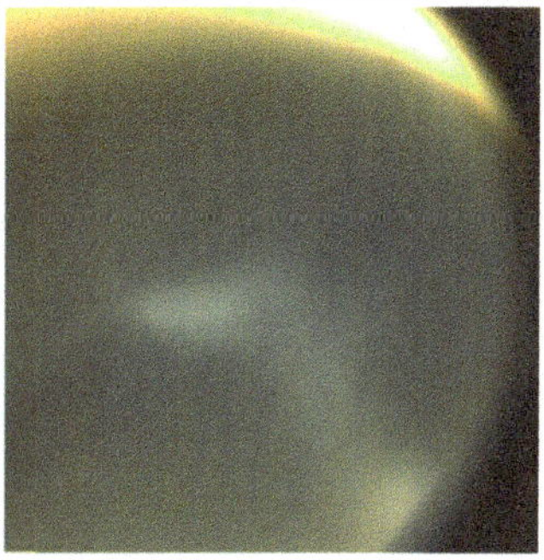 Primate
Detachment	Separation of the posterior vitreous from the retinal internal limiting membrane	
Floaters/debris	Fibrillar or cellular condensates within the vitreous	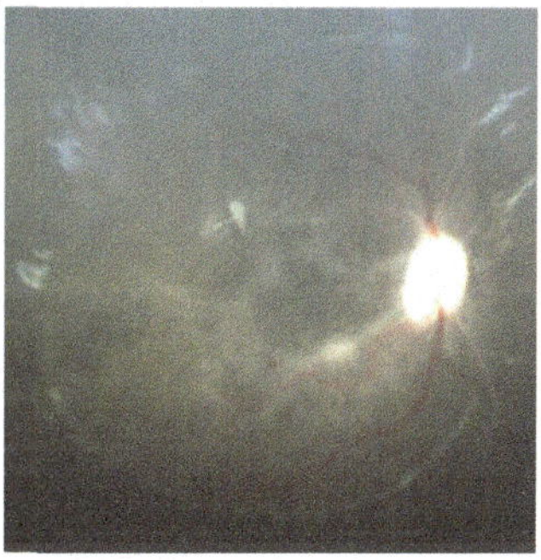 Primate. Vitreal traction bands, petechial retinal hemorrhage, and macular degeneration also present
		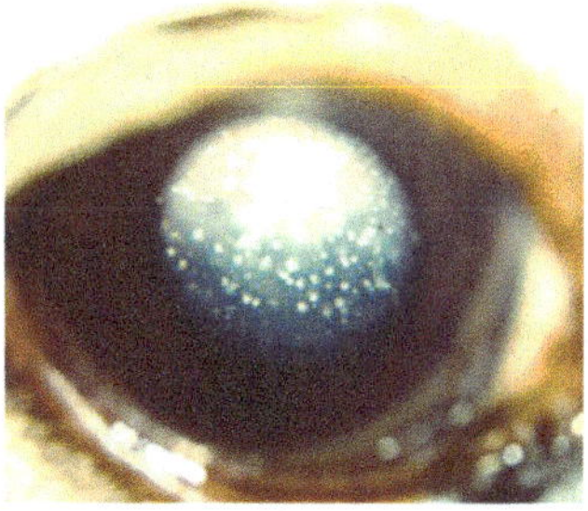 Dog. A suspension of calcium-lipid complexes referred to as asteroid hyalosis

(continued)

Vitreous		
Observation	Definition	Photo + legend
		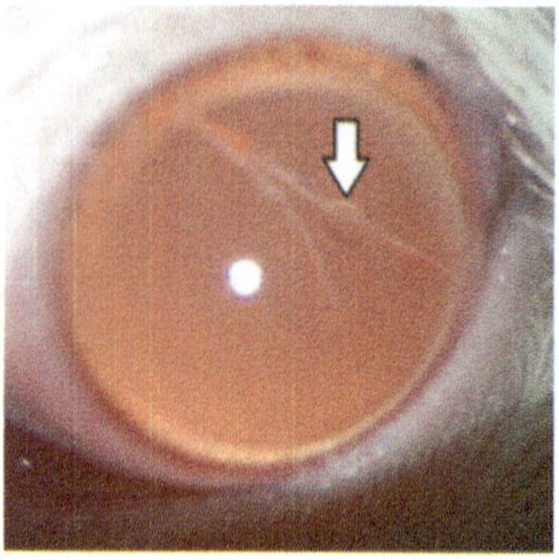 Rat. Transient vacuole located against the posterior lens capsule and associated with regressing hyaloid vasculature
Haze	Reduced transparency of the vitreous, may be caused by cells, increase in protein, or exogenously introduced material See Chap. 5 for scoring	 Primate
		 Primate. Petechial retinal hemorrhages and perivascular sheathing also present

(continued)

Vitreous		
Observation	Definition	Photo + legend
Hemorrhage	Blood within the vitreous. Origin may be the retina or uveal tissue, or from rupture of a persistent, patent hyaloid artery	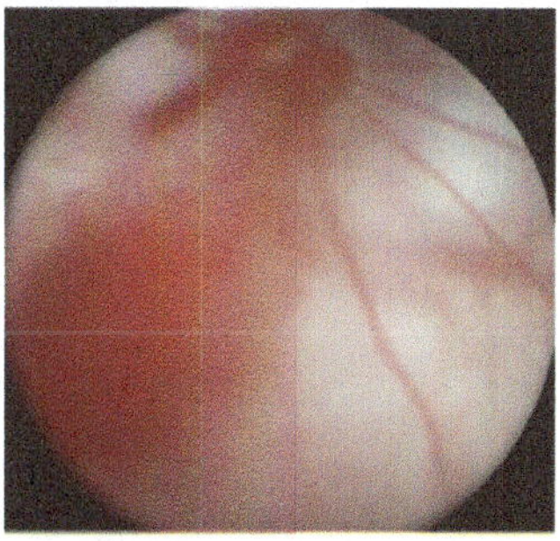 Rat
		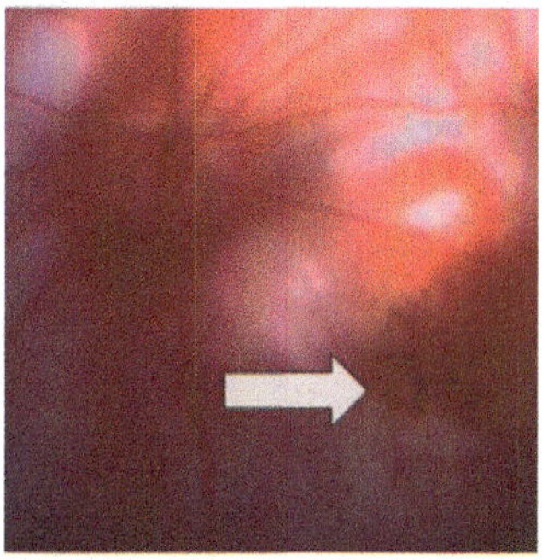 Rat. RBCs on posterior lens capsule from previous vitreous hemorrhage
		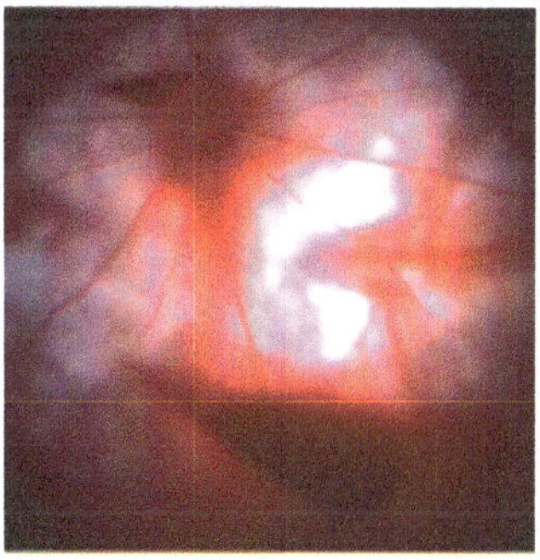 Rat

(continued)

Vitreous		
Observation	Definition	Photo + legend
		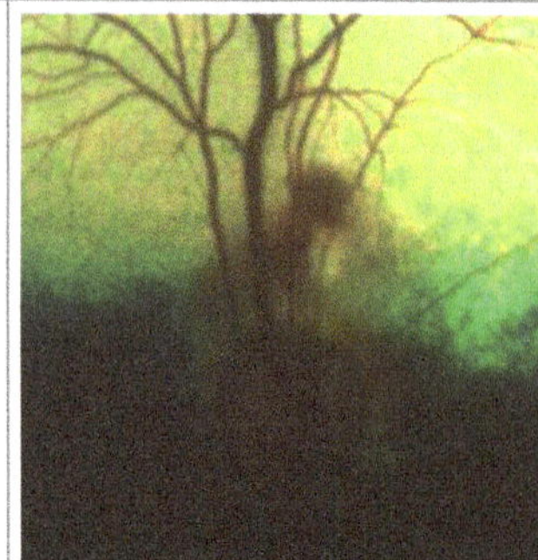 Dog
		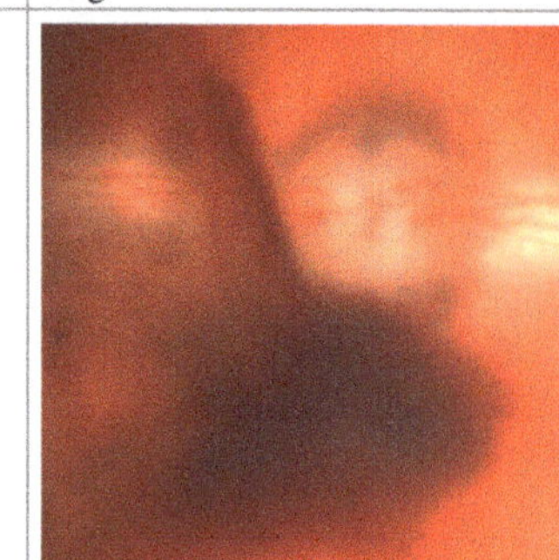 Rabbit
Persistent hyaloid artery	Postnatal persistence of the hyaloid vasculature may or may not be patent	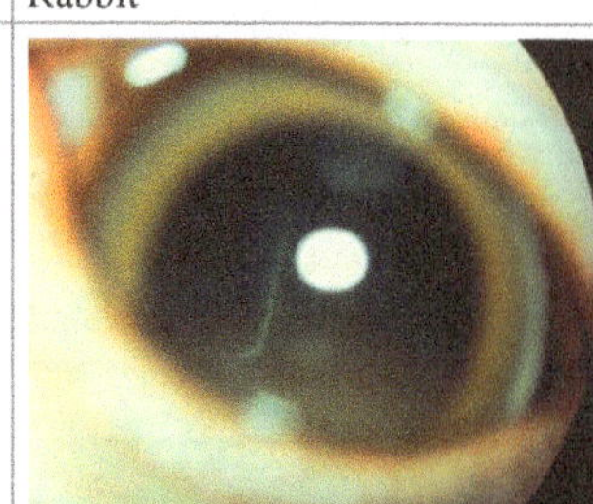 Primate. Nonpatent hyaloid artery
		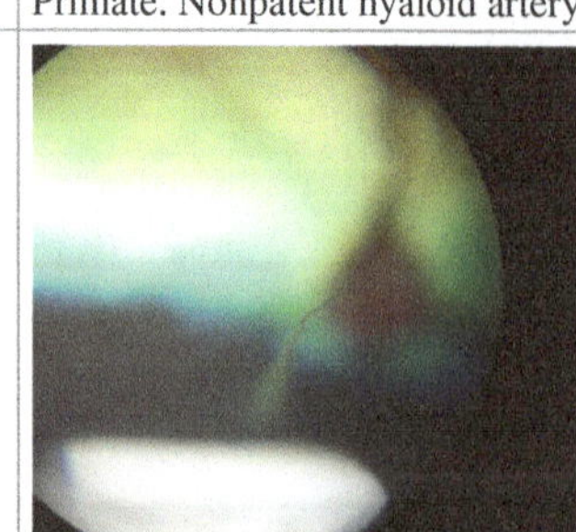 Dog. Partially patent hyaloid artery

(continued)

Vitreous		
Observation	Definition	Photo + legend
		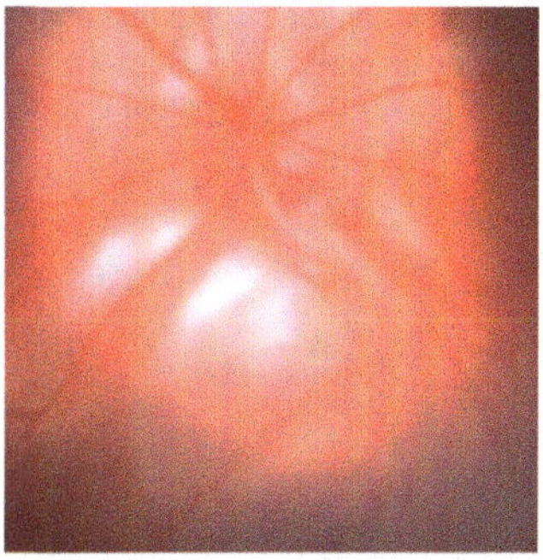 Mouse. Patent hyaloid artery
		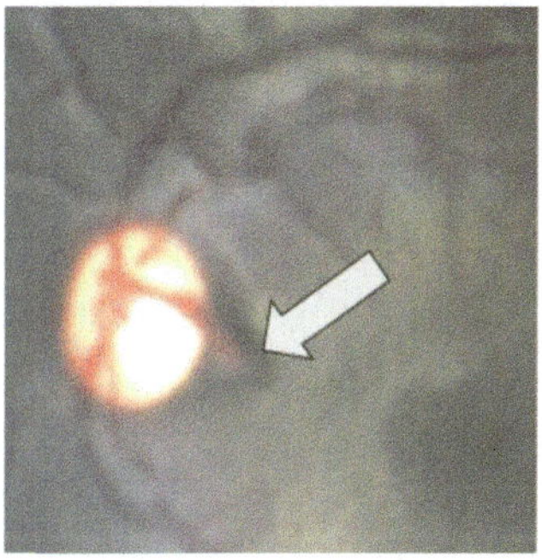 Primate. Patent hyaloid artery
		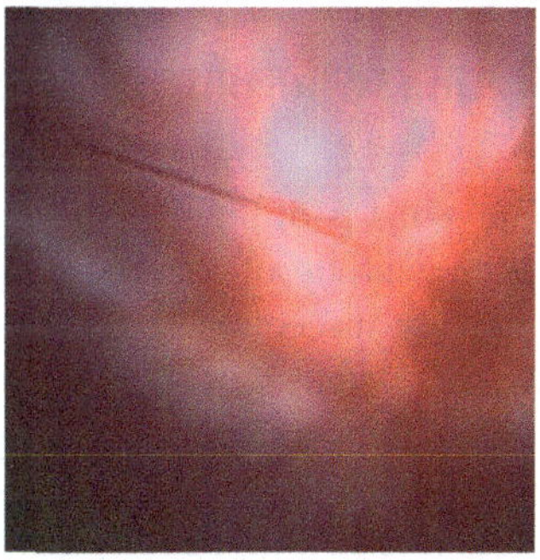 Rat. Patent hyaloid artery
Persistent hyperplastic vitreous	Postnatal persistence of the tunica vasculosa lentis with hyperplasia, possibly including fibrosis and pigmentation	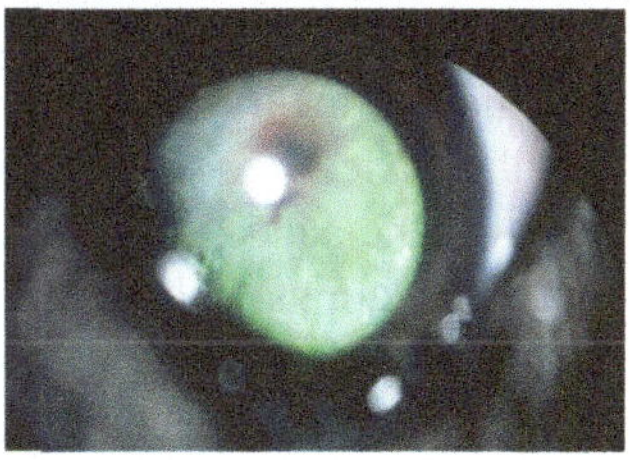 Dog

(continued)

Vitreous		
Observation	Definition	Photo + legend
Persistent tunica vasculosa lentis (PTVL)	Postnatal persistence of the tunica vasculosa lentis may or may not be patent	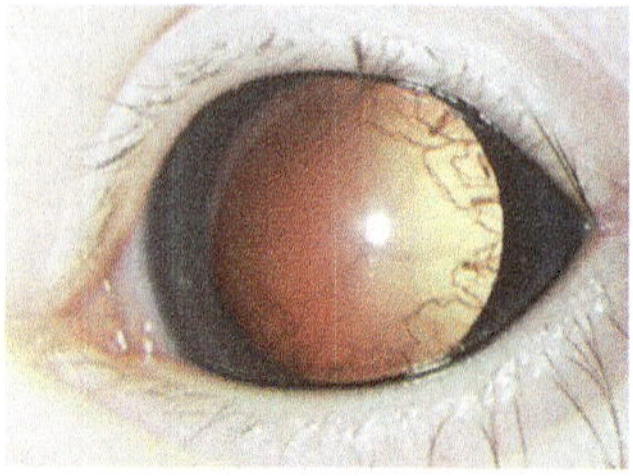 Primate. Anterior PTVL
		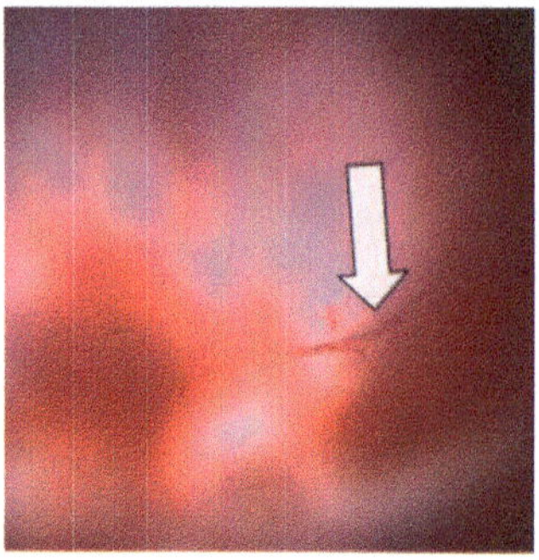 Rat. Patent PTVL

Retina, Choroid, and Optic Nerve

The retina is of high significance on ocular toxicology examination. The three primary neurons of the retina (photoreceptor, bipolar cell, and ganglion cell) are uniquely susceptible to toxicological or inflammatory insult. Continuous regeneration of phototransduction cascade proteins and daily turnover of light-sensitive disks within the photoreceptors makes this cell-type one of the most metabolically demanding within the body. Alterations in blood flow, oxygenation, and nutrient delivery or presences of compounds which significantly interfere with these processes can result in photoreceptor dysfunction and death, which in great enough numbers can lead to blindness. The axons of ganglion cells extend the entire distance from the eye to the brain making them uniquely susceptible to elevation of intraocular pressure, which in ocular toxicology studies might result as a sequela of persistent uveitis changes occluding the aqueous humor outflow pathways. Death of ganglion cells results in the manifestations of the clinical disease of glaucoma.

The recommended terminology described in this section covers the fundus evaluation, notably, retina, choroid, and optic nerve. Many of the terms are species- and/or strain-specific, and strong knowledge of background changes is important to adequately differentiate test item-related effects from normal variation. The intent of this terminology is to be as precise as possible; however, in some situations it may not be possible to differentiate between retinal and choroidal changes. Histopathologic evaluation may be required to precisely identify the exact location of a particular finding within the retinal layers or if affecting retina and underlying choroid. The unique tapetum lucidum structure found in some species (such as dogs, cats, and ferrets) is being described as a separate entity due to its appearance, location, and history of being a possible test item target. The only common laboratory animal species with a macula lutea are NHP; as this region, being of critical importance for high visual acuity, is of strong translational interest in human clinical trials, it warrants additional discussion within the call tables.

Historically an incidental finding in subset of purpose-bred cynomolgus or rhesus macaques, showing clinically as a frequently bilateral anomaly of the temporal optic nerve head, has been described as "bilateral optic nerve atrophy (BOA)." Although the details of progression (if any) and etiology have yet to be definitively described, for the purposes of harmonization efforts, it is recommended that this observation be categorized as "optic nerve hypoplasia."

Location: superior, inferior, temporal, nasal (alternatively quadrants may be used—superotemporal, inferotemporal, inferonasal, superonasal), central, peripheral, peripapillary, foveal, macular, vascular arcades, tapetal, or nontapetal.

Size: millimeter/centimeter scale (depending on species) or relative to optic nerve head (ONH) widths (for instance, "said lesion is approximately three ONH widths").

Extent: minimal, mild, moderate, or severe.

Retina		
Observation	Definition	Photo + legend
Aneurysm	Localized blood-filled outpocket (dilation) in the wall of a blood vessel	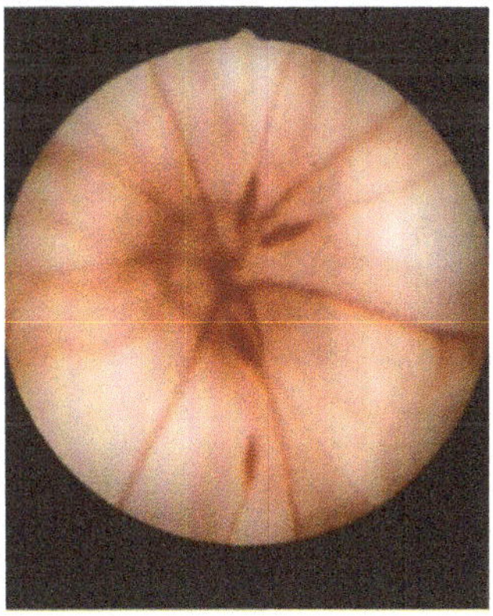 Rat (photo courtesy of David Wilkie)

(continued)

Retina		
Observation	Definition	Photo + legend
Degeneration	Deterioration of the retina with the progressive and eventual death of the cells of the retina Synonym: Atrophy, scar	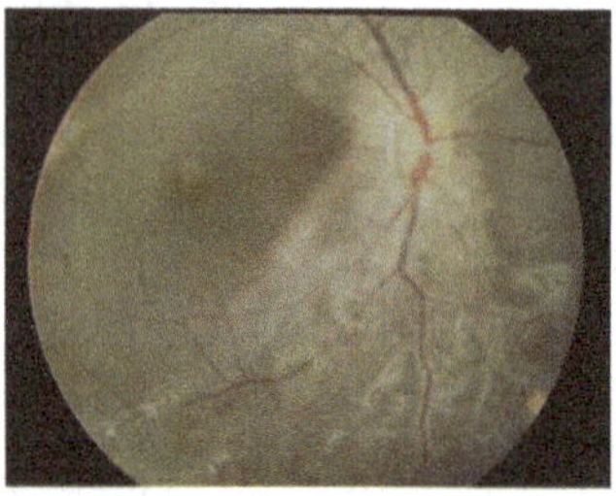 Primate
		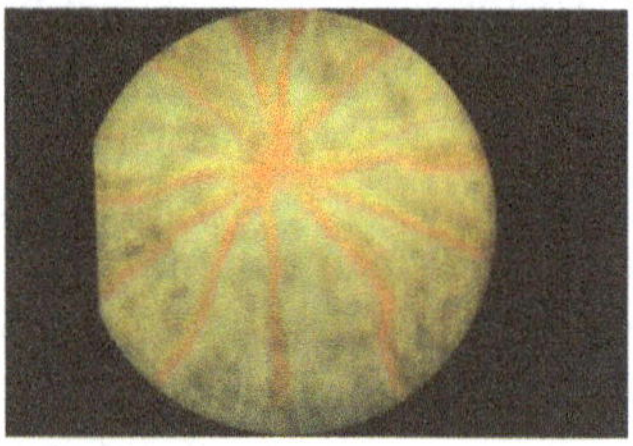 Rat. Light-induced retinal degeneration
		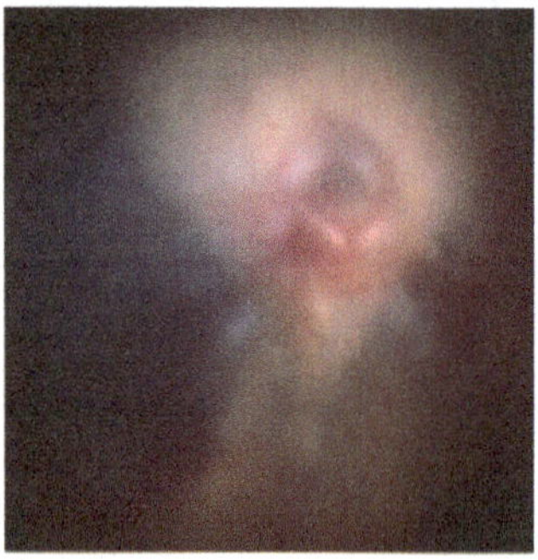 Mouse
		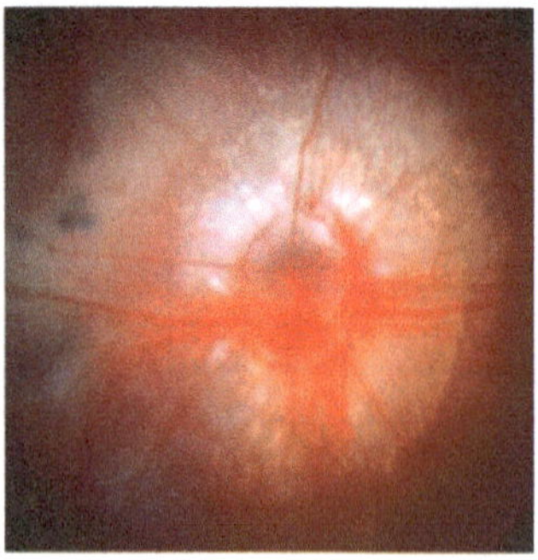 Mouse. Retinal degeneration, hemorrhage, and fundus hyperreflectivity

(continued)

Retina

Observation	Definition	Photo + legend
		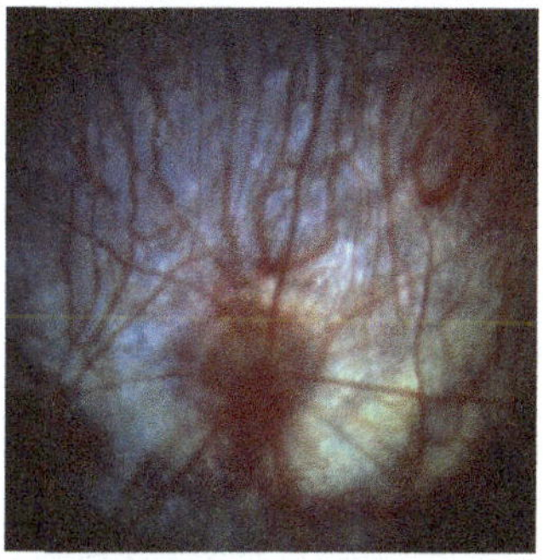 Rat. Retinal degeneration
Detachment	Separation of the neurosensory retina from the underlying pigment epithelium Synonym: Retinal separation	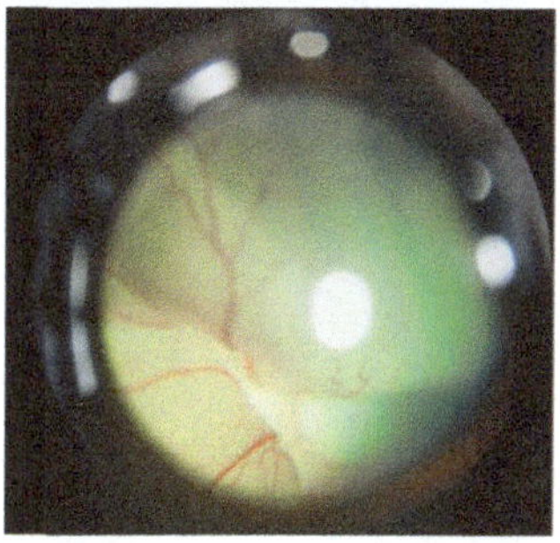 Dog
		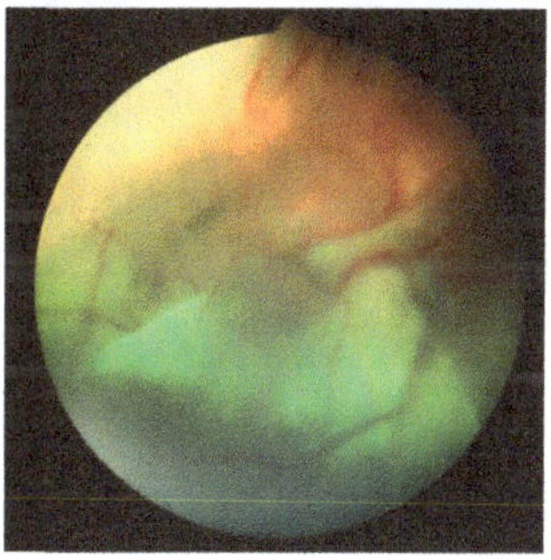 Dog

(continued)

Retina		
Observation	Definition	Photo + legend
		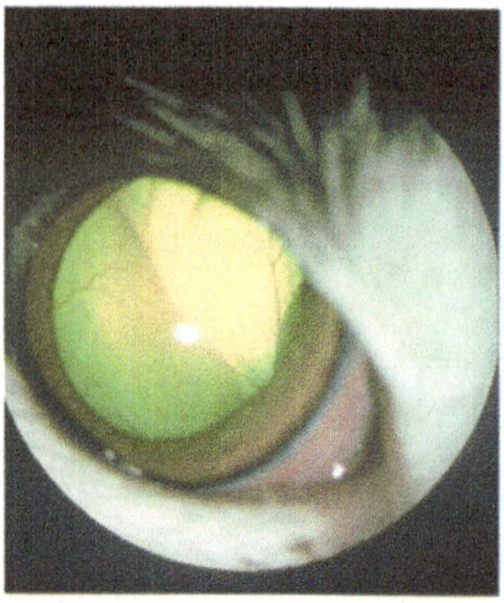 Cat
		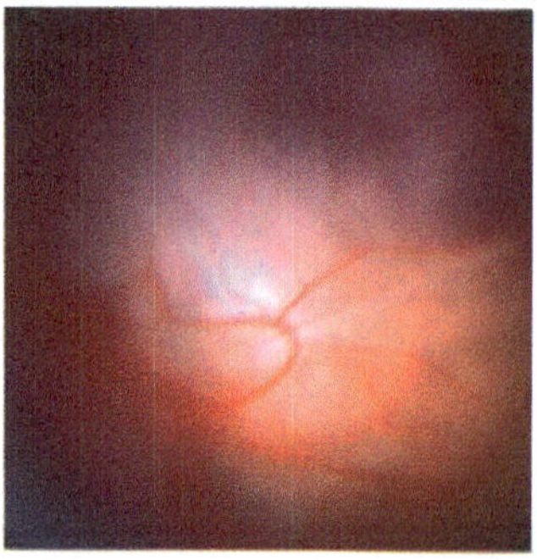 Mouse
		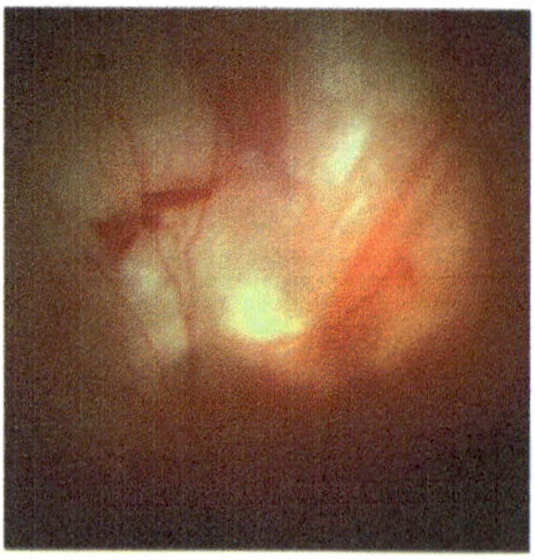 Rat. Note also retinal hemorrhage

(continued)

Retina		
Observation	Definition	Photo + legend
		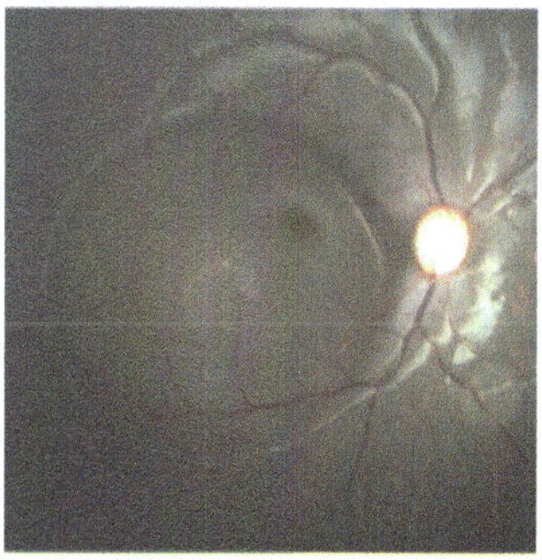 Primate. Transient retinal detachment resulting from submacular injection
Fold	Abnormal development or differentiation of the retina. In rodents may occur as chorioretinal dysplasia Synonym: Choroidal atrophy, choroidal hypoplasia, retinal dysplasia	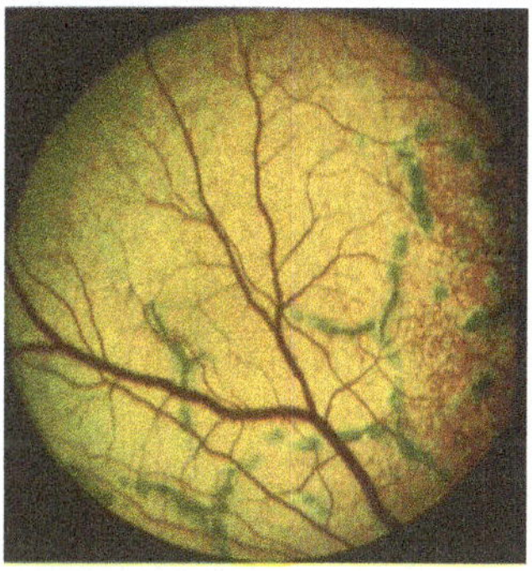 Dog. Retinal folds
		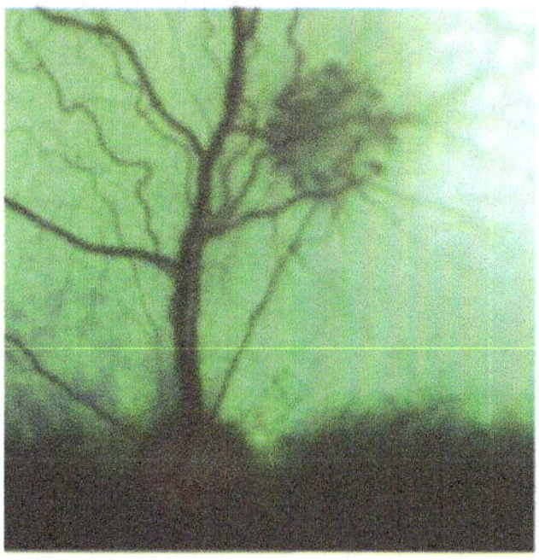 Dog. Retinal folds, multifocal

(continued)

Retina		
Observation	Definition	Photo + legend
		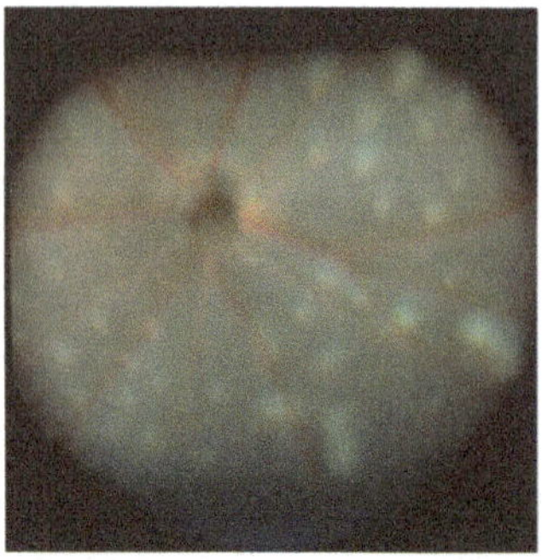 Hamster. Retinal folds
		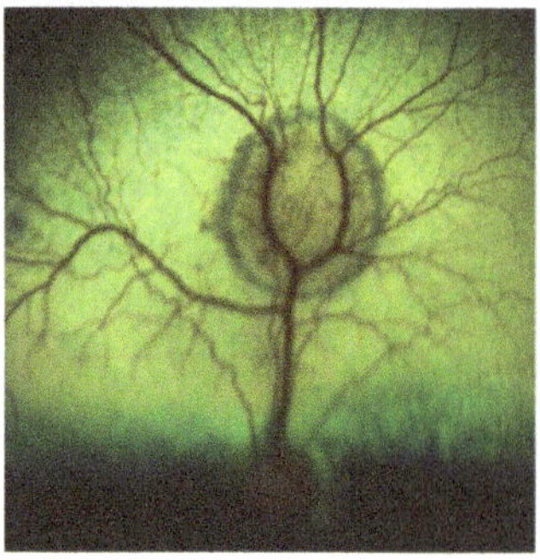 Dog. Retinal folds, geographic
Fundus hazy view	Fundus visualization impaired by opacities in the cornea, anterior chamber, lens, or vitreous	
Fundus not visible	Fundus detail not visible due to opacities in the cornea, anterior chamber, lens, or vitreous	
Haze	Indistinct loss of transparency within the retina, often due to edema and/or retinal inflammation Synonym: Edema	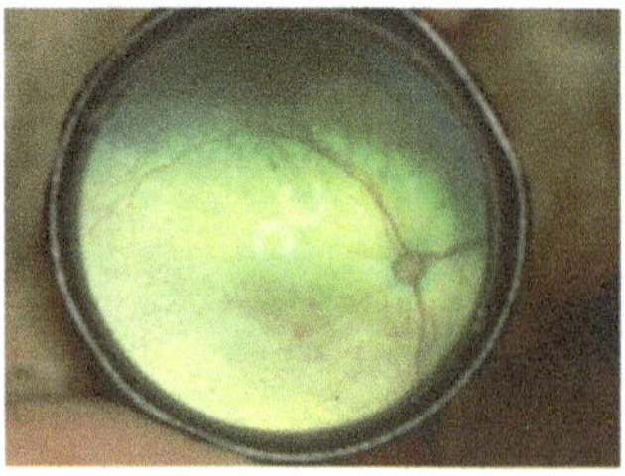 Cat

(continued)

Retina		
Observation	Definition	Photo + legend
		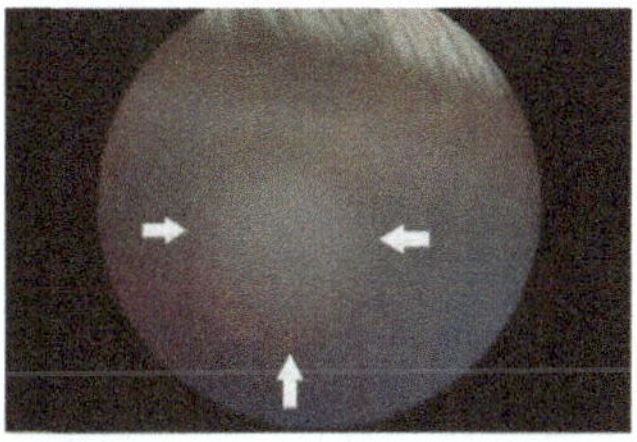 Rabbit
Hemorrhage	Extravascular blood within the retina or subretinal space Specify as preretinal, intraretinal, or subretinal	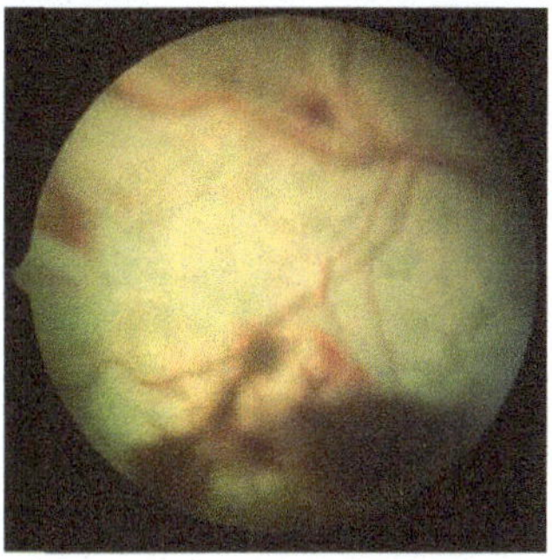 Dog. Preretinal and intraretinal
		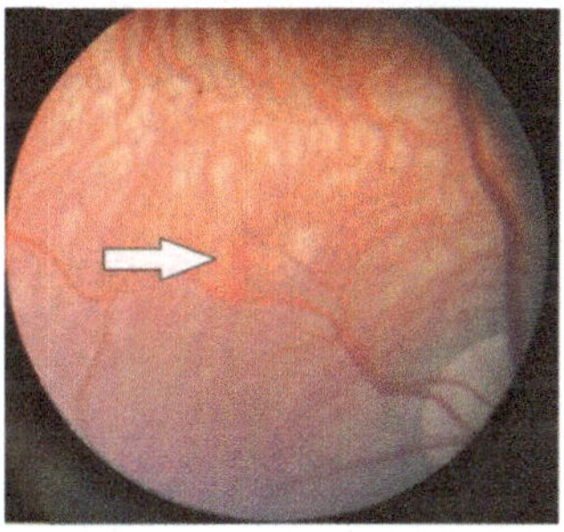 Pig. Preretinal
		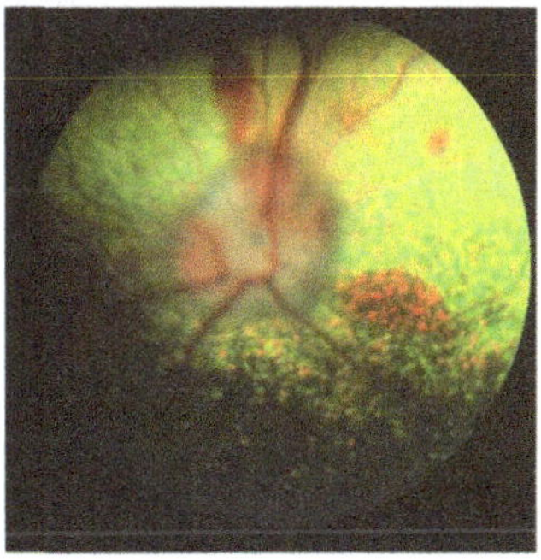 Dog. Preretinal

(continued)

Retina		
Observation	Definition	Photo + legend
		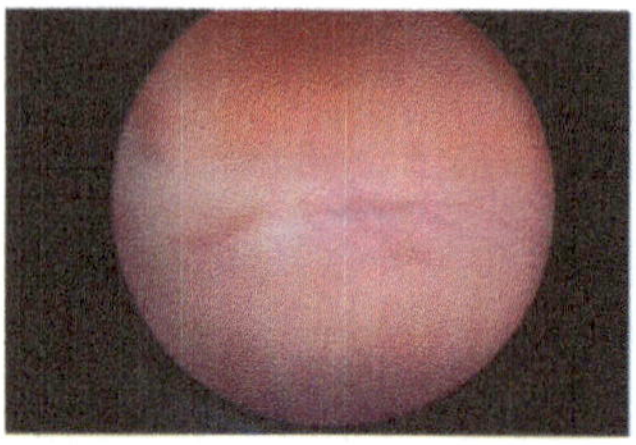 Rabbit
		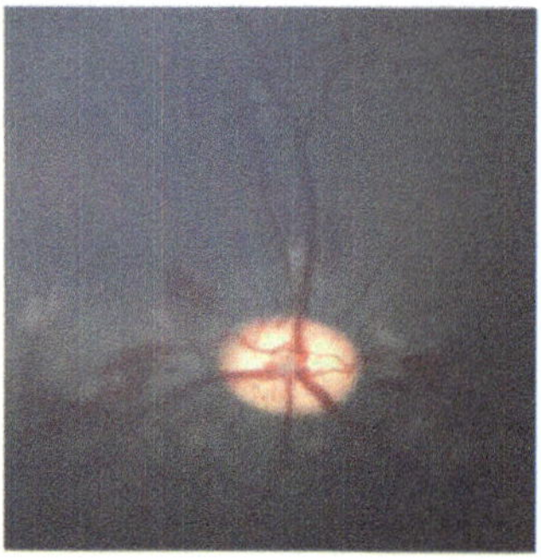 Pig
Hole/tear	Hole in the retina, revealing the underlying retinal pigment epithelium	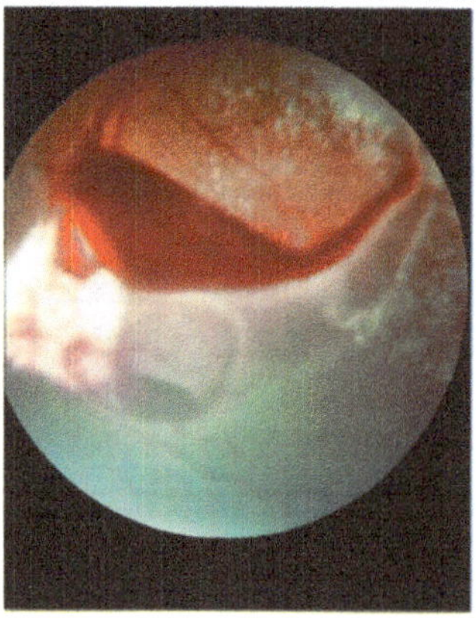 Dog. Retinal tear and hemorrhage

(continued)

Retina		
Observation	Definition	Photo + legend
		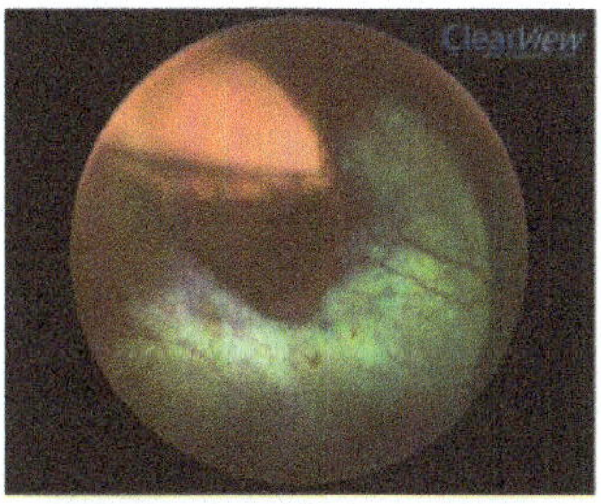 Dog. Retinal tear
		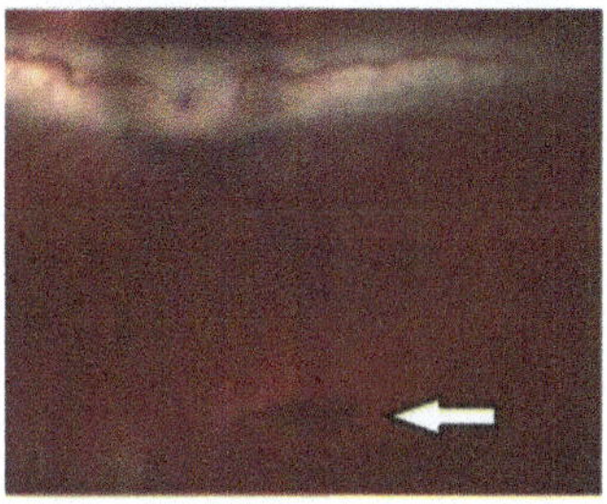 Rabbit. Retinal hole
Opacity	Complete lack of transparency due to accumulation of cells or other material Histopathology required to elucidate. Specify as preretinal, intraretinal, subretinal	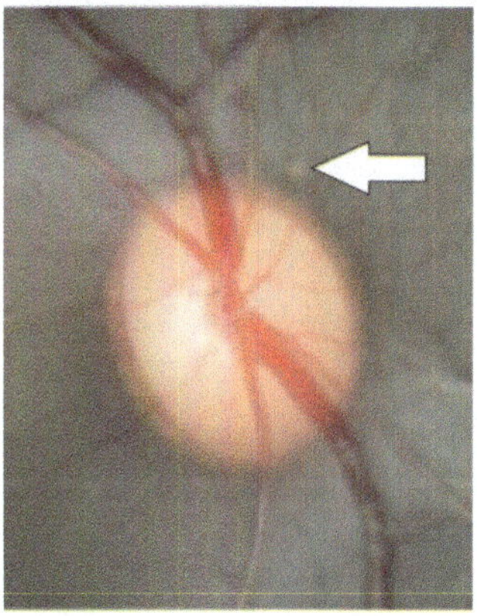 Primate. Retinal opacity, peripapillary
Perivascular sheathing	Lack of transparency adjacent to retinal vasculature due to accumulation of cells or other material. Commonly begins in periphery Synonym: Perivascular opacity, retinal cuffing, vasculitis	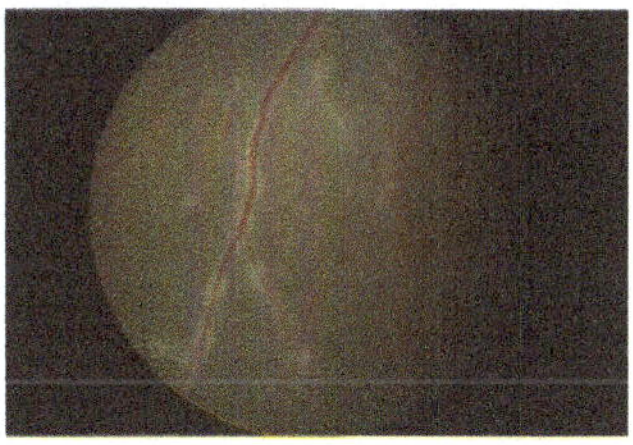 Primate

(continued)

Retina		
Observation	Definition	Photo + legend
		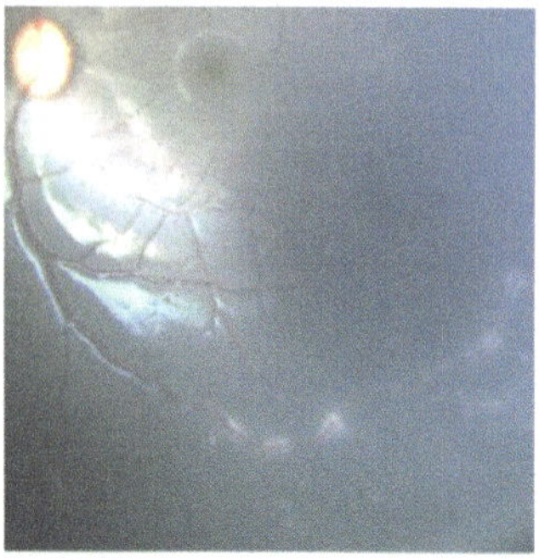 Primate
Scar	Area of presumed fibrosis within retina, usually well-defined, may be associated with thinning Synonym: Fibrosis	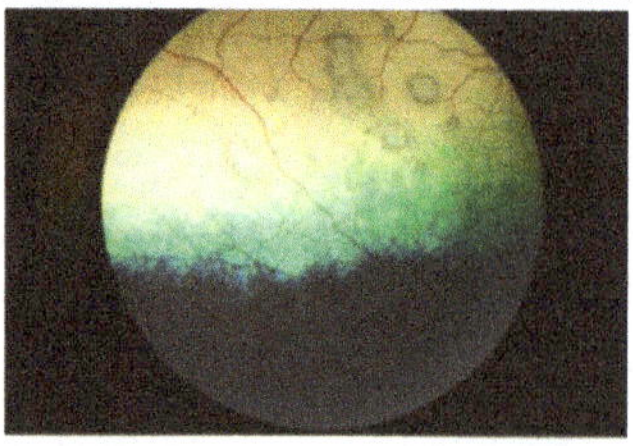 Dog. Retinal scar, multifocal
		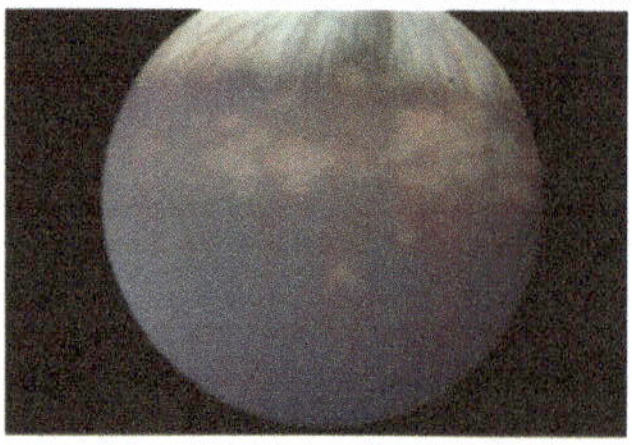 Rabbit. Retinal scar, multifocal
Vascular attenuation	Reduced diameter of retinal vasculature	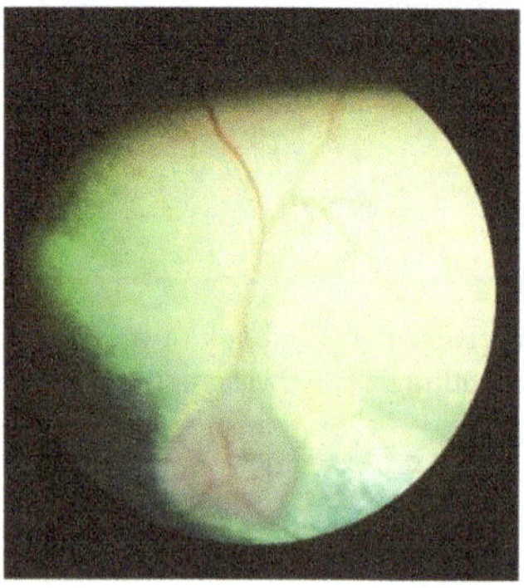 Dog. Tapetal hyperreflectivity, and optic nerve atrophy also present

(continued)

Retina		
Observation	Definition	Photo + legend
		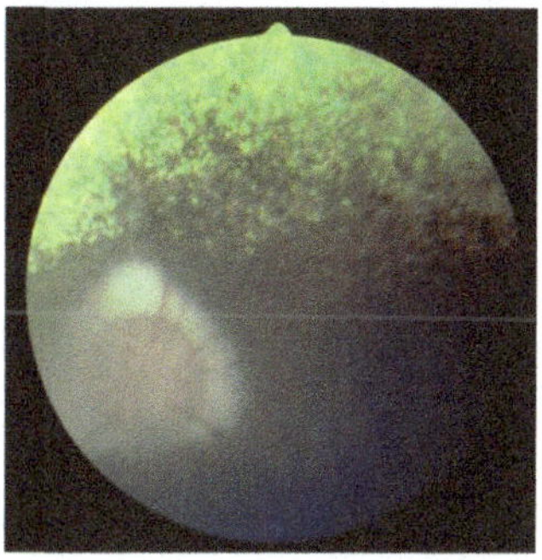 Dog. Optic nerve atrophy also present
Vascular congestion	Increased diameter of retinal vessels	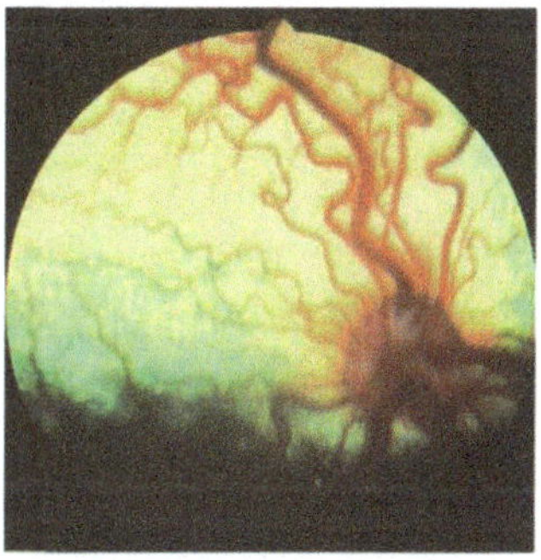 Dog. Note also vascular tortuosity
Vascular tortuosity	Increased vessel sinuosity, often accompanied by vessel congestion	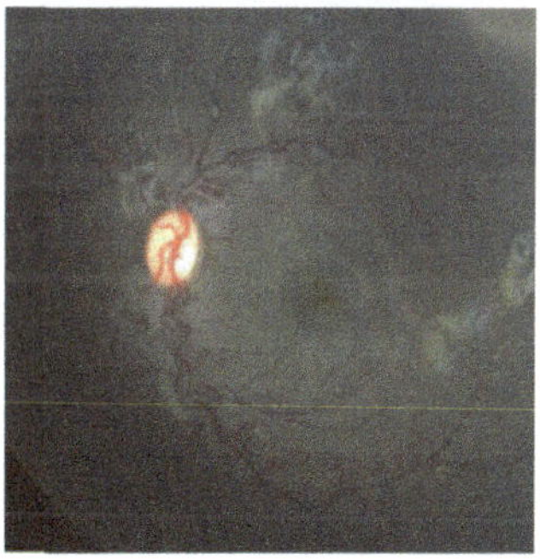 Primate

(continued)

Retina

Observation	Definition	Photo + legend
		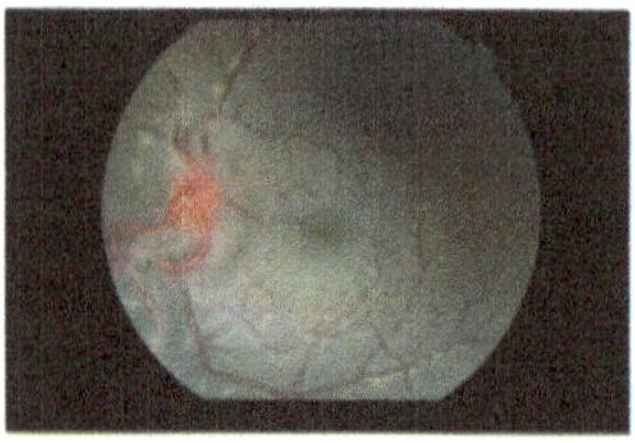 Primate. Vascular anomaly, increased tortuosity and congestion
		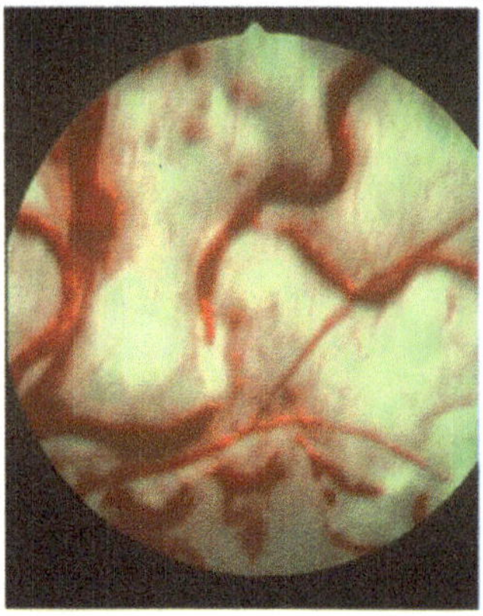 Dog. Note also vascular congestion and retinal hemorrhage
		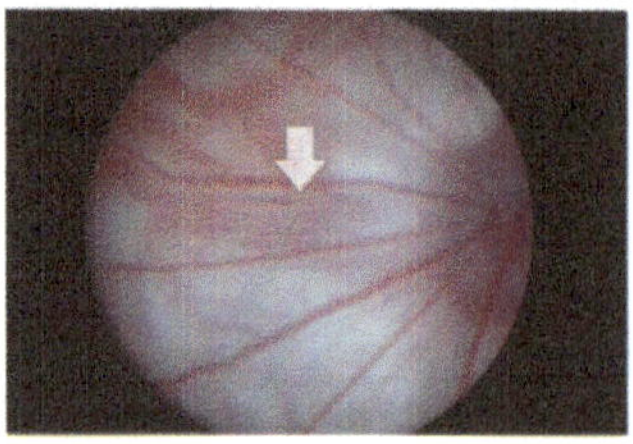 Rat. Retinal myelin (arrow)

Choroid/retinal pigment epithelium (RPE)

Observation	Definition	Photo + legend
Opacity		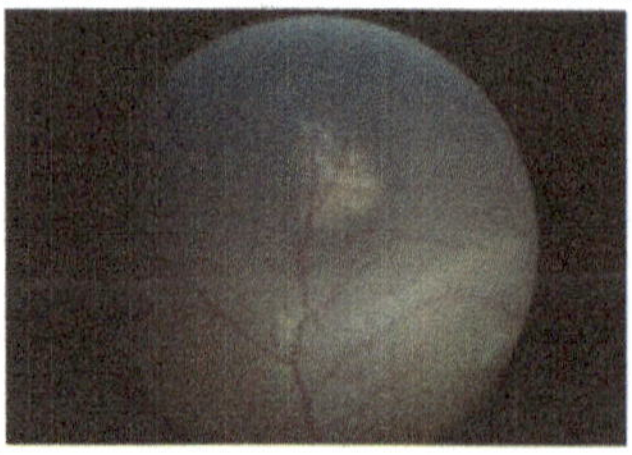 Primate. Subretinal opacity

(continued)

Choroid/retinal pigment epithelium (RPE)		
Observation	Definition	Photo + legend
Atrophy	Mostly occurring in young albino rat strains resulting in atrophy of the choroid and outer retina causing one or more "white bands" (representing increased visualization of the underlying sclera). Retinal hemorrhage is seen early in the disease Synonym: Chorioretinal dysplasia, choroidal hypoplasia	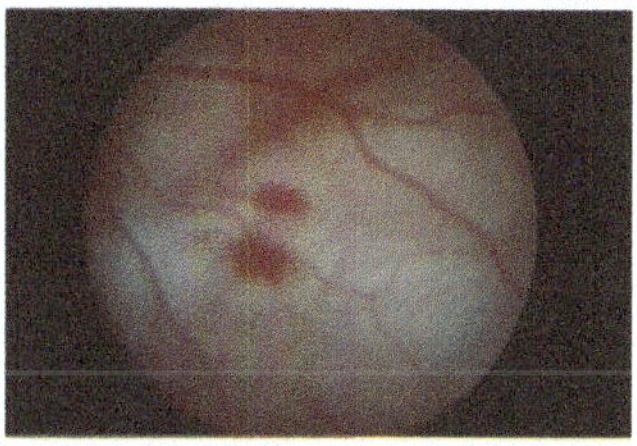 Rat. Developing chorioretinal atrophy and intraretinal hemorrhages
		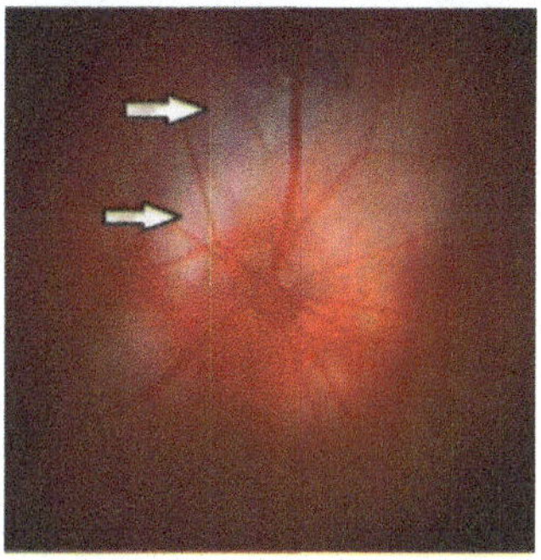 Mouse
		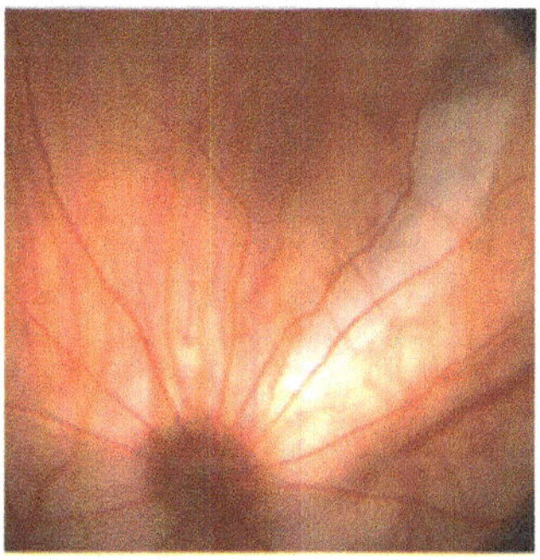 Rat
		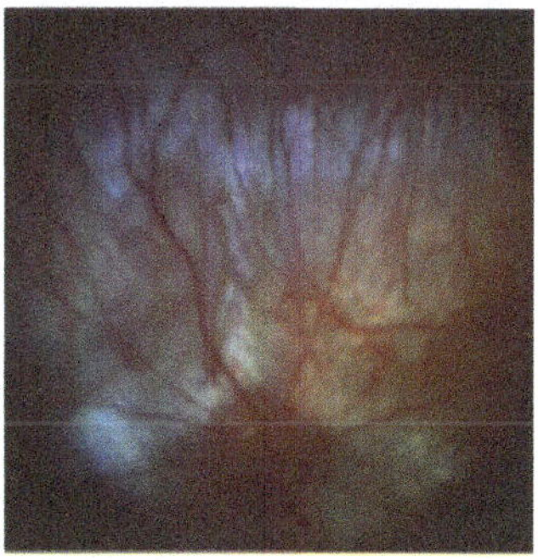 Rat

(continued)

Choroid/retinal pigment epithelium (RPE)		
Observation	Definition	Photo + legend
		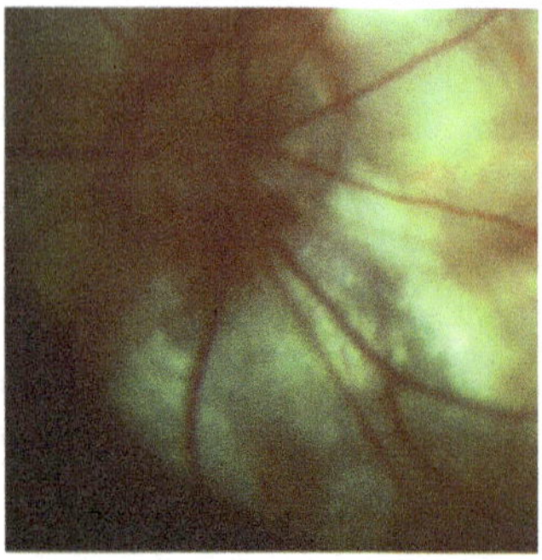 Rat
Coloboma	Congenital developmental abnormality. Cleft or defect in normal continuity of the choroid and/or RPE	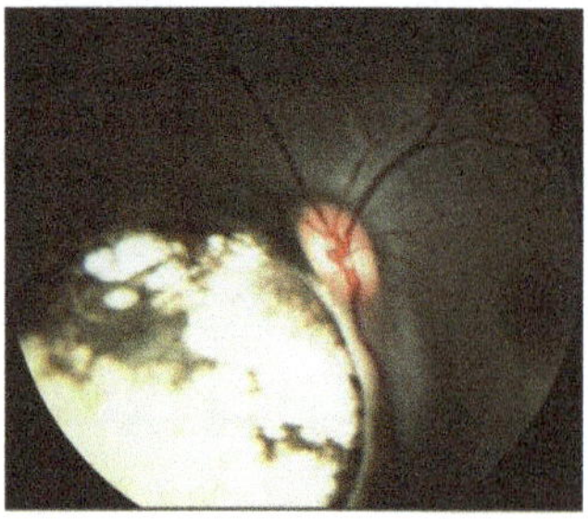 Primate
		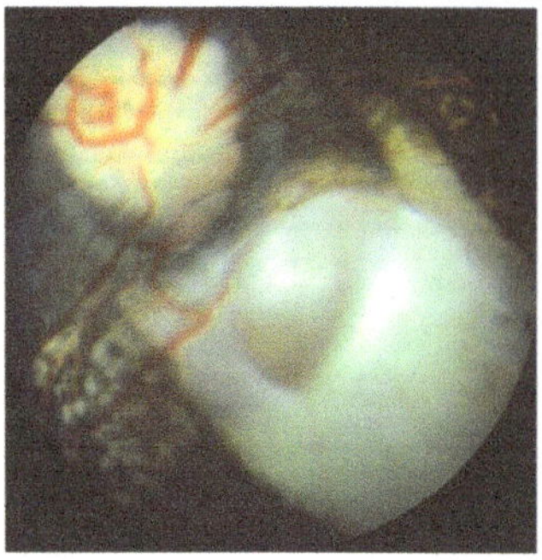 Dog

(continued)

Choroid/retinal pigment epithelium (RPE)		
Observation	Definition	Photo + legend
		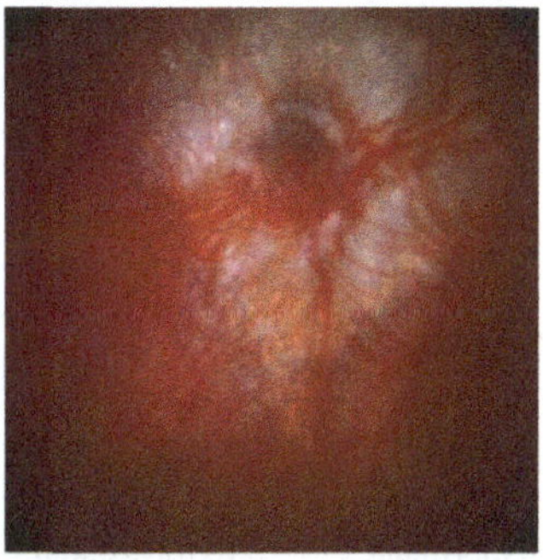 Mouse. Chorioretinal coloboma with atrophy
		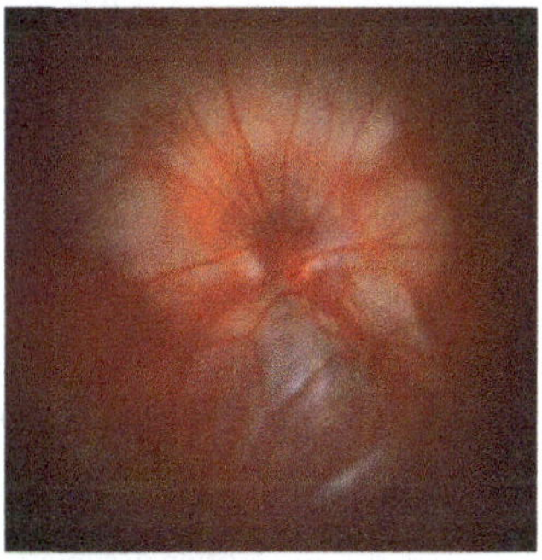 Mouse. Chorioretinal coloboma
Depigmentation	Whitish foci in pigmented fundus. Unknown origin and may be congenital Synonyms: Retinal scar, retinal hypopigmentation, pigment irregular	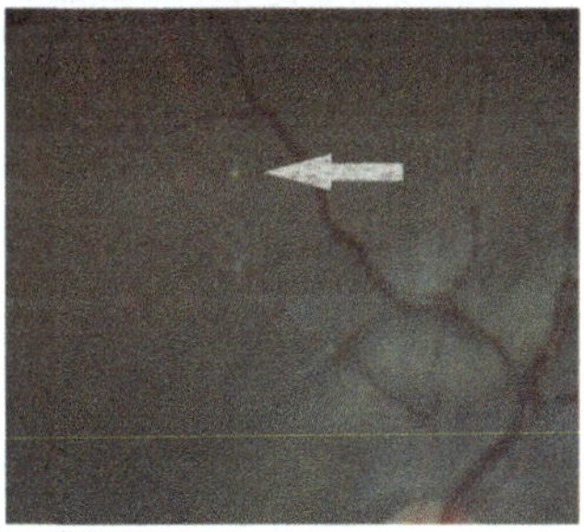 Primate. Retinal depigmentation, focal

(continued)

Choroid/retinal pigment epithelium (RPE)		
Observation	Definition	Photo + legend
		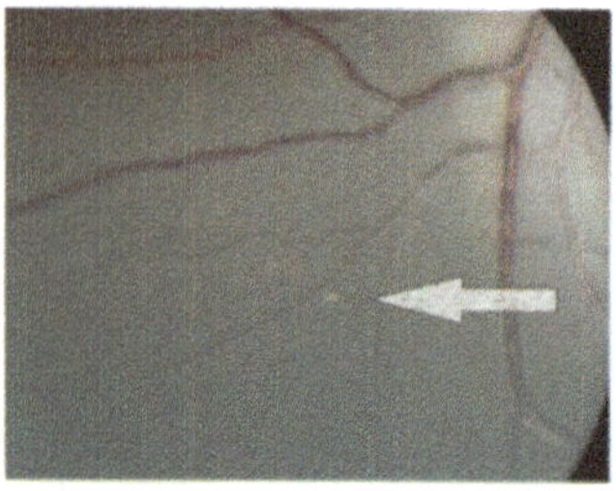 Primate. Retinal depigmentation, focal
Hemorrhage	Extravascular blood within the retina, subretinal space, or choroid	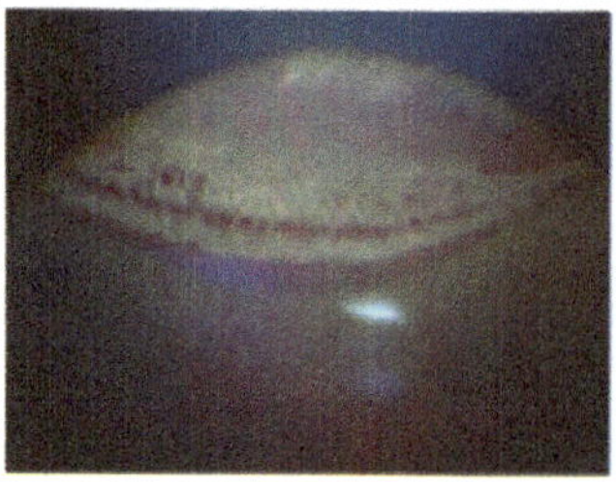 Rabbit. Chorioretinal hemorrhage
Hyperpigmentation	Darker area(s) secondary to increase in pigmentation Synonym: Retinal scar	
Hypopigmentation	Reduced pigmentation of the RPE, often associated with increased visualization of the underlying choroidal vasculature	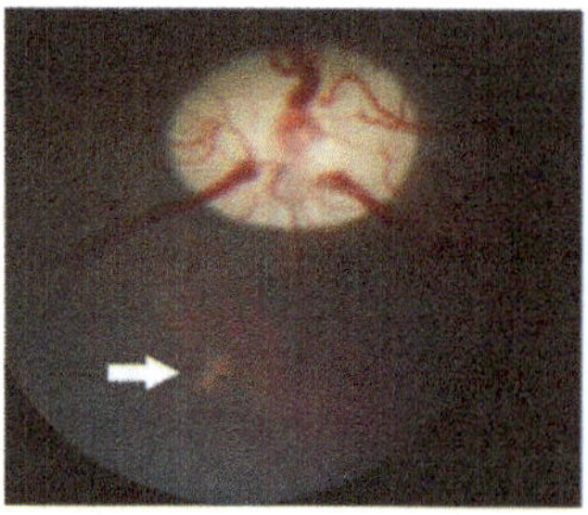 Pig
		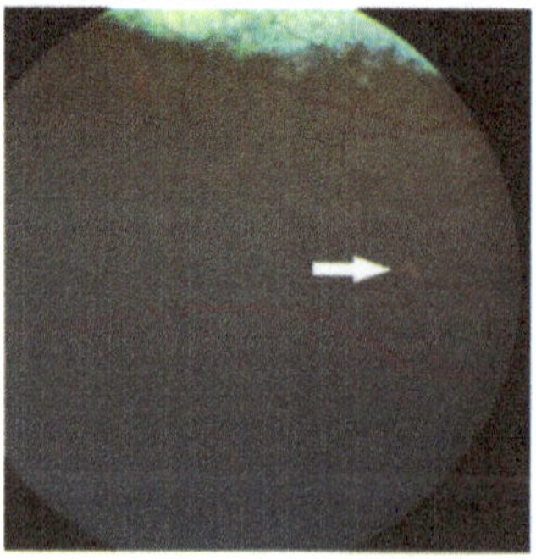 Dog

(continued)

Choroid/retinal pigment epithelium (RPE)		
Observation	Definition	Photo + legend
Pigment irregular	Common background change in pigmented species where the RPE and/or choroidal pigmentation is not uniform. May also occur secondary to previous inflammation Synonym: Pigment variation	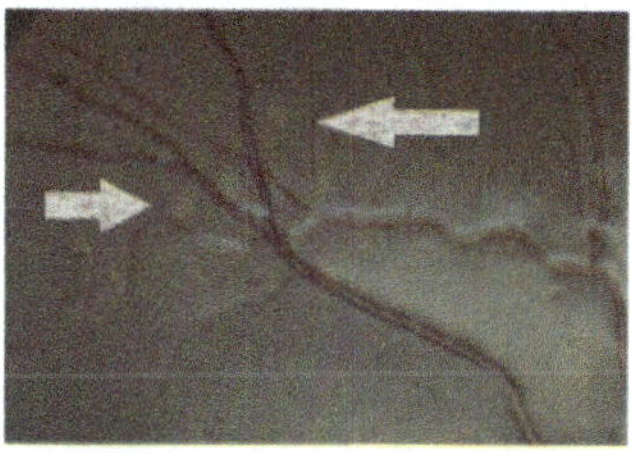 Primate
		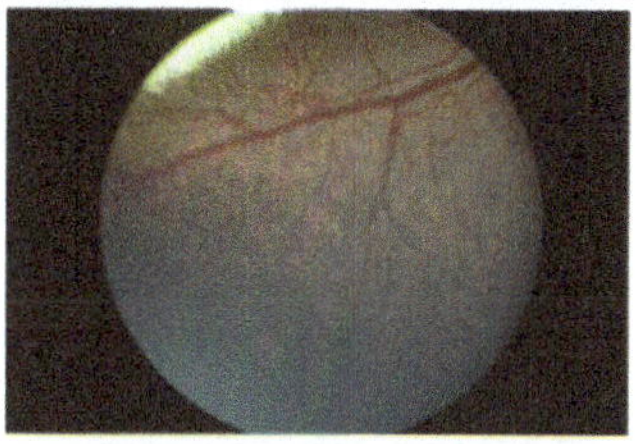 Dog. Retinal irregular pigmentation
Scar	Area of presumed fibrosis, usually well-defined	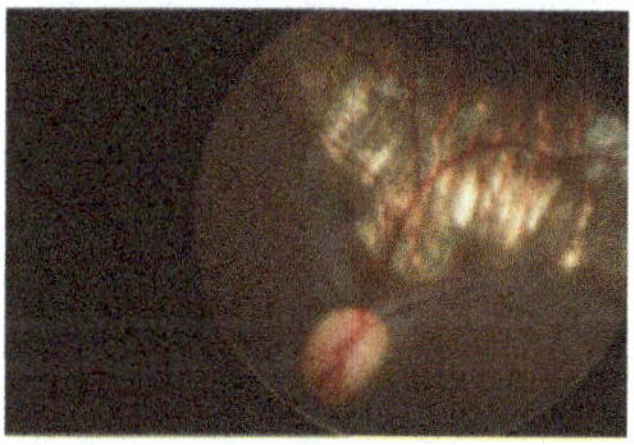 Primate. Chorioretinal scar
		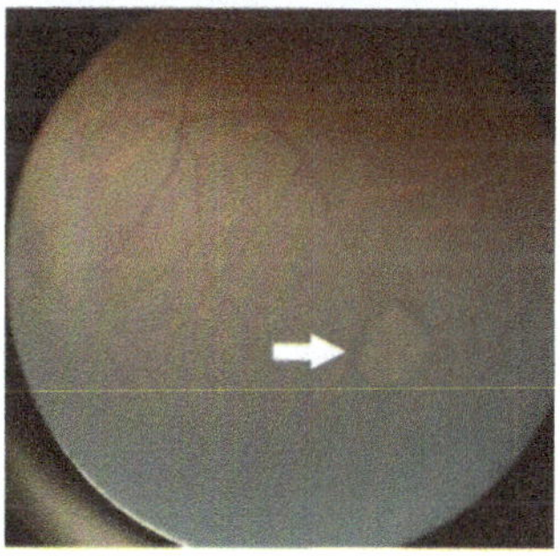 Primate. Chorioretinal scar, focal

(continued)

Choroid/retinal pigment epithelium (RPE)

Observation	Definition	Photo + legend
		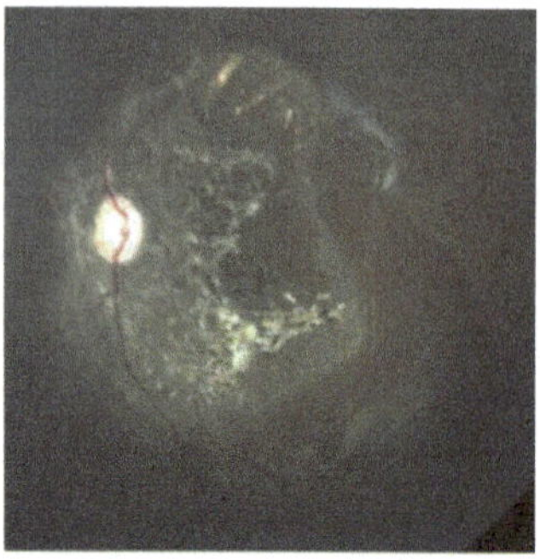 Chorioretinal scar, multifocal
		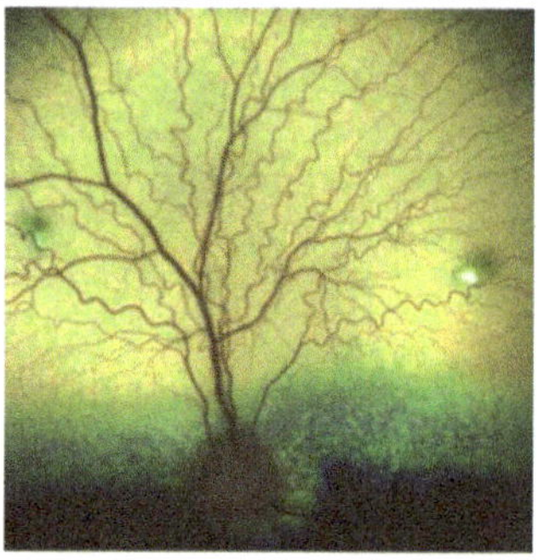 Dog. Chorioretinal scar, multifocal
		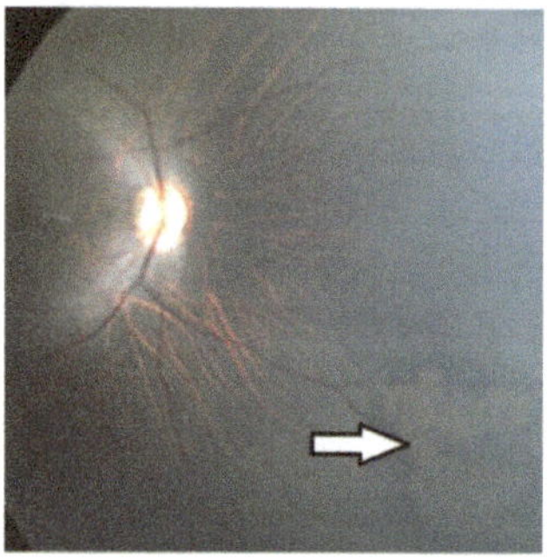 Primate. Chorioretinal scar, focal

Tapetum		
Observation	Definition	Photo + legend
Altered reflectivity	Usually associated with retinal degeneration or atrophy causing increased light reflectivity Synonym: Retinal degeneration, retinal atrophy	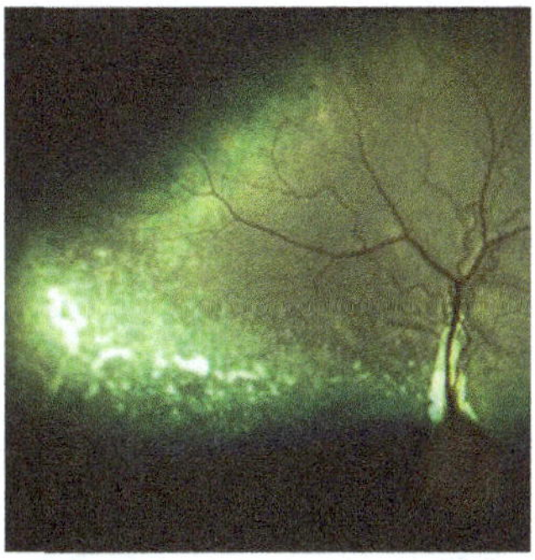 Dog
		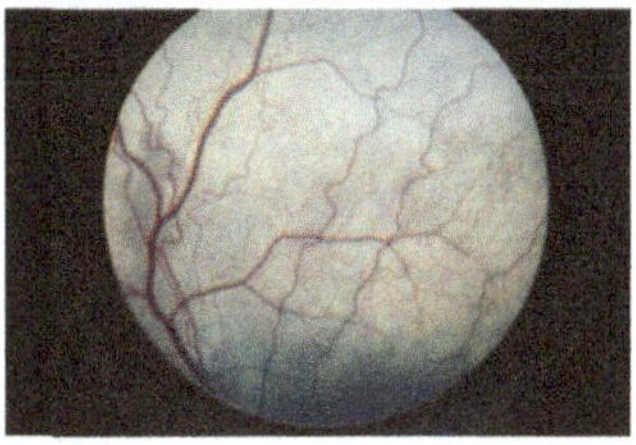 Dog
		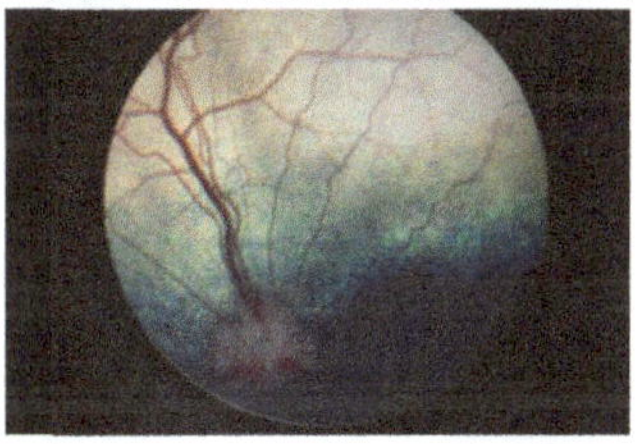 Dog
		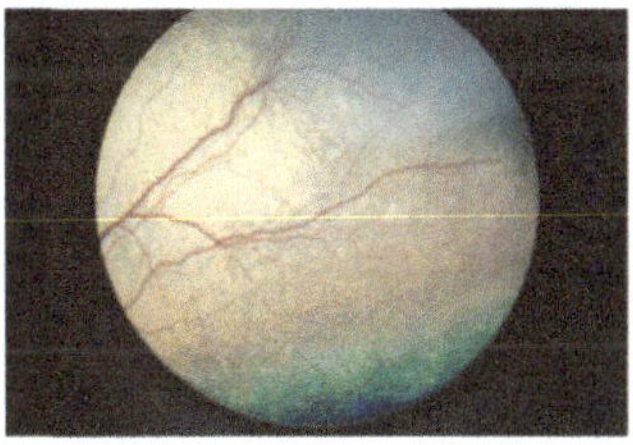 Dog

(continued)

Tapetum		
Observation	Definition	Photo + legend
Hypoplasia	Incomplete development of the tapetum	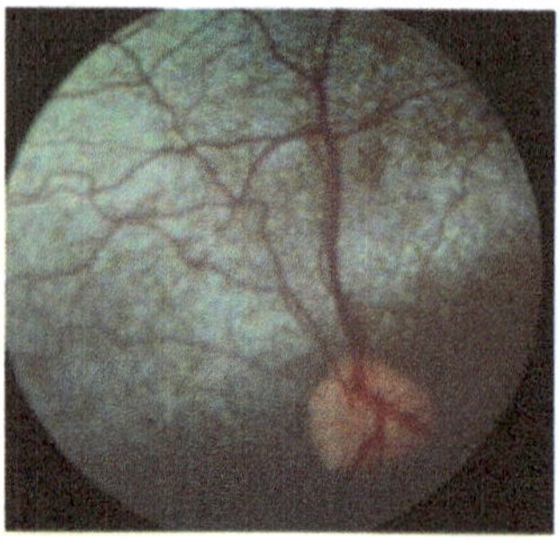 Dog
Hyperpigmentation	Increased pigment (most commonly melanin, other pigments possible)	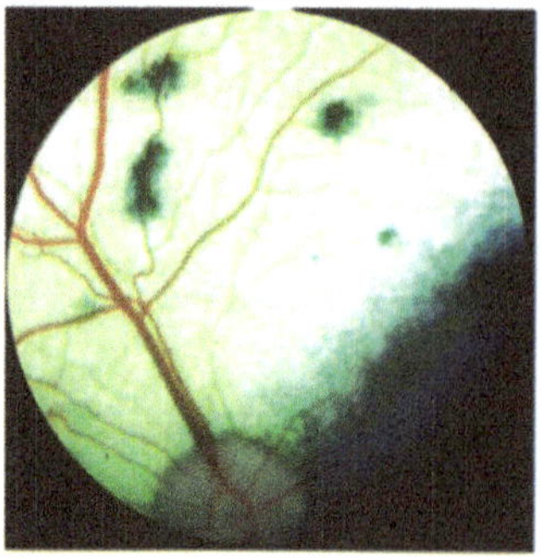 Dog
		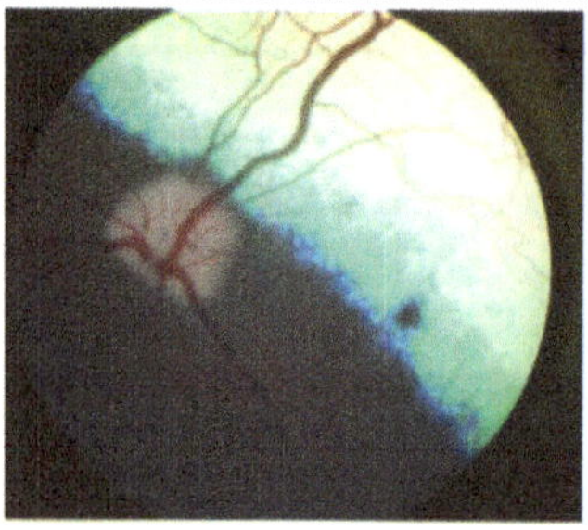 Dog

(continued)

Macula/fovea		
Observation	Definition	Photo + legend
Coloboma		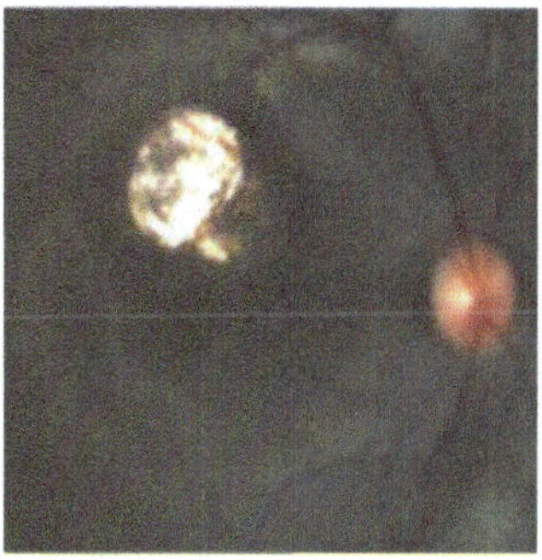 Primate
Degeneration	Loss of retinal cells in the macular/ foveal area	
Depigmentation	Areas of depigmentation, commonly very small	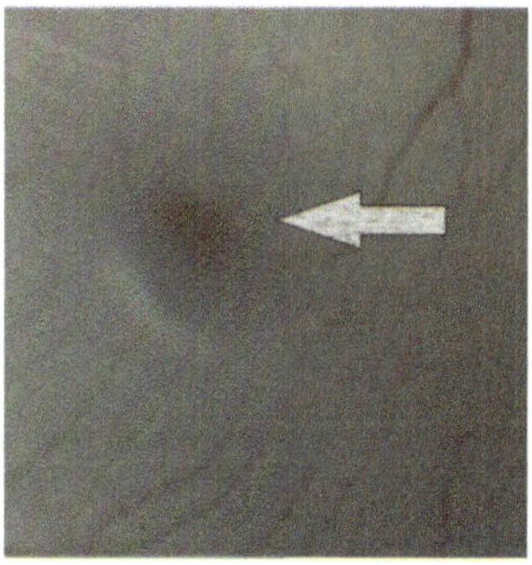 Primate
		 Primate

(continued)

Macula/fovea		
Observation	Definition	Photo + legend
		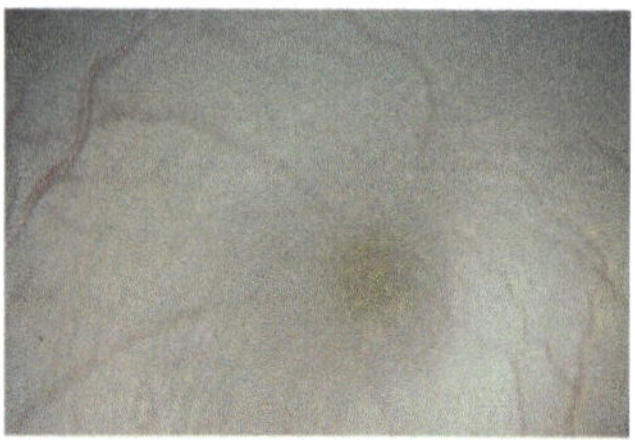 Primate
Edema/haze	Indistinct loss of transparency within the macula, often due to edema and/or retinal inflammation	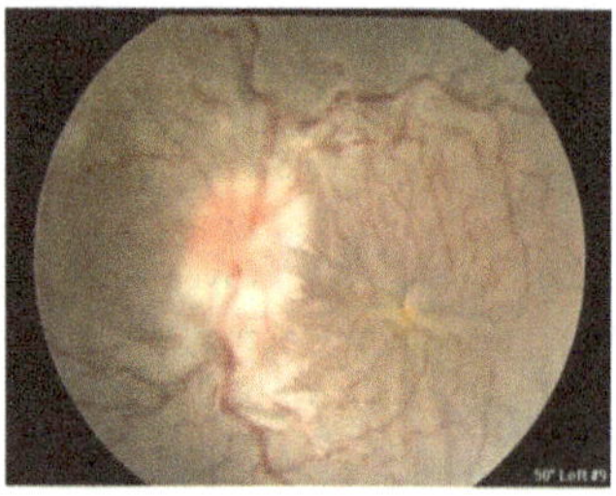 This image also illustrates optic neuritis, retinal vascular congestion and tortuosity, retinal edema, and retinal folds
Hemorrhage	Extravascular blood	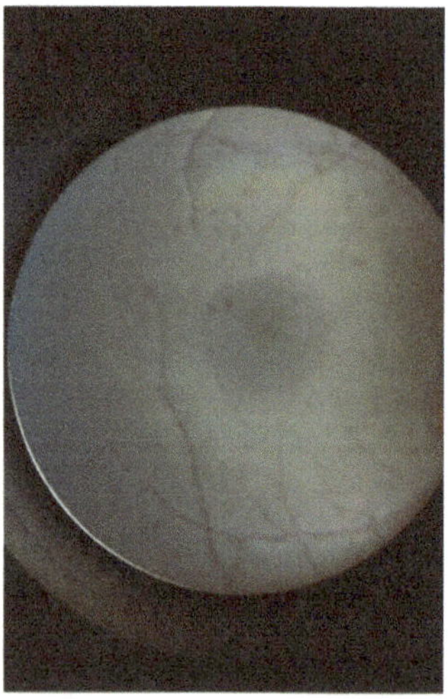 Primate. Parafoveal hemorrhage

(continued)

Macula/fovea		
Observation	Definition	Photo + legend
		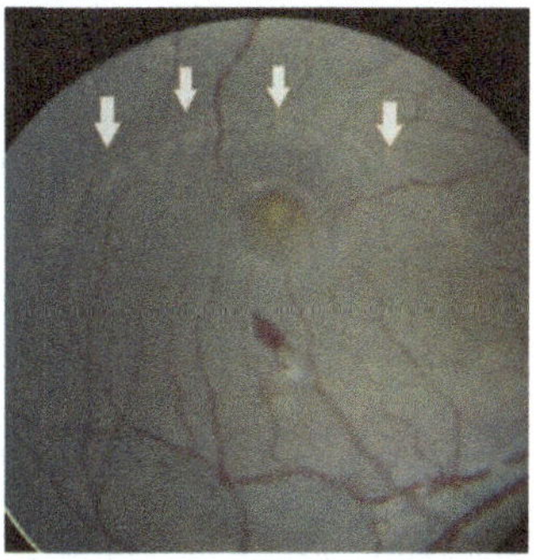 Primate. Macular hemorrhage and irregular pigmentation (arrows)
Hole/tear	Retinal hole in the macular/foveal area	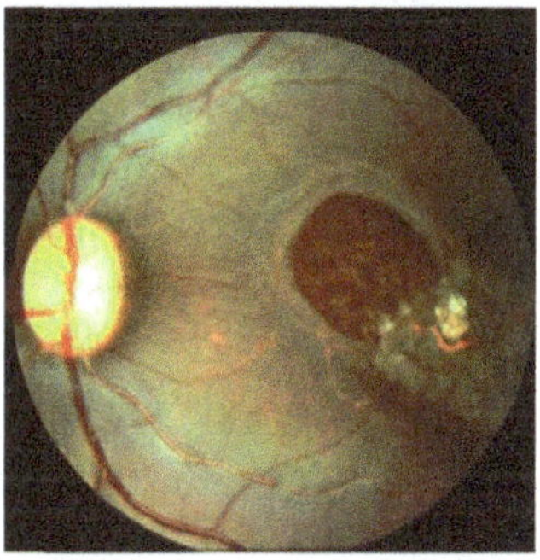 Primate
Hyperpigmentation	Increased pigment (most commonly melanin, other pigments possible). May also refer to benign hyperpigmentation	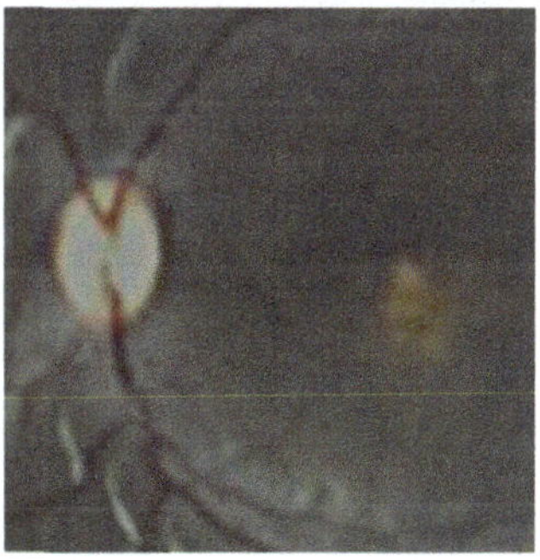

(continued)

Macula/fovea		
Observation	Definition	Photo + legend
Opacity	May include the drusen-like opacities (white hyaline deposits on Bruch's membrane of the RPE) or other type of opacities that may require histopathology to determine etiology Synonym: Drusen, deposits, precipitates	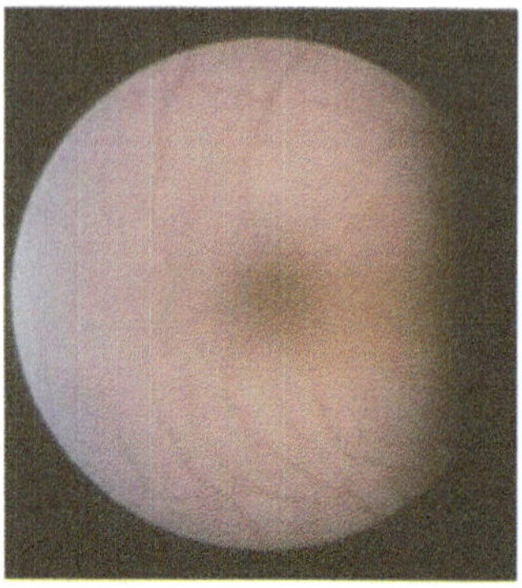 Primate
		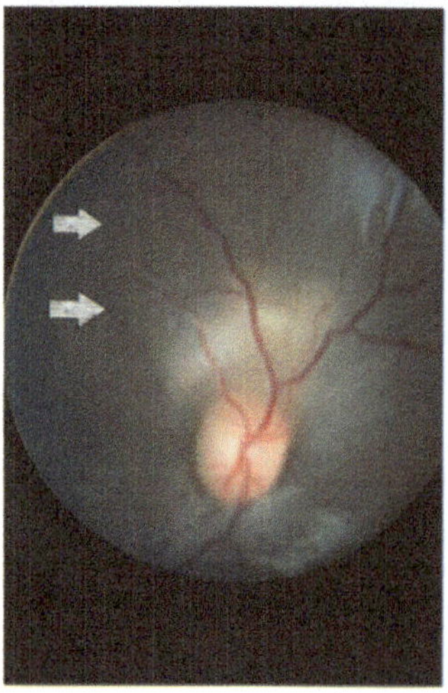 Primate. Subretinal mass with retinal elevation (arrows)
		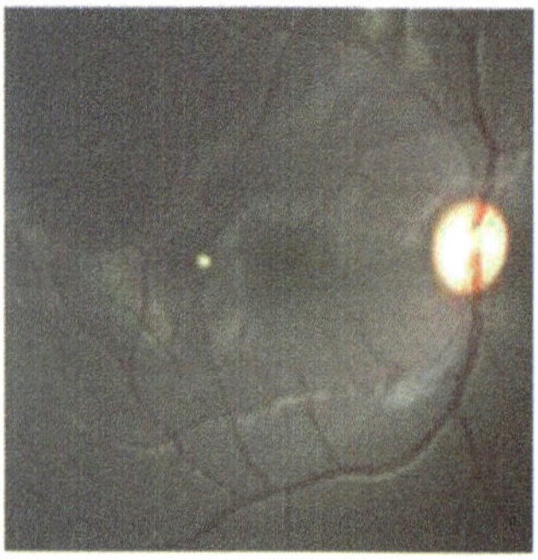 Primate

(continued)

Macula/fovea		
Observation	Definition	Photo + legend
Pigment irregular	Common background change in pigmented species where the RPE and/or choroidal pigmentation is not uniform. May also occur secondary to previous inflammation Synonym: Pigment variation	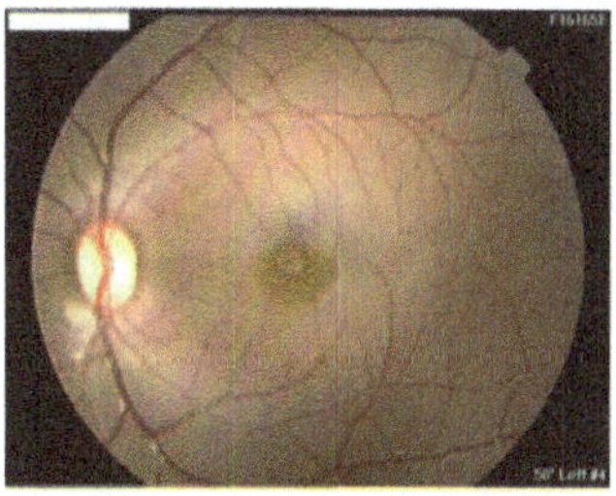 Primate
		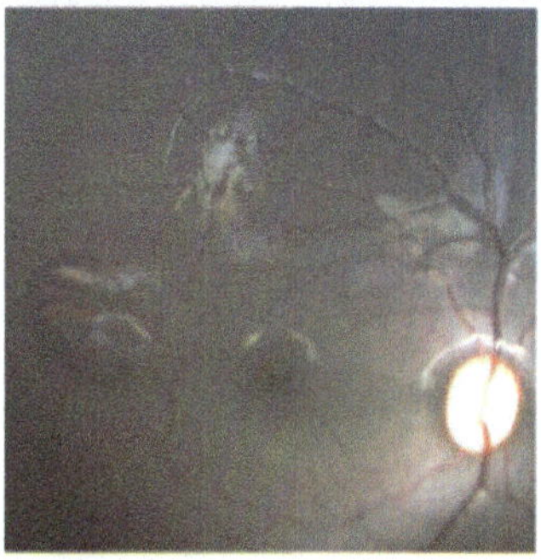 Primate
Scar	Area of presumed fibrosis within retina, usually well-defined, may be associated with thinning	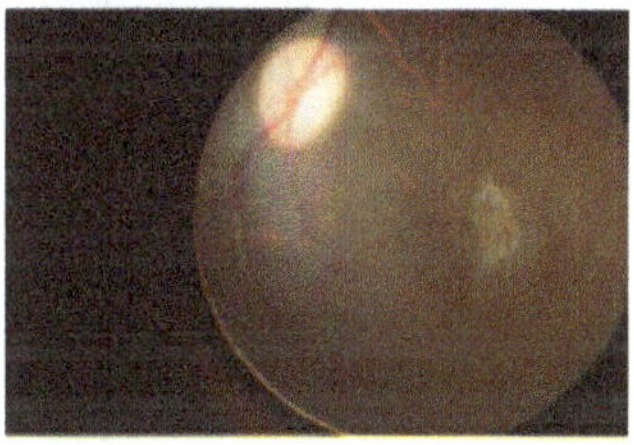 Primate
		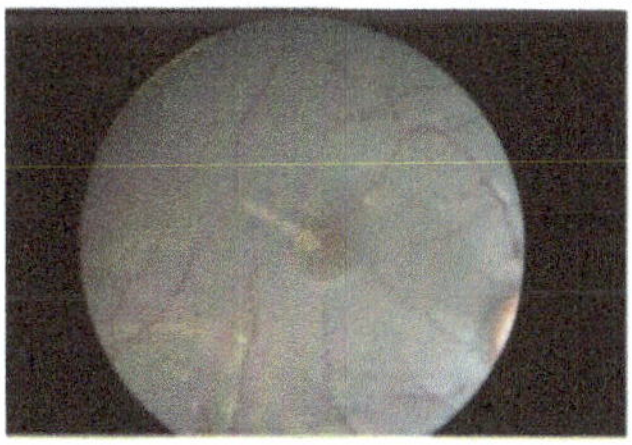 Primate. Macula/fovea scar, multifocal

(continued)

Optic nerve		
Observation	Definition	Photo + legend
Atrophy	End stage degeneration of optic nerve cells, associated with impaired vision	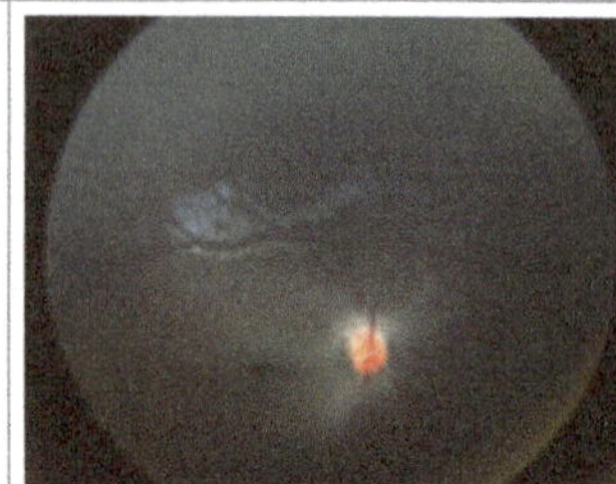
		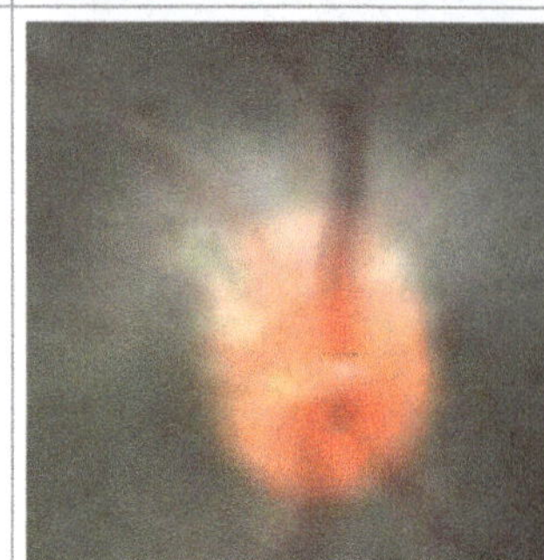 Primate, low and high magnification
Coloboma	Congenital cleft or defect in normal continuity of the optic nerve	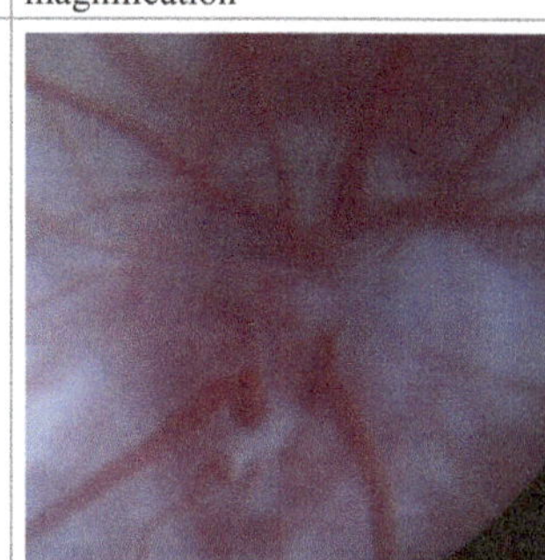 Rat

(continued)

Optic nerve		
Observation	Definition	Photo + legend
		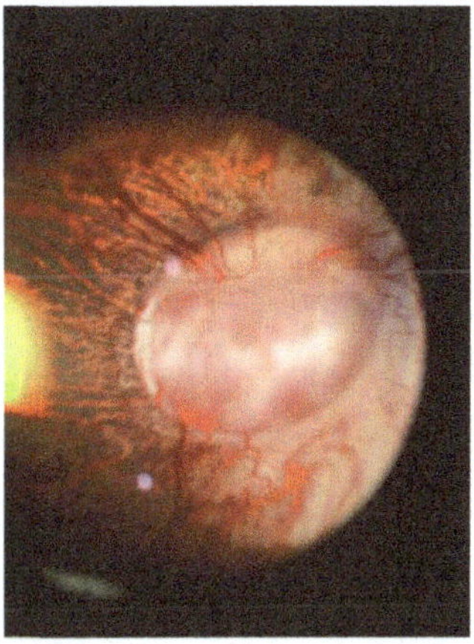 Dog
		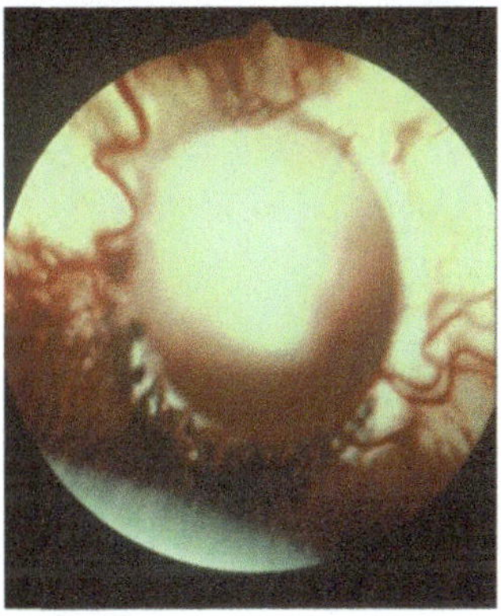 Dog
		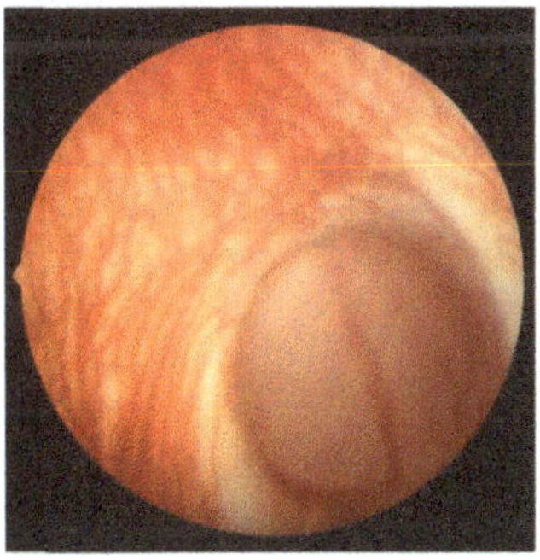 Rabbit

Optic nerve		
Observation	Definition	Photo + legend
		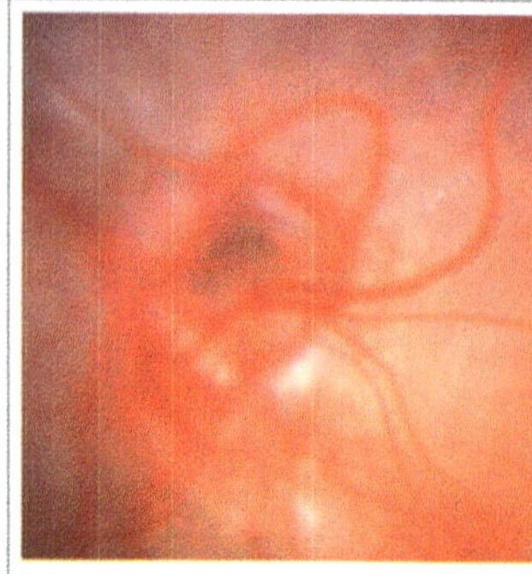 Mouse
		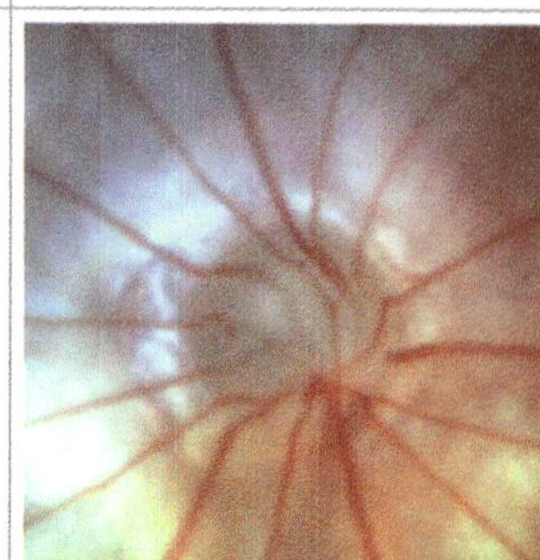 Rat
		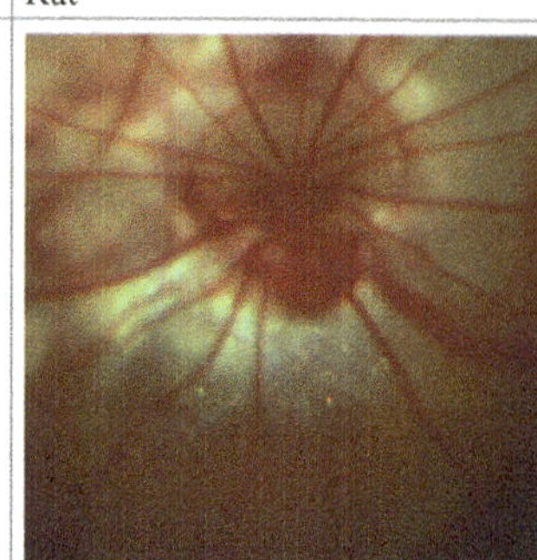 Rat

(continued)

Optic nerve		
Observation	Definition	Photo + legend
Cupping	Enlarged and deepened optic cup such as noted with chronic glaucoma	
Defect resulting in exposed scleral ring around the optic nerve	Congenital peripapillary absence of choroid and RPE. Normal variant Synonym: Conus	
Hyaloid remnant	Remnant of hyaloid vasculature attached to optic nerve	See example in vitreous section above
Hyperemia	Congestion/hyperemia of optic nerve head. Often associated with swelling	
Hypoplasia	Congenitally small optic disc may be regional or diffuse. Vision may or may not be affected. In primates, characterized by pallor of the temporal optic nerve head, in more severe forms a notable structural defect and/or scleral show may be present. This condition is presumed to be congenital/developmental and non- or very slowly progressive without notable behavioral and functional impairment. It may be bilateral, not necessarily symmetrical Synonym: Bilateral optic atrophy in primates	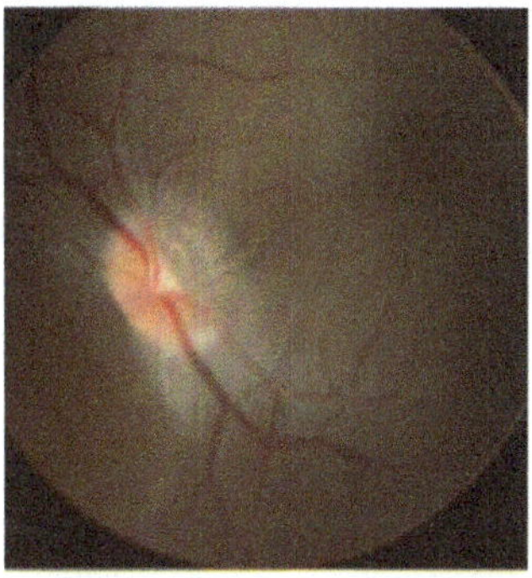 Primate
		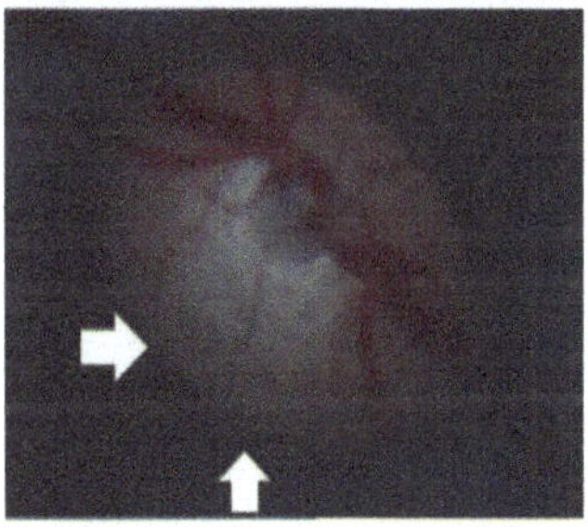 Primate
		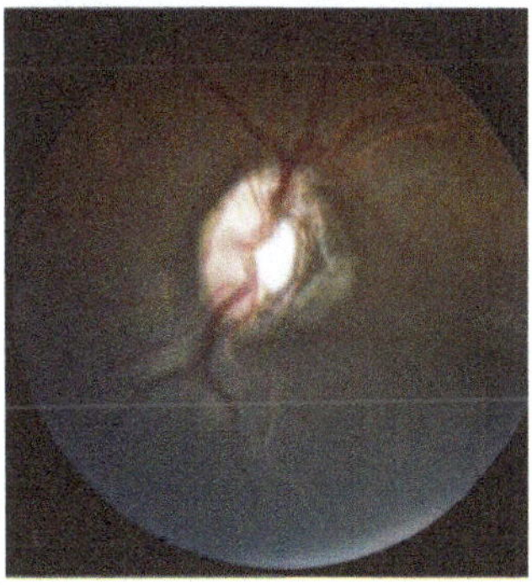 Primate

(continued)

Optic nerve		
Observation	Definition	Photo + legend
		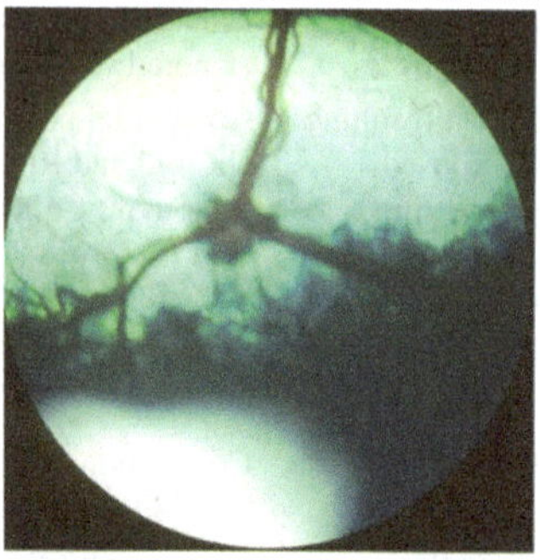 Dog
Mass	Space occupying area by cells or other material. May include benign proliferation of oliodendroglial cells, neurons, or myelinated axons	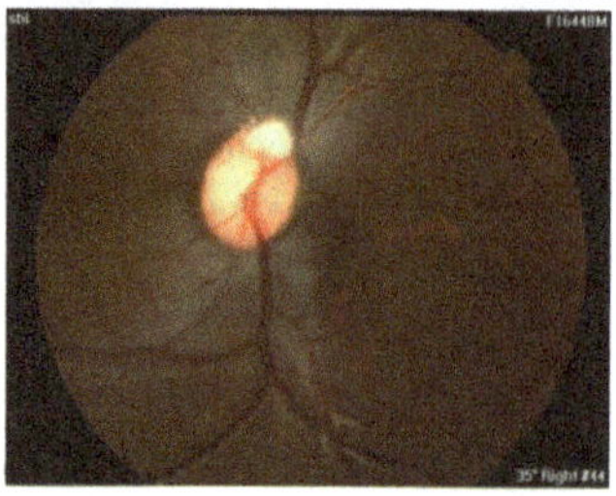 Primate
Micropapilla	Congenitally small optic disc with an otherwise normal appearance and no vision deficit. May be clinically indistinguishable from optic nerve hypoplasia (above) without assessment of vision and pupillary light reflexes that are normal here. May be unilateral	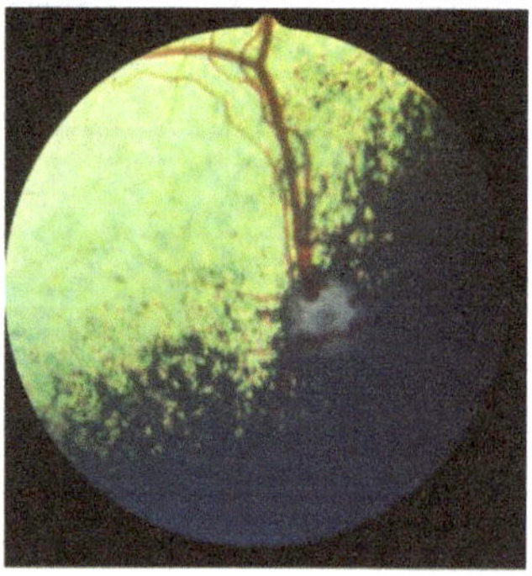 Dog
Myelin, deficient	Acquired loss of myelin around the optic disc, may be progressive	

(continued)

Optic nerve		
Observation	Definition	Photo + legend
Myelination, excessive	An incidental background finding with myelination of nerve fibers extending into the optic disc and adjacent retina	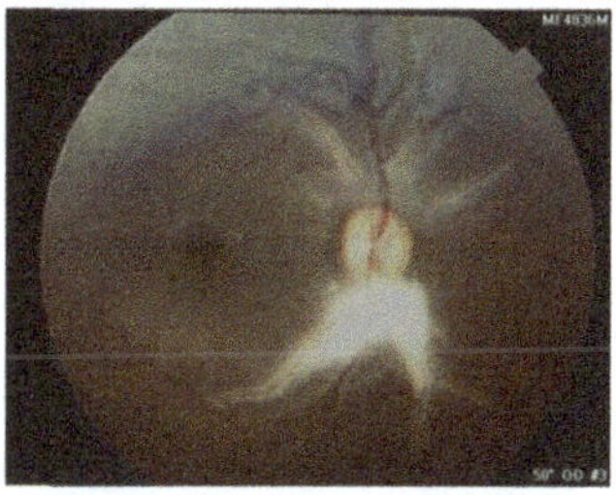 Primate
		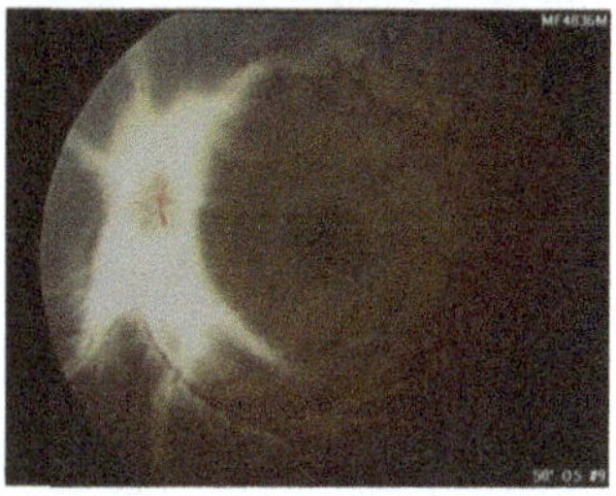 Primate
		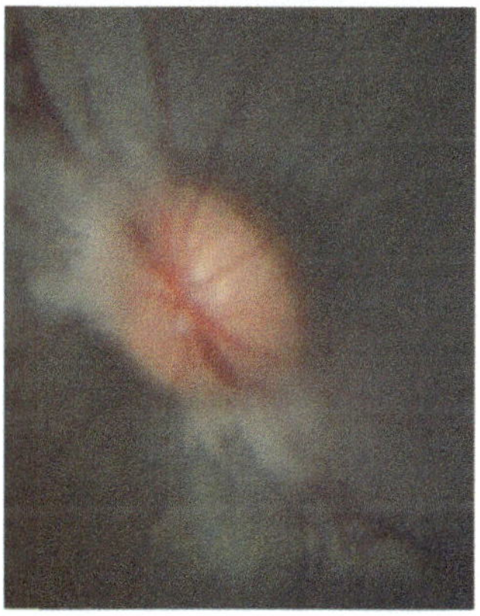 Primate
		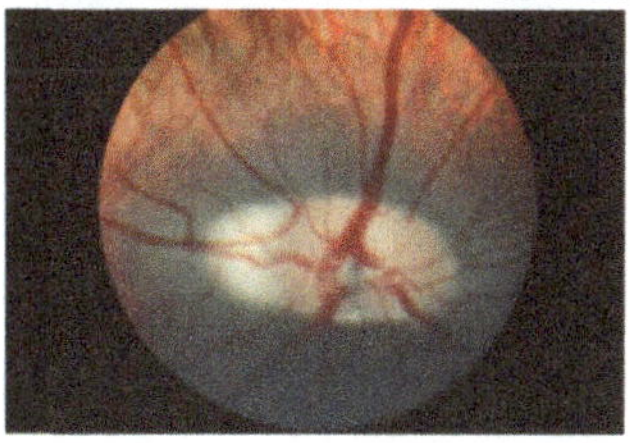 Pig

(continued)

Optic nerve		
Observation	Definition	Photo + legend
Swelling	Enlarged optic nerve head with hazy margins	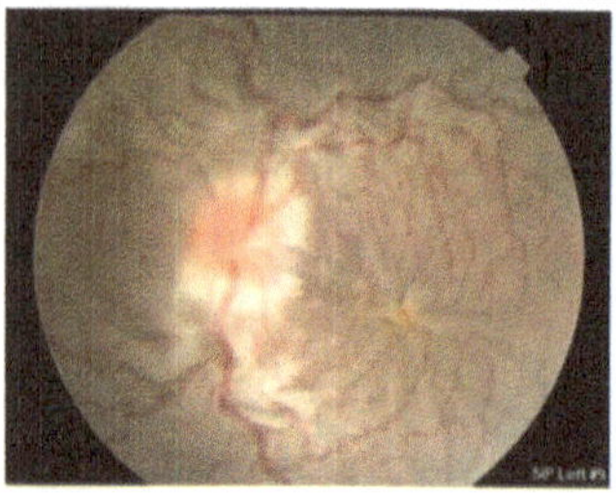 Primate. Blinding optic neuritis and retinitis
		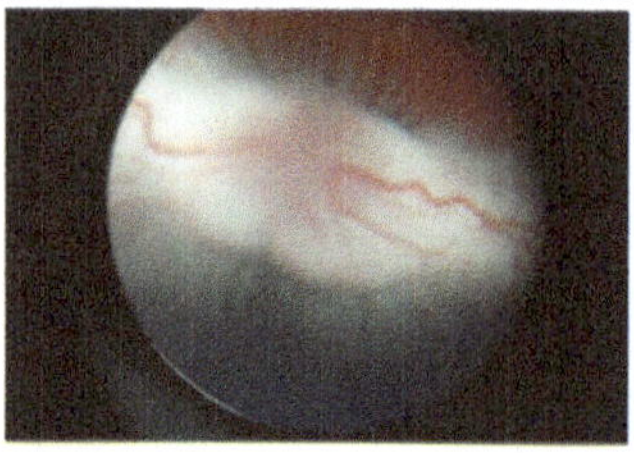 Rabbit
		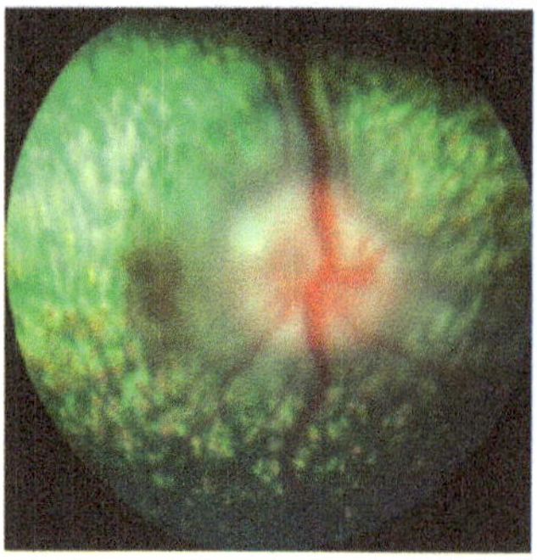 Dog

Neuro-Ophthalmology

Neuro-ophthalmology focuses on study of the nervous system components that affect vision, control of eye movements, and pupillary reflexes. Visual impairment or vision loss due to injury to the brain or optic nerves, which transmit visual signals from the eyes to the brain, may occur on ocular or general toxicology studies. Such injury can be caused by trauma, inflammation, vascular conditions, tumors, toxicities, and infections. Fortunately, neuro-ophthalmologic findings of notable consideration are infrequently encountered during preclinical ocular toxicology assessments. The significant role of the cranial nerves and ocular function necessitates consideration of several key findings. Species-specific conditions regarding neuro-ophthalmology are not common. Pathologic processes to occur include afferent visual system disorders (e.g., optic neuritis, optic neuropathy, papilledema, brain tumors, and vascular conditions) and efferent visual system disorders (e.g., anisocoria, ophthalmoplegia, ptosis, nystagmus, and blepharospasm). Neurotropic drugs, toxins, and some foods can affect metabolic processes needed to maintain the integrity of the visual system, ocular function, and underlying structural components. Pigmented epithelial cells, glial cells, and vascular components of the afferent visual pathway are all susceptible to the effects of drugs, toxins, and some foods. This table highlights the most common clinical neuro-ophthalmological findings in laboratory species.

Location: superior, inferior, temporal, or nasal.

Extent: minimal, mild, moderate, or severe.

Neuro-ophthalmology		
Observation	Definition	Photo + legend
Anisocoria	Pupils of unequal size. Specify which pupil is abnormal compared to the normal eye and whether it is larger or smaller than in the fellow eye	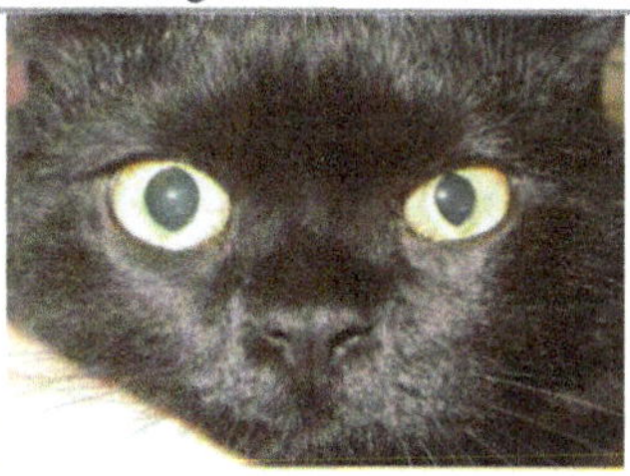 Cat
Miosis	Contraction of the pupil/the state of the pupil being contracted. In abnormal state, the pupil may be resistant to dilation (from uveitis effects)	See left pupil in photo above
Mydriasis	Dilation of the pupil. In the abnormal state, the pupil may fail to constrict from pharmacologic blockade, synechia, defects in the iris (especially involving the pupil), and increased intraocular pressure	
Nystagmus	Rhythmic and involuntary movement of the eyes, described as pendular or by direction of the fast phase of the ocular movement	

Normal examples		
Species	Description	Photo + legend
Dog	Excessive myelin	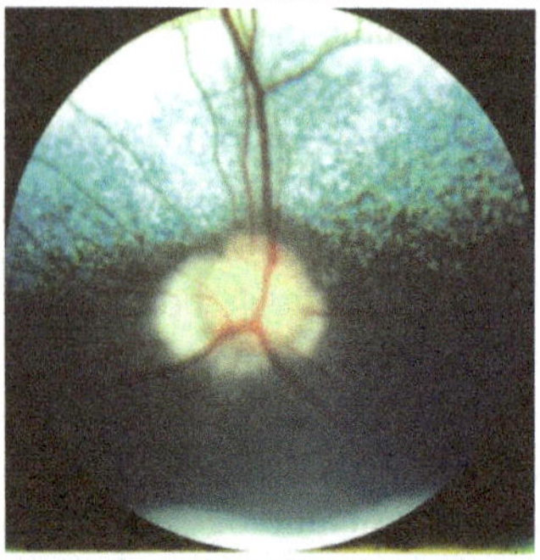
Dog	Subalbinotic fundus	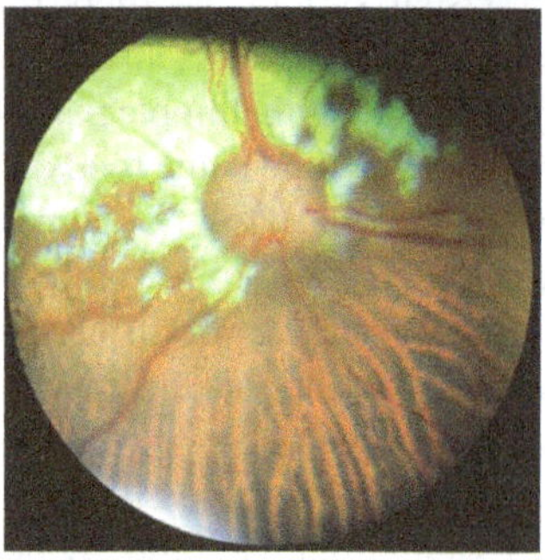
Dog		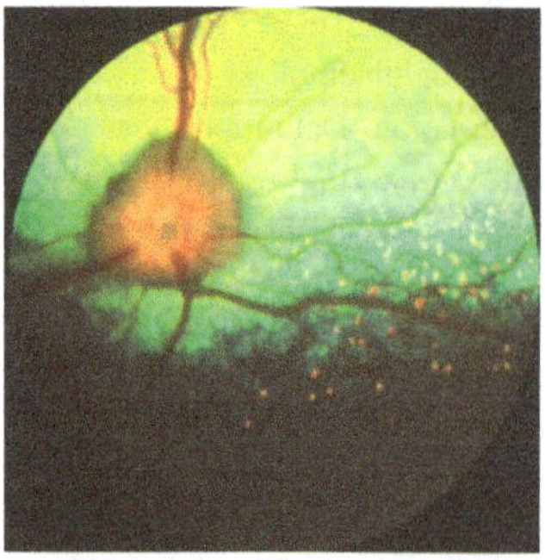
Gottingen minipig		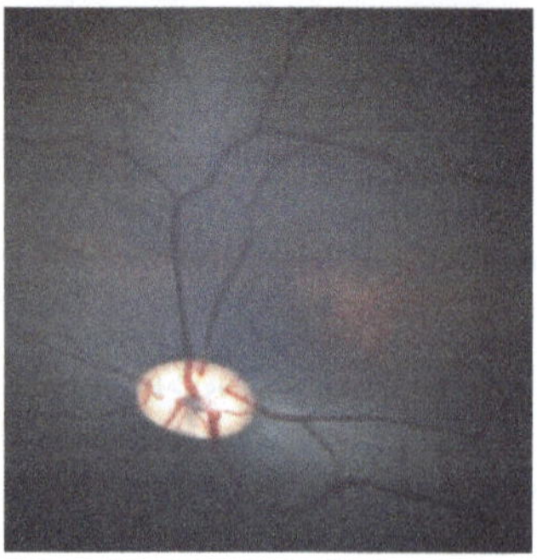

(continued)

Normal examples		
Species	Description	Photo + legend
Guinea pig, albino		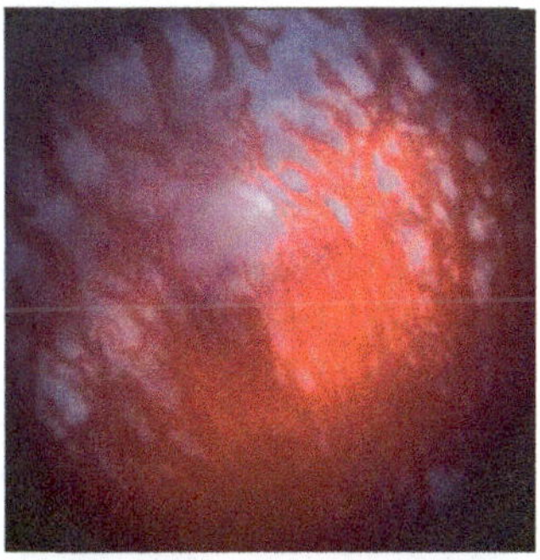
Guinea pig, pigmented		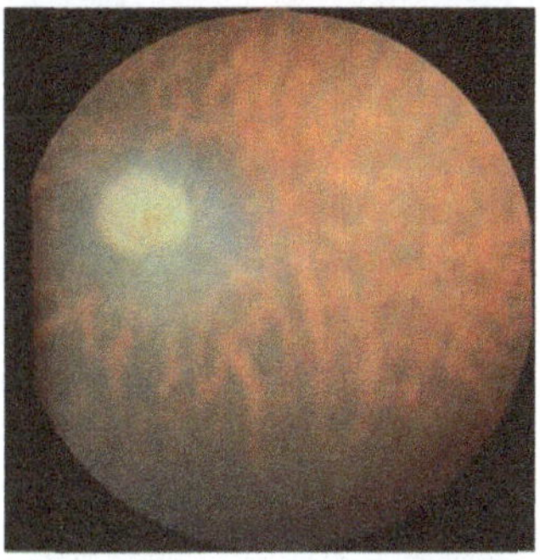
Hamster		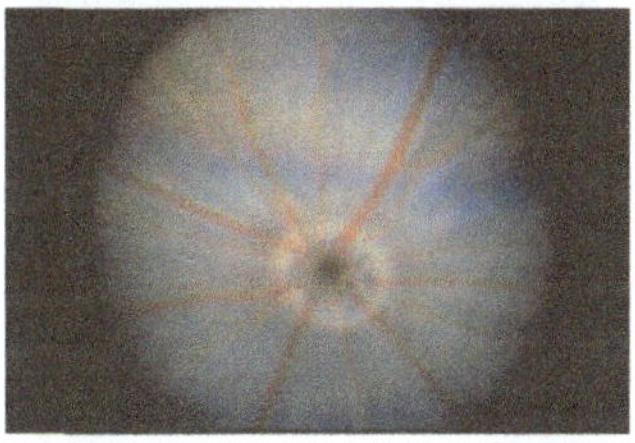
Mouse		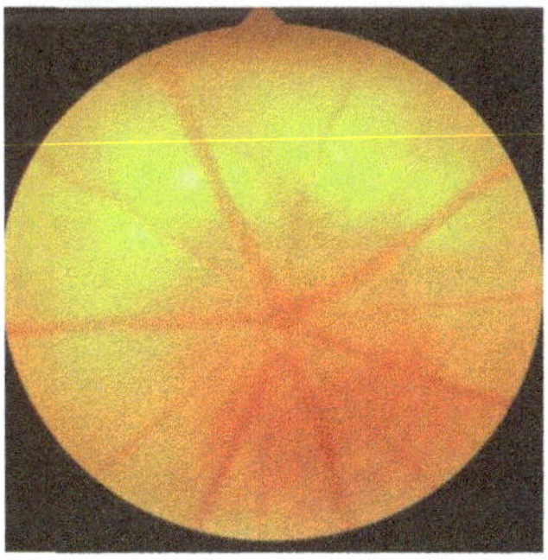

(continued)

Normal examples		
Species	Description	Photo + legend
Primate	Preretinal vessel loop, normal variation	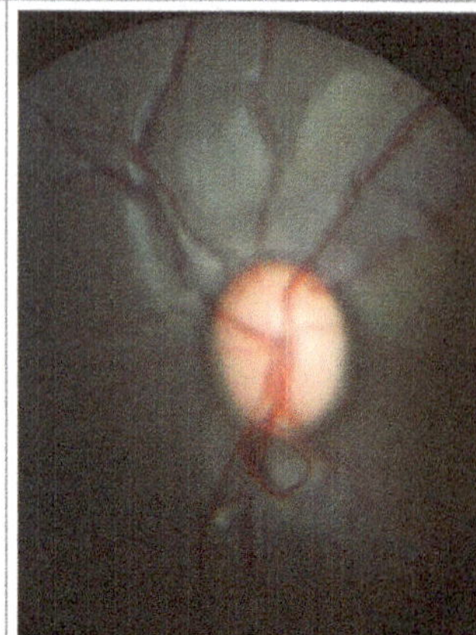
		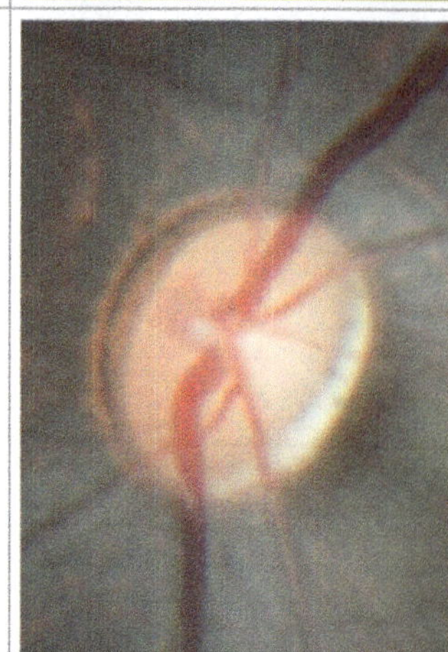
Primate	Optic nerve head vascular loop	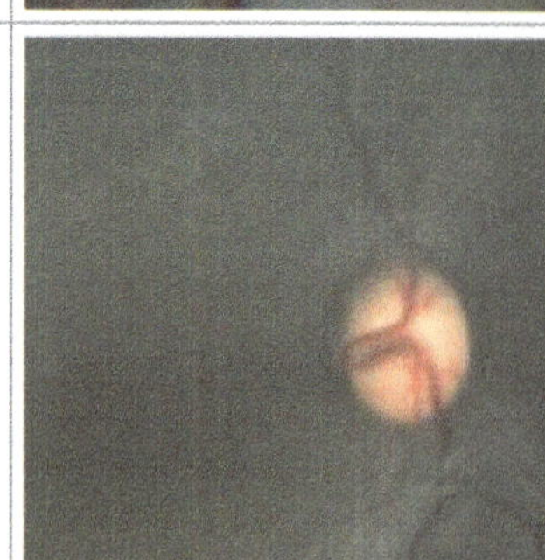

(continued)

Normal examples		
Species	Description	Photo + legend
Primate		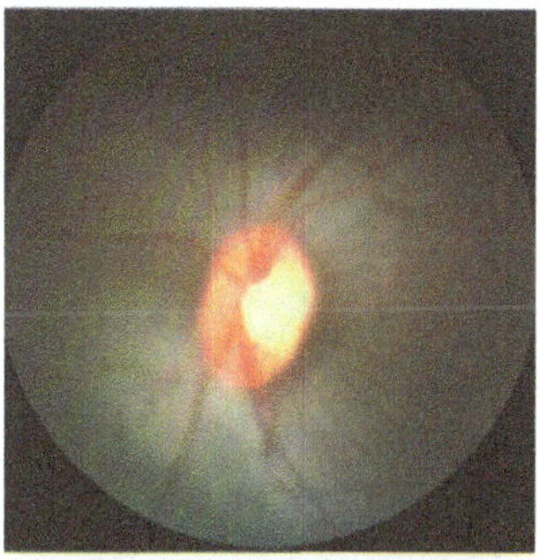
Primate	Hypopigmentation with choroidal vessels visible	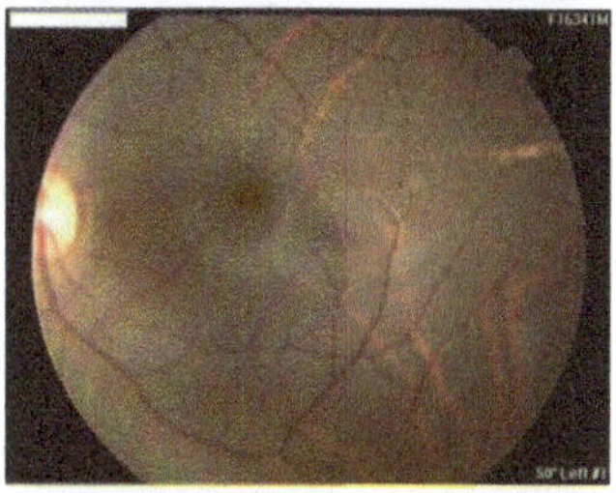
Primate	Normal pigment variation temporal	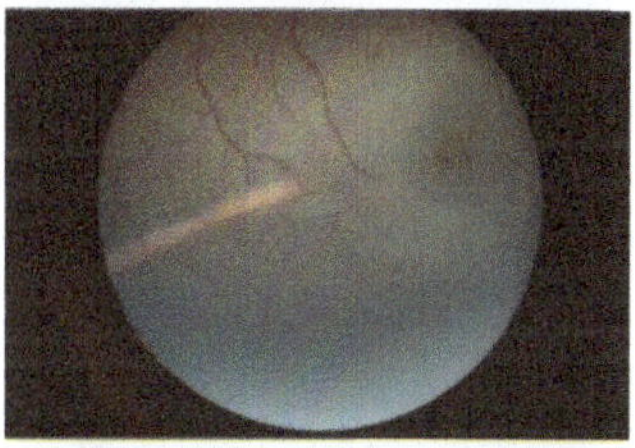
Primate	Peripapillary myelin	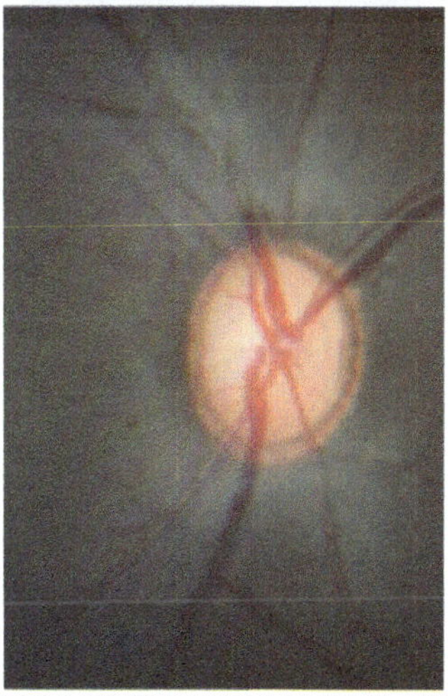

(continued)

Normal examples		
Species	Description	Photo + legend
Primate, Aotes		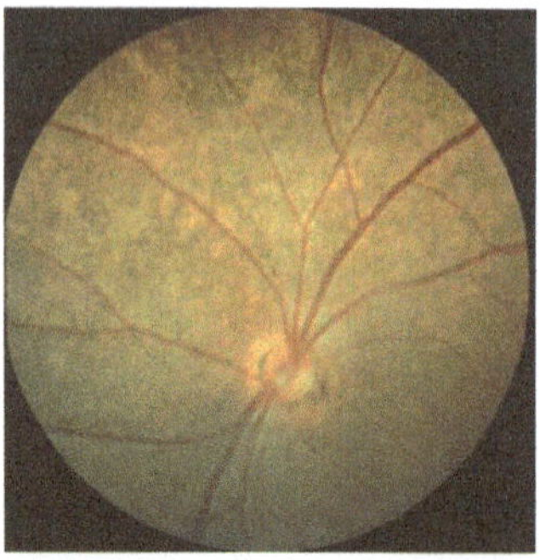
Primate, Cynomolgus	Normal degree of RPE and choroidal hypopigmentation allowing visualization of choroidal vasculature	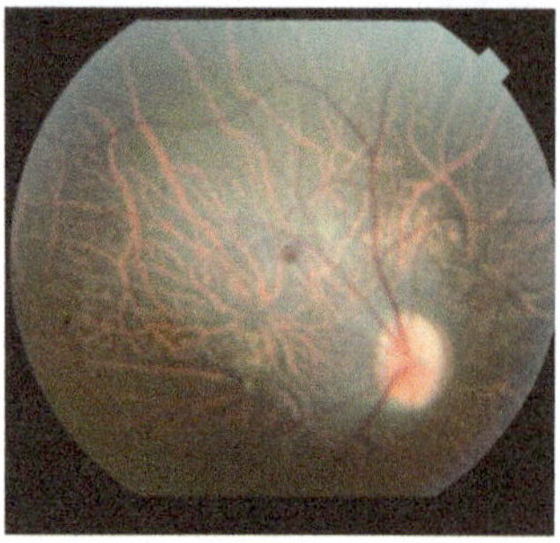 (Courtesy of Randy Sharp)
Primate, rhesus macaque		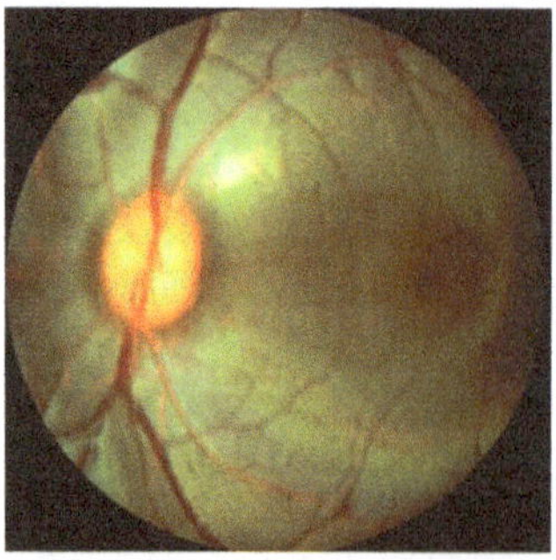
Rabbit		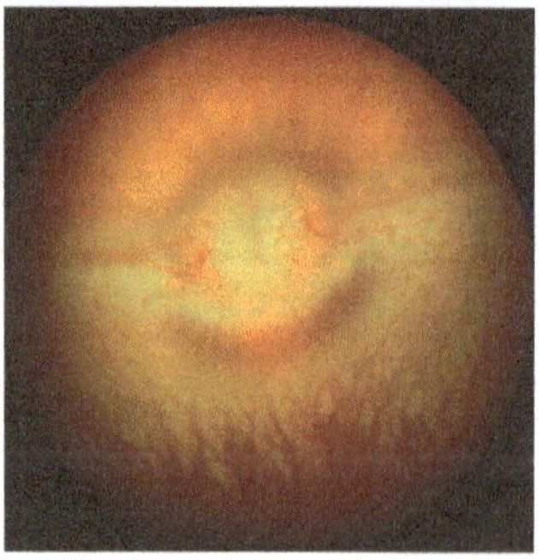

(continued)

Normal examples		
Species	Description	Photo + legend
Rabbit		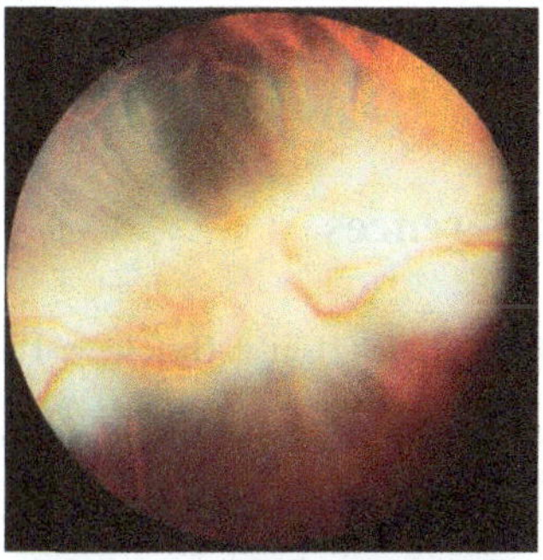
Rabbit	"Lens dimples," faint round depressions that can be seen on high magnification in some rabbits	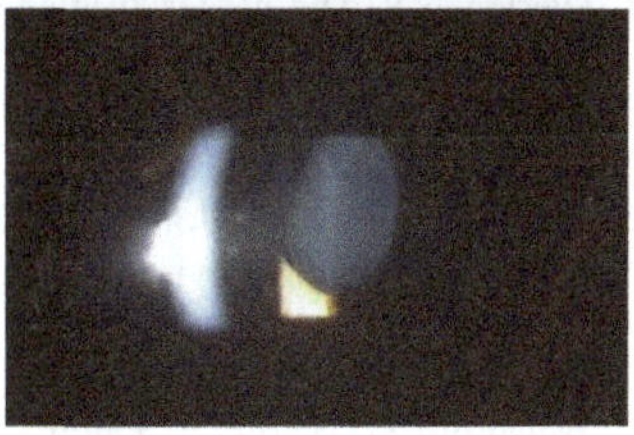 Slit lamp image. The subcapsular vertical anterior suture line is also visible
Rat, pigmented		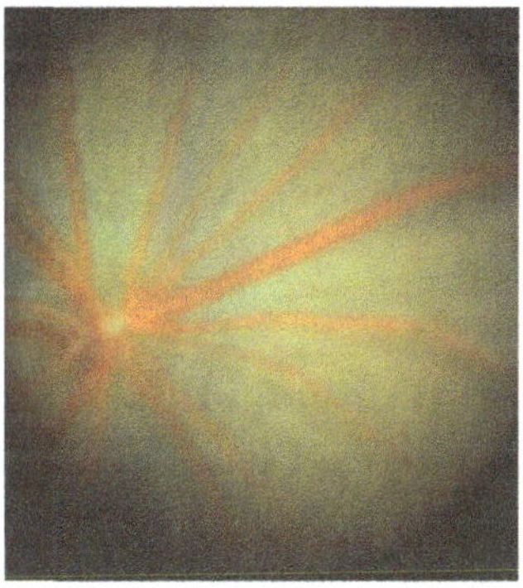

Conclusions

This chapter provides a comprehensive list of terminology recommended for description of findings observed on ocular toxicology assessments. The ultimate goal of this effort at harmonization of terminology used on preclinical safety studies is development of a common lexicon acceptable for submission with SEND-compliant reporting and via other global computerized reporting initiatives. The power of this lexicon harmonization arises when a common "language" is used to ensure effective and efficient communication of study observations between investigators within the field, across investigators of different fields, and ultimately to the global regulatory bodies that make final approval decisions based on these data.

Acknowledgments The authors wish to thank Drs. David Wilkie, Roy Bellhorn, and Randy Sharp for generously providing images, Dr. Craig Zwickle (Chair SEND CT) for a detail discussion regarding the SEND terminology approval process, and Dr. John Vahle (Member INHAND GESC) for providing a historical perspective of the INHAND effort.

References

1. Van Herck H, et al. Histological changes in the orbital region of rats after orbital puncture. Lab Anim. 1992;26(1):53–8.
2. Timm KI. Orbital venous anatomy of the rat. Lab Anim Sci. 1979;29(5):636–8.
3. Timm KI. Orbital venous anatomy of the Mongolian gerbil with comparison to the mouse, hamster and rat. Lab Anim Sci. 1989;39(3):262–4.
4. Djeridane Y. The harderian gland of desert rodents: a histological and ultrastructural study. J Anat. 1992;180(Pt 3):465–80.
5. Djeridane Y. Comparative histological and ultrastructural studies of the harderian gland of rodents. Microsc Res Tech. 1996;34(1):28–38.
6. Bhatt PN, Percy DH, Jonas AM. Characterization of the virus of sialodacryoadenitis of rats: a member of the coronavirus group. J Infect Dis. 1972;126(2):123–30.
7. Jacoby RO, Bhatt PN, Jonas AM. Pathogenesis of sialodacryoadenitis in gnotobiotic rats. Vet Pathol. 1975;12:196.
8. Weisbroth SH, Peress N. Ophthalmic lesions and dacryoadenitis: a naturally occurring aspect of sialodacryoadenitis virus infection of the laboratory rat. Lab Anim Sci. 1977;27(4):466–73.
9. Percy DH, et al. Comparison of strain susceptibility to experimental sialodacryoadenitis in rats. Lab Anim Sci. 1984;34(3):255–60.
10. Percy DH, Wojcinski ZW, Schunk MK. Sequential changes in the harderian and exorbital lacrimal glands in Wistar rats infected with sialodacryoadenitis virus. Vet Pathol. 1989;26(3):238–45.
11. Burling K, et al. Anatomy of the rabbit nasolacrimal duct and its clinical implications. Vet Comp Ophthalmol. 1991;1(1):33–40.

For Additional Information of the SEND and INHAND Initiatives, Please See These Additional Resources:

https://www.goreni.org/
https://www.fda.gov/ScienceResearch/SpecialTopics/CriticalPathInitiative/ucm076689.htm
https://www.cdisc.org/standards

Chapter 4
Spontaneous Incidence of Ocular Abnormalities in Laboratory Animals

Brian C. Gilger, Michael H. Brown, Robert J. Munger, Joshua T. Bartoe, Martin Bussieres, and Cynthia S. Cook

Abstract This chapter provides incidence data on spontaneous ophthalmic abnormalities in the most commonly used species in toxicological and pharmacokinetic drug research. This data can be used to better differentiate test article-related ocular findings from background incidental lesions to enhance interpretation of ophthalmic findings, improve speed of drug development, reduce the number of studies that need to be repeated, and thus reduce the overall number of animals used in toxicology research and drug development.

Keywords Incidence · Spontaneous · Ocular lesions · Laboratory animal · Ophthalmology · Ocular toxicology

Introduction

Understanding the incidence of spontaneous ocular lesions in laboratory animals is critical for interpretation of, and differentiation from, test article effects that may develop over the course of a toxicology study. Furthermore, critical information,

---

Endorsed by the American College of Veterinary Ophthalmologists (ACVO).

B. C. Gilger (✉) · J. T. Bartoe
MPI Research Ophthalmology Services, 54943 N Main St., Mattawan MI, USA
e-mail: bgilger@ncsu.edu

M. H. Brown
Animal Eye Center of New Jersey, Little Falls, NJ, USA

R. J. Munger
Animal Ophthalmology Clinic, Dallas, TX, USA

M. Bussieres
V&O Services Inc., Saint-Lazare, QC, Canada
e-mail: mb@eyelab.ca

C. S. Cook
Veterinary Vision, Inc., San Carlos, CA, USA
e-mail: Cook1@VeterinaryVision.com

B. C. Gilger et al. (eds.), *Standards for Ocular Toxicology and Inflammation*,
https://doi.org/10.1007/978-3-319-78364-2_4

such as the types of lesions, age of development, and sex predilection, are also important during interpretation of study findings. There have been several publications describing incidence of ocular lesions in various laboratory animals, but large-scale data collection of such lesions for the most common laboratory animals in toxicology studies has not been done. Understanding the incidence rates of spontaneous disease may also permit use of lower group numbers, and better interpretation of data may eliminate the need to repeat studies—both important to help better achieve guidelines to reduce, refine, and replace (i.e., 3 R's) use of animals in research [1].

For this chapter, the authors contacted the largest and most influential contract research organizations (CROs) in North America to provide data on ophthalmic examinations performed by veterinary ophthalmologists in the past 5 years during their pre-study examinations and for their control groups throughout toxicological and pharmacokinetic studies. Ophthalmic data from the most common animal species used in toxicology studies was provided for the incidence data analysis, including data from mice, rats, rabbits, beagle dogs, and cynomolgus monkeys. We purposely avoided collecting incidence data in animals from different animal suppliers to avoid the potential commercial conflicts that may be associated with analysis of this type of data. There are many other animals that are commonly used in toxicology studies that were not included in this report because of low numbers of examinations; this includes many individual strains of rodents, guinea pigs, cats, hamsters, pigs, and others. For those species, we have reviewed the literature with regard to occurrence but have no data regarding incidence.

The purpose of this study is to provide incidence data on ophthalmic abnormalities in the most commonly used species in toxicological and pharmacokinetic drug research to better differentiate test article-related ocular findings from background incidental lesions. The overall goal is to enhance interpretation of ophthalmic findings, improve and speed up the development of drugs, reduce the number of studies that need to be repeated, and thus reduce the overall number of animals used in toxicology research and drug development.

Rodents

Rodents are the most common species used for toxicological research and drug development. This is primarily due to their low-cost (permitting large group numbers), ease of handling and treatment, and large amount of historical data on rodent physiology, pharmacology, and genetic uniformity. We have collected ophthalmic incidence data on nearly 40,000 rodents, including albino strains: CD-1 mouse, Sprague-Dawley rat, the CD rat, the Wistar rat, and the pigmented Long-Evans rat.

CD-1 Mice

The CD-1 mice strains (also referred to as "Swiss mice") are outbred albino mice originally derived from mice imported from Switzerland in 1926. The CD-1 mice are generally used for toxicological and pharmacology research [2, 3]. We report on ophthalmic lesion incidence data from 5300 CD-1 mice, ranging in age from 1 to 12 weeks of age (Table 4.1). The most common spontaneous ophthalmic lesions observed were persistent hyaloid artery (3.97%), retinal degeneration (1.71%), and bilateral (1.17%) or unilateral (0.64%) cataract. Other relatively common findings were corneal dystrophy (0.58%) and iris coloboma (0.46%) (Table 4.1). These results are similar to a recent histologic study of spontaneous eye lesions of 3456 CD-1 mice from a CRO in Scotland [4]. In this histologic study, the most common histologic ocular findings were cataract, retinal atrophy, and corneal degeneration [4]. In another study focusing on spontaneous eye disease observed on ophthalmic examinations in young CD-1 mice (4–5 weeks; $n = 2953$), the most common lesions were also cataract, retinal degeneration, iris coloboma, and corneal disease [5]. A survey of corneal opacities in a variety of mouse strains identified a 4.3% incidence in CD-1 mice [6].

Sprague-Dawley Rat

This common, albino, outbred rat strain was established in 1925 by Robert Dawley [7]. We report on ophthalmic lesion incidence data from 25,312 Sprague-Dawley (SD) rats, ranging in age from 1 to 12 weeks of age (Table 4.2). The most common spontaneous ophthalmic lesions were bilateral corneal dystrophy (9.11%) and unilateral vitreous hemorrhage (0.47%) (likely from persistent hyaloid arteries, although may not have been visible due to hemorrhage). The corneal dystrophy is more frequent in males and seems to increase in frequency with age. Other frequent lesions (but less than 0.15% incidence) were unilateral or bilateral cataract and hyphema (Table 4.2). Our results were similar, but lower in incidence, to a study of 800 young SD rats (3–6 weeks of age) in which the most common spontaneous ocular lesions were corneal dystrophy (up to 75.2% in males) and vitreous hemorrhage (up to 5.4% in males) [8]. Another survey of 8-week-old SD rats revealed that more than 70% of animals had corneal opacities with male animals being more frequently affected [9]. Sprague-Dawley and Wistar rats were previously noted to have a higher incidence of corneal opacities than Lewis rats. In a study of 3000 SD rats in France, the most common spontaneous ophthalmic lesions were corneal dystrophy, cataract, PPM, and hyaloid remnant [10]. Although retinal lesions were relatively uncommon in our cohort of animals, another study evaluating specifically spontaneous retinal lesions in 6000 SD rats found focal linear retinopathy and coloboma as the most common findings, although incidence was not reported [11]. Ultrastructural lesions of retinal degeneration in the SD rat has been described [12].

Table 4.1 Incidence of spontaneous ocular lesions in CD-1 mice[a]

			Number of animals examined with lesion												
Sex	Age (weeks)	Total # examined	No ocular lesions (bilateral)	Corneal crystals/ dystrophy (bilateral)	Corneal crystals/ dystrophy (unilateral)	Cataract (bilateral)	Cataract (unilateral)	Hyphema (unilateral)	Iris coloboma (unilateral)	Persistent hyaloid (unilateral)	Phthisis bulbi (bilateral)	Phthisis bulbi (unilateral)	Chorioretinal hypoplasia (unilateral or bilateral)	Retinal atrophy (unilateral or bilateral)	Retinal hemorrhage (unilateral)
Female	1	10	10	0	0	0	0	0	0	0	0	0	0	0	0
	6	34	21	0	0	0	0	0	0	6	0	2	1	4	0
	7	2131	2032	12	1	4	14	0	5	67	0	4	1	40	0
	8	148	138	1	0	2	0	0	0	0	0	1	0	0	0
	9	256	254	1	0	0	17	0	0	4	0	0	1	1	0
	12	210	210	0	0	0	0	0	0	0	0	0	0	0	0
Total female		2789	2665	14	1	6	31	0	5	77	0	7	3	45	0
	% of total #		95.55	0.50	0.04	0.22	1.11	0.00	0.18	2.76	0.00	0.25	0.11	1.61	0.00
	Incidence per 1000		955.5	5.0	0.4	2.2	11.1	0.0	1.8	27.6	0.0	2.5	1.1	16.1	0.0
Male	1	10	10	0	0	0	0	0	0	0	0	0	0	0	0
	6	37	21	0	0	0	0	0	0	14	0	0	1	1	0
	7	1721	1329	12	2	46	2	1	17	76	1	6	2	35	1
	8	276	255	3	0	6	0	0	0	8	2	0	1	0	0
	9	256	246	0	0	4	0	0	0	5	0	0	1	0	0
	12	211	207	2	0	0	1	0	0	0	0	0		0	0
Total male		2511	2068	17	2	56	3	1	17	103	3	6	5	36	1

	% of total #	82.36	0.68	0.08	2.23	0.12	0.05	0.68	4.10	0.12	0.24	0.24	1.43	0.05
	Incidence per 1000	823.6	6.8	0.8	22.3	1.2	0.5	6.8	41.0	1.2	2.4	2.4	14.3	0.5
Total CD-1 Mice	5300	4733	31	3	62	34	1	22	180	3	13	8	81	1
% of total #		89.30	0.58	0.06	1.17	0.64	0.02	0.46	3.80	0.06	0.27	0.17	1.71	0.02
Incidence per 1000		893.0	5.8	0.6	11.7	6.4	0.2	4.6	38.0	0.6	2.7	1.7	17.1	0.2

[a]Data contributed from CRL-Wil Ohio; MPI Research

Table 4.2 Incidence of spontaneous ocular lesions in Sprague-Dawley rats[a]

			Number of animals examined with lesion															
Sex	Age (weeks)	Total # examined	No ocular lesions (bilateral)	Corneal crystals/ dystrophy (bilateral)	Corneal crystals/ dystrophy (unilateral)	Cataract (bilateral)	Cataract (unilateral)	Hyphema (bilateral)	Hyphema (unilateral)	Persistent hyaloid (unilateral)	Vitreous hemorrhage (unilateral)	Persistent pupillary membrane (unilateral)	Phthisis bulbi (unilateral)	Buphthalmia (unilateral)	Retinal hemorrhage (unilateral)	Blepharitis (unilateral)	Retinal degeneration (unilateral)	Coloboma/retina/ optic nerve (unilateral)
Female	1	121	117	2	0	0	1	0	0	0	0	0	0	0	0	0	0	0
	4	530	528	0	0	0	0	0	0	0	3	0	0	0	0	0	0	0
	5	975	889	32	0	0	0	0	0	0	7	0	0	0	0	0	0	0
	6	1638	1587	98	0	0	0	0	0	2	15	0	0	0	0	0	0	3
	7	6722	5977	674	1	11	9	0	8	3	13	0	3	1	1	0	0	0
	8	1269	1171	56	0	0	0	0	0	0	10	0	2	0	0	0	0	0
	9	676	640	29	0	1	0	0	0	0	3	1	0	0	0	0	0	2
	10	113	87	25	0	0	0	0	0	0	1	0	0	0	0	0	0	0
	11	419	379	37	0	0	0	0	1	0	0	0	0	0	0	0	0	0
	12	113	102	11	0	0	0	0	0	0	0	0	0	0	0	0	0	0
Total female		12,576	11,477	964	1	12	10	0	9	5	52	1	5	1	1	0	0	5
	% of total #		91.26	7.67	0.01	0.10	0.08	0.00	0.08	0.04	0.45	0.01	0.04	0.01	0.01	0.00	0.00	0.04
	Incidence per 1000		912.6	76.7	0.1	1.0	0.8	0.0	0.8	0.4	4.5	0.1	0.4	0.1	0.1	0.0	0.0	0.4

Male	1	125	106	12	0	0	0	0	0	0	0	1	0	0	1	0	0	0
	4	530	521	1	0	0	0	0	0	0	8	0	0	0	0	0	0	0
	5	1025	936	80	0	1	0	0	0	4	10	3	0	0	0	0	0	0
	6	1497	1212	25	0	1	0	0	1	8	1	0	0	0	0	0	0	1
	7	6769	5685	919	0	16	9	1	11	3	21	0	1	0	0	0	0	4
	8	1462	1239	100	0	0	3	2	1	0	12	0	0	0	0	1	0	0
	9	623	468	57	0	0	3	0	1	1	1	1	0	0	0	1	0	1
	10	402	269	97	0	0	1	0	1	4	0	0	0	0	0	1	2	0
	11	303	244	51	0	1	0	0	3	0	0	0	0	0	0	0	0	0
	12	0	0	0	0	0	0	0	0	0	0	0	0	0	0	0	0	0
Total male		12,736	10,680	1342	0	19	16	3	18	20	53	5	1	0	1	3	2	6
	% of total #		83.86	10.54	0.00	0.15	0.13	0.02	0.17	0.16	0.50	0.04	0.01	0.00	0.01	0.03	0.02	0.06
	Incidence per 1000		838.6	105.4	0.0	1.5	1.3	0.2	1.7	1.6	5.0	0.4	0.1	0.0	0.1	0.3	0.2	0.6
Total SD rat		25,312	22,157	2306	1	31	26	3	27	25	105	6	6	1	2	3	2	11
% of total #			87.54	9.11	0.00	0.12	0.10	0.01	0.12	0.10	0.47	0.02	0.02	0.00	0.01	0.01	0.01	0.05
Incidence per 1000			875.4	91.1	0.0	1.2	1.0	0.1	1.2	1.0	4.7	0.2	0.2	0.0	0.1	0.1	0.1	0.5

[a]Data contributed from CRL-Wil Ohio; Envigo, MPI Research

CD Rats

The CD rat is derived from the Sprague-Dawley rat and was developed by Charles River Inc. [13, 14] We evaluated the ophthalmic examination results from 4159 CD rats that ranged from 6 to greater than 13 weeks of age (Table 4.3). The most common abnormalities observed in CD rats included vitreous hemorrhage (3.1%), corneal dystrophy (2.7%), chorioretinal hypoplasia (1.9%), retinal degeneration (1.5%), persistent hyaloid (1.5%), and cataract (1.1%) (Table 4.3). In a study comparing the ocular findings in the CD vs SD rat over 2 years (n = 120 rats/strain), SD rats had a higher percentage of corneal opacity (especially older male rats), while the CD rats had a higher percentage of cataracts compared to the SD rats at 24 months of age [14]. The rat data in our study did not extend to 24 months of age, but in our dataset, the SD rats also had a higher percentage of corneal dystrophy (9.1% vs 2.7%) and lower percentage of cataract (0.12% vs 1.1%) compared to CD rats.

Wistar Rats

The Wistar rat is an albino outbred rat originally developed by Helen King and is considered the first standardized laboratory rat. Our ophthalmic findings in 3029 rats revealed the most common ocular lesions to be corneal dystrophy (40.03%) and choroidal hypoplasia (1.6%) (Table 4.4). Corneal dystrophy has been noted previously in 33-day-old Wistar rats when a shipment of 33-day-old rats where both eyes of 40 of 43 males and 26 of 29 female rats were affected [15]. Corneal and lens opacities have been previously described in the Wistar rat [1, 16]. Corneal dystrophy lesions in the Wistar rat appear much more common than that observed in the SD (9.1%) and CD (2.7%) rats.

Long-Evans Rats

This pigmented rat was developed by Long and Evans in 1915 by crossing a Wistar and a wild-type rat. Our dataset is based on ophthalmic examinations of 2232, 12-week-old Long-Evans rats. The only common ophthalmic lesion noted was corneal dystrophy (47.7%), although persistent hyaloid artery (1.3%) and retinal dysplasia (1.5%) were the next most common lesions observed (Table 4.5). The incidence of corneal dystrophy is similar that observed in the Wistar rat, which is expected since the Long-Evans is derived from the Wistar rat. Intraocular hemorrhage has been previously described as a spontaneous finding in the Long-Evans rat [17]. An increased rate of occurrence of corneal lesions initiated by general anesthesia was seen in the Wistar, Long-Evans, and Fischer 344 rats compared with Sprague-Dawley and Lewis rats [18].

Table 4.3 Incidence of spontaneous ocular lesions in CD rats[a]

			Number of animals examined with lesion															
Sex	Age (weeks)	Total # examined	No ocular lesions (bilateral)	Corneal crystals/dystrophy (bilateral)	Corneal crystals/dystrophy (unilateral)	Keratitis (unilateral or bilateral)	Cataract (unilateral or bilateral)	Hyphema (unilateral or bilateral)	Persistent hyaloid (unilateral or bilateral)	Vitreous hemorrhage (unilateral)	Persistent pupillary membrane (unilateral)	Phthisis bulbi/ microphthalmia (unilateral)	Iritis/uveitis (unilateral)	Iris coloboma (unilateral)	Retinal hemorrhage (unilateral or bilateral)	Chorioretinal hypoplasia (unilateral or bilateral)	Retinal degeneration (unilateral or bilateral)	Retinal dysplasia (unilateral or bilateral)	Coloboma optic nerve/retina (unilateral or bilateral)
Female	2	30	28	0	0	0	0	0	1	0	0	0	0	0	1	0	0	0	0
	5	30	24	0	0	0	0	1	0	0	0	0	0	0	0	4	1	0	0
	6	159	97	18	17	0	0	1	1	5	0	1	0	1	2	9	2	3	1
	7	1184	1010	15	22	6	3	12	19	26	0	0	8	0	4	34	14	3	6
	8	102	80	0	0	0	0	2	5	5	0	0	0	0	1	4	3	0	2
	9	156	150	0	0	0	0	0	0	1	0	0	0	0	0	3	2	0	0
	10	194	162	7	8	2	6	0	0	3	0	0	0	0	1	1	2	0	1
	12	88	80	0	1	0	2	0	0	0	1	0	0	0	0	1	3	0	0
	13	7	7	0	0	0	0	0	0	0	0	0	0	0	0	0	0	0	0
	>13	53	48	0	0	1	1	0	0	2	0	0	0	0	0	0	0	0	0
Total female		2003	1686	40	48	9	12	0	26	42	1	1	8	1	9	56	27	6	10
	% of total #		84.17	2.00	2.40	0.45	0.60	0.00	1.30	2.49	0.05	0.05	0.40	0.05	0.53	140.00	1.62	15.00	0.60
	Incidence per 1000		841.7	20.0	24.0	4.5	6.0	0.0	13.0	24.9	0.5	0.5	4.0	0.5	5.3	1400.0	16.2	150.0	6.0

(continued)

Table 4.3 (continued)

			Number of animals examined with lesion																
Sex	Age (weeks)	Total # examined	No ocular lesions (bilateral)	Corneal crystals/dystrophy (bilateral)	Corneal crystals/dystrophy (unilateral)	Keratitis (unilateral or bilateral)	Cataract (unilateral or bilateral)	Hyphema (unilateral or bilateral)	Persistent hyaloid (unilateral or bilateral)	Vitreous hemorrhage (unilateral)	Persistent pupillary membrane (unilateral)	Phthisis bulbi/ microphthalmia (unilateral)	Iritis/uveitis (unilateral)	Iris coloboma (unilateral)	Retinal hemorrhage (unilateral or bilateral)	Chorioretinal hypoplasia (unilateral or bilateral)	Retinal degeneration (unilateral or bilateral)	Retinal dysplasia (unilateral or bilateral)	Coloboma optic nerve/retina (unilateral or bilateral)
Male	2	36	36	0	0	0	0	0	0	0	0	0	0	0	0	0	0	0	0
	5	53	46	0	0	0	0	0	1	1	0	0	0	0	0	3	0	0	2
	6	205	99	32	31	0	4	3	4	11	0	0	2	0	3	10	1	3	1
	7	1136	927	28	24	0	17	17	23	30	2	2	11	0	6	32	11	1	5
	8	150	110	2	3	0	3	2	4	8	0	0	4	0	3	6	4	0	1
	9	422	387	7	6	0	9	0	0	2	0	0	0	0	1	4	2	3	1
	10	45	38	0	0	0	0	0	1	3	0	0	0	0	0	3	0	0	0
	13	16	11	0	0	0	0	0	2	3	0	0	0	0	0	0	0	0	0
	>13	93	86	0	0	0	0	0	0	5	0	0	0	0	0	1	0	0	0
Total male		2156	1740	69	64	0	33	22	35	63	2	2	17	0	13	59	18	7	10
	% of total #		80.71	3.20	2.97	0.00	1.53	1.02	1.62	3.62	0.09	0.09	0.79	0.00	0.75	85.51	1.06	10.14	14.49
	Incidence per 1000		807.1	32.0	29.7	0.0	15.3	10.2	16.2	36.2	0.9	0.9	7.9	0.0	7.5	855.1	10.6	101.4	144.9
Total CD rats		4159	3404	109	112	9	45	22	61	105	3	3	25	1	22	115			
% of total #			81.85	2.62	2.69	0.26	1.08	0.53	1.47	3.08	0.07	0.07	0.60	0.02	0.65	3.42	45		20
Incidence per 1000			818.5	26.2	26.9	2.6	10.8	5.3	14.7	30.8	0.7	0.7	6.0	0.2	6.5	34.2	1.34		0.59

Table 4.4 Incidence of spontaneous ocular lesions in Wistar rats[a]

Sex	Age (weeks)	Total # examined	Number of animals examined with lesion: No ocular lesions (bilateral)	Corneal crystals/ dystrophy (bilateral)	Cataract (unilateral or bilateral)	Hyphema (unilateral or bilateral)	Persistent hyaloid (unilateral or bilateral)	Vitreous hemorrhage (unilateral)	Persistent pupillary membrane (unilateral)	Retinal degeneration (unilateral or bilateral)	Choroidal hypoplasia (unilateral or bilateral)
Female	6	189	48	139	0	0	1	2	3	0	0
	7	322	161	137	2	1	2	2	2	0	11
	8	429	273	156	0	0	0	1	1	0	0
	9	182	178	3	0	0	0	0	0	1	0
	10	108	31	78	0	0	0	0	0	0	0
	11	77	38	39	0	0	0	0	0	0	0
	12	203	203	0	0	0	0	0	0	0	0
Total female		1510	932	552	2	1	3	5	6	1	11
	% of total #		61.72	36.56	0.13	0.18	0.20	0.54	0.40	0.11	1.99
	Incidence per 1000		617.2	365.6	1.3	1.8	2.0	5.4	4.0	1.1	19.9
Male	5	76	7	69	0	0	0	0	0	0	0
	6	211	40	97	0	0	1	2	5	0	1
	7	320	118	141	1	3	5	4	3	0	4
	8	258	188	147	0	0	1	0	3	0	2
	9	274	228	40	0	0	0	1	0	0	0
	10	108	30	78	0	0	0	0	0	0	0
	11	78	19	58	0	0	0	0	0	0	1
	12	194	193	0	0	0	0	1	0	0	0
Total male		1519	823	630	1	3	7	8	11	0	8

(continued)

Table 4.4 (continued)

			Number of animals examined with lesion								
Sex	Age (weeks)	Total # examined	No ocular lesions (bilateral)	Corneal crystals/ dystrophy (bilateral)	Cataract (unilateral or bilateral)	Hyphema (unilateral or bilateral)	Persistent hyaloid (unilateral or bilateral)	Vitreous hemorrhage (unilateral)	Persistent pupillary membrane (unilateral)	Retinal degeneration (unilateral or bilateral)	Choroidal hypoplasia (unilateral or bilateral)
	% of total #		54.18	41.47	0.07	0.20	0.46	0.97	0.72	0.00	1.27
	Incidence per 1000		541.8	414.7	0.7	2.0	4.6	9.7	7.2	0.0	12.7
Total Wistar rats		3029	1755	1182	3	4	10	13	17	1	19
% of total #			57.94	39.02	0.10	0.13	0.33	0.74	0.56	0.06	1.61
Incidence per 1000			579.4	390.2	1.0	1.3	3.3	7.4	5.6	0.6	16.1

[a]Data contributed from Envigo, MPI Research

Table 4.5 Incidence of spontaneous ocular lesions in Long-Evans rats[a]

			Number of animals examined with lesion									
Sex	Age (week)	Total # examined	No ocular lesions (bilateral)	Corneal crystals/ dystrophy (bilateral)	Cataract (unilateral or bilateral)	Corneal scar (unilateral)	Persistent hyaloid (unilateral)	Vitreous hemorrhage (unilateral)	Persistent pupillary membrane (unilateral)	Retinal hemorrhage (unilateral)	Retinal degeneration (unilateral)	Retinal dysplasia (unilateral)
Female	12	1663	543	1033	13	5	25	8	2	1	8	23
Total female		1663	543	1033	13	5	25	8	2	1	8	23
	% of total #	32.65		62.12	0.78	0.92	1.50	1.47	0.12	0.18	1.47	2.23
	Incidence per 1000	326.5		621.2	7.8	9.2	15.0	14.7	1.2	1.8	14.7	22.3
Male	12	569	491	31	7	10	3	4	0	1	12	10
Total male		569	491	31	7	10	3	4	0	1	12	10
	% of total #		86.29	5.45	1.23	1.76	0.53	0.70	0.00	0.18	2.11	1.76
	Incidence per 1000		862.9	54.5	12.3	17.6	5.3	7.0	0.0	1.8	21.1	17.6
Total Long-Evans rats		2232	1034	1064	20	15	28	12	2	2	20	33
% of total #			46.33	47.67	0.90	1.45	1.25	0.54	0.09	0.09	0.9	1.48
Incidence per 1000			463.3	476.7	9.0	14.5	12.5	5.4	0.9	0.9	9.0	14.8

[a]Data contributed from CRL Horsham

Other Rodent Species

Comparison with other published surveys is challenging because of the many potential variables that are often not identified in the published reports. These include variability in examiners, age of animals, and terminology used. In rodents, "corneal degeneration" and "corneal dystrophy" are often used interchangeably to describe spontaneous corneal opacities. There are many strains of rodents that are bred specifically for induction of ocular abnormalities, including lacrimal, corneal, lens, and retinal diseases. As these strains are not used in toxicology screening studies, they have not been considered here. However, some rodent strains do develop spontaneous ocular lesions, as the C57Bl/6J mouse (pigmented), which develop congenital ocular malformations (microphthalmia, anterior segment dysgenesis) corneal opacities, lens opacities, and retinal degeneration [19–22]. The BALB/c mouse (albino) has reported to develop spontaneous microphthalmia and cataract, hyaloid vessel remnant, corneal opacity, cataract, and corneal ulcer [6, 23–25]. The ICR (Institute of Cancer Research) mouse (albino) has been reported to have hyaloid vessel remnant, retinal degeneration, corneal opacity, cataract, and anisocoria [24]. The C3H mouse (pigmented) and CF1 mouse (albino) develop spontaneous corneal opacity [6], while the Fischer 344 is known to develop corneal dystrophy [3, 4, 26, 27]. Also, the Shumiya Cataract Rat (SCR) strain rat, as its name implies, develops cataract [28]. Use of a strain known to have a background spontaneous incidence of abnormalities would be expected to be associated with a lower threshold for test article-induced affect.

Guinea Pig

We did not collect incidence data on the guinea pig. Furthermore, there is very little published information in the guinea pig regarding ocular disease despite their popularity as pets and research animals. Most reports in the literature refer to congenital, acquired infectious or age-related conditions. Anophthalmos is reported as an inherited trait in guinea pigs [29]. Conformational eyelid abnormalities to include trichiasis and entropion have been reported. Keratitis and corneal ulcers may then occur secondarily. Blepharitis and keratitis have been associated with the Shealey strain (HSV-1 Sh) [30]. In one study, 5–7% of guinea pigs have some form of conjunctival disease secondary to eyelid conformation, trauma, embryologic malformations, nutrition, and infectious disease [31]. Conjunctivitis secondary to vitamins C deficiency (scurvy) and subconjunctival fat deposition may occur ("fatty eye", "pea eye") to cause conjunctival swellings. Dermoids have been reported involving the cornea and conjunctiva [32, 33].

Williams and Sullivan reported cataracts as the most common ocular abnormality in the guinea pig, affecting up to 17% of one population [31]. Cataracts may be inherited, diabetic, nutritional, or age-related. Inherited cataracts have been proposed in the Abyssinian and English shorthair, although no mode of inheritance has been identified [34]. Congenital cataracts in the Abyssinian are frequently associated with microphthalmos [34]. The N13 strain of laboratory guinea pig has a congenital nuclear cataract secondary to a mutation in the ζ crystalline gene [34, 35]. Rapidly progressive cataracts have been noted in diabetic guinea pigs, although no experimental evidence to support a cause and effect relationship has been reported.

Heterotopic bone formation is osseous metaplasia within the ciliary body and may appear as a white, irregular mass in the ciliary body region [36]. The white material may exhibit varying degrees of vascularization and may extend through the iris and continue circumferentially in the anterior chamber. Causes of this condition include renal insufficiency and dietary factors which may contribute elevated levels of ascorbic acid in the aqueous humor or ciliary body. Osseous choristoma formation has been reported to cause secondary glaucoma [37, 38].

There is little reported information regarding abnormalities of the guinea pig retina. The type of retinal vascular pattern of the guinea pig is controversial. Clinically, the retina appears anangiotic, but histologically there are vessels leaving the optic disc margin and extending slightly into the retina consistent with a paurangiotic retinal vascular pattern. A spontaneous disorder of rod function as characterized by electroretinography has been reported [39].

Hamster

We did not collect incidence data on the hamster. Hamsters lack a tapetum and have a holangiotic vascular pattern [40]. The retina is rod dominated and supports their nocturnal lifestyle. Reports of ophthalmic disease are rare in the veterinary literature. Conjunctivitis, keratoconjunctivitis sicca, eyelid melanoma, and retinal dysplasia are noted [41]. Congenital orbital disease in the hamsters is primarily related to anophthalmic Syrian whites. These hamsters are homozygous for the Wh gene and are born without identifiable eyes [42]. Affected homozygotes are blind, sterile, and deaf and have a shorter life expectancy. Exophthalmos may occur secondary to a retrobulbar abscess, sialodacryoadenitis, trauma, facial vein thrombosis, and orbital neoplasia. Entropion is reported in Syrian and dwarf breeds. Acquired ophthalmic disease is common in the hamster. Keratoconjunctivitis sicca has been reported and may be immune mediated [43, 44]. Cataracts are common in the hamster and are most commonly associated with age and diabetes [45]. Glaucoma has been reported in a cohort of Djungarian hamster at 11 months of age.

Retinal dysplasia was diagnosed in 2% of Syrian hamsters in one study [41]. The dysplastic lesions were detected during ophthalmoscopic examinations between 6 weeks and 9 months of age. Ophthalmoscopically, the dysplastic foci varied from retinal streaks to small circular areas of cream-colored depigmentation. Blindness or other apparent visual defects were not seen. Histologic examination of the affected hamsters revealed focal dysplasias limited to the retina and characterized as rosette-like structures composed of elements of the photoreceptor layer, outer limiting membrane, and outer nuclear layer. Retinopathy has been associated with diabetes in Chinese Hamsters [45].

Rabbits

Rabbits are among the most common laboratory animal for ophthalmic studies, with New Zealand White (NZW) and Dutch Belted (DB) rabbits likely the most commonly used. Our data is from ophthalmic examinations of 218 NZW and 870 DB rabbits, for a total of 1088 rabbits ranging in age from 13 to 53 weeks (Table 4.6). The only abnormalities observed in NZW rabbits in our dataset was unilateral conjunctivitis or conjunctival hyperemia (Table 4.6A). More abnormalities were observed in DB rabbits compared to NZW rabbits in our dataset; the most common of which in DB rabbits was corneal dystrophy (0.57%) and unilateral conjunctivitis or conjunctival hyperemia (0.57%) (Table 4.6B). In a recent review of ocular lesions in laboratory rabbits, a much higher percentage of rabbits had spontaneous ocular lesions (9.6%) compared to our data, with most lesions found in the corneal and lens [46]. Another study evaluating spontaneous ocular lesions in NZW rabbits only, an incidence of ocular lesions of 9.6% was also found, with a finding of cataracts in 1.9% of rabbits [47]; this contrasts our dataset, where no lens lesions were observed. An additional study, by Munger et al. [48], found a 5.7% incidence of spontaneous cataracts in NZW rabbits suggesting an autosomal recessive mode of inheritance [48]. One possible cause of the relatively few spontaneous lesions observed in our dataset may partially be due to the fact that many of the rabbits were prescreened for ophthalmic abnormalities at their source prior to shipment to the study sites. In addition, the rabbits in our survey were examined prior to study initiation and were probably younger than in other surveys. The incidence of spontaneous cataracts in rabbits has been shown to increase in older populations [49].

Beagles

In our data, 2559 laboratory beagles were examined ranging in age from less than 20–62 weeks. Compared to rodents, the overall incidence of spontaneous ophthalmic lesions was low. The most common ocular lesions included optic nerve hypoplasia (0.6%), retinal dysplasia (0.4%), and other lesions such as persistent pupillary membrane, retinal atrophy, and cataract (all less than 0.25%) (Table 4.7). In a histologic review of the spontaneous lesions in 266 beagles (8–15 months of age), only 1 male dog had an eye lesion (0.7%) [50]. In two other studies evaluating incidence of spontaneous lesions in more than 1000 laboratory beagles, there was no ocular lesions described [51, 52].

Table 4.6 Incidence of spontaneous ocular lesions in rabbits[a]

Sex	Age (weeks)	Total # examined	Number of animals examined with lesion: No ocular lesions (bilateral)	Corneal crystals/ dystrophy (unilateral)	Conjunctivitis/hyperemia (unilateral or bilateral)	Chorioretinitis (unilateral)	Retinal atrophy focal (unilateral)	Retinal detachment (unilateral)
(A) New Zealand white rabbits								
Female	23	22	22	0	0	0	0	0
	24	65	60	0	5	0	0	0
	25	1	1	0	0	0	0	0
	28	1	1	0	0	0	0	0
	30	2	2	0	0	0	0	0
	32	1	1	0	0	0	0	0
Total female		92	87	0	5	0	0	0
	% of total #		94.57	0.0	5.43	0.0	0.0	0.0
	Incidence per 1000		945.7	0.0	54.3	0.0	0.0	0.0
Male	20	22	22	0	0	0	0	0
	24	58	57	0	1	0	0	0
	25	2	2	0	0	0	0	0
	26	15	15	0	0	0	0	0
	53	29	29	0	0	0	0	0
Total male		126	125	0	1	0	0	0
	% of total #		99.21	0.0	0.79	0.0	0.0	0.0
	Incidence per 1000		992.1	0	7.9	0.0	0.0	0.0
Total NZW		218	212	0	6	0	0	0
% of total #			97.25	0.0	2.75	0.0	0.0	0.0
Incidence per 1000			972.5	0	27.5	0	0	0

(continued)

Table 4.6 (continued)

Sex	Age (weeks)	Total # examined	Number of animals examined with lesion: No ocular lesions (bilateral)	Corneal crystals/dystrophy (unilateral)	Conjunctivitis/hyperemia (unilateral or bilateral)	Chorioretinitis (unilateral)	Retinal atrophy focal (unilateral)	Retinal detachment (unilateral)
(B) Dutch belted rabbits								
Female	13	18	17	1	0	0	0	0
	16	23	23	0	0	0	0	0
	23	2	2	0	0	0	0	0
	24	379	377	0	1	0	0	1
	28	10	10	0	0	0	0	0
Total female		432	429	1	1	0	0	1
	% of total #		99.31	0.23	0.23	0.0	0.0	0.23
	Incidence per 1000		993.1	2.3	2.3	0.0	0.0	
Male	13	18	17	0	0	1	0	0
	24	386	384	0	1	0	1	0
	25	12	12	0	0	0	0	0
	26	11	5	4	2	0	0	0
	28	10	10	0	0	0	0	0
	32	1	1	0	0	0	0	0
Total male		438	429	4	3	1	1	0
	% of total #		97.95	0.91	0.68	0.23	0.23	0.0
	Incidence per 1000		979.5	9.1	6.8	2.3	2.3	0.0
Total DB		870	858	5	5	1	1	1
% of total #			98.62	0.57	0.46	0.11	0.11	0.11
Incidence per 1000			98.2	5.7	4.6	1.1	1.1	1.1

[a]Data contributed from MPI Research and Powered Research

Table 4.7 Incidence of spontaneous ocular lesions in Laboratory Beagles[a]

			Number of animals examined with lesion													
Sex	Age (week)	Total # examined	No ocular lesions (bilateral)	Cataract (bilateral)	Cataract (unilateral)	Keratitis (unilateral or bilateral)	Prolapsed nictitans gland (unilateral)	Persistent hyaloid (unilateral)	Persistent pupillary membrane (unilateral)	Conjunctivitis (unilateral)	Chorioretinitis (unilateral)	Retinal atrophy (focal) (unilateral)	Retinal dysplasia (unilateral)	Optic nerve coloboma (unilateral)	Optic nerve hypoplasia (unilateral)	Irregular retinal/ choroidal pigmentation (unilateral)
Female	<20	41	41	0	0	0	0	0	0	0	0	0	0	0	0	0
	22	127	123	0	1	0	0	0	0	0	0	0	0	0	0	3
	23	54	52	0	0	0	0	0	0	0	1	0	1	0	0	0
	24	109	100	0	0	0	0	2	2	0	1	0	0	0	0	0
	25	85	82	0	0	0	0	0	0	0	0	0	1	0	2	0
	26	53	51	0	1	0	0	0	0	0	0	0	0	0	0	0
	27	215	202	1	2	1	0	0	0	0	0	0	1	0	2	3
	28	92	92	0	0	0	0	0	0	0	0	0	0	0	0	0
	29	89	89	0	0	0	0	0	0	0	0	0	0	0	0	0
	30	163	163	0	0	0	0	0	0	0	0	0	0	0	0	0
	31	57	57	0	0	0	0	0	0	0	0	0	0	0	0	0
	37	37	37	0	0	0	0	0	0	0	0	0	0	0	0	0
	38	22	22	0	0	0	0	0	0	0	0	0	0	0	0	0
	41	22	22	0	0	0	0	0	0	0	0	0	0	0	0	0
	43	75	75	0	0	0	0	0	0	0	0	0	0	0	0	0
	44	39	38	0	1	0	0	0	0	0	0	0	0	0	0	0
	62	11	11	0	0	0	0	0	0	0	0	0	0	0	0	0
Total female		1250	1216	1	4	0	0	2	2	0	2	2	3	0	4	6

(continued)

Table 4.7 (continued)

Sex	Age (week)	Total # examined	No ocular lesions (bilateral)	Cataract (bilateral)	Cataract (unilateral)	Keratitis (unilateral or bilateral)	Prolapsed nictitans gland (unilateral)	Persistent hyaloid (unilateral)	Persistent pupillary membrane (unilateral)	Conjunctivitis (unilateral)	Chorioretinitis (unilateral)	Retinal atrophy (focal) (unilateral)	Retinal dysplasia (unilateral)	Optic nerve coloboma (unilateral)	Optic nerve hypoplasia (unilateral)	Irregular retinal/ choroidal pigmentation (unilateral)
			Number of animals examined with lesion													
	% of total #		97.28	0.08	0.32	0.00	0.00	0.16	0.16	0.00	0.16	0.16	0.24	0.00	0.33	0.49
	Incidence per 1000		972.8	0.8	3.2	0.0	0.0	1.6	1.6	0.0	1.6	1.6	2.4	0.0	3.3	4.9
Male	<20	38	38	0	0	0	0	0	0	0	0	1	2	0	2	0
	22	108	107	0	0	0	0	0	0	0	0	0	1	0	0	0
	23	56	53	0	0	0	0	1	0	0	0	0	0	0	2	0
	24	133	129	0	0	0	0	0	0	0	0	0	1	0	3	0
	25	70	68	0	0	0	0	0	0	0	0	0	1	0	1	0
	26	134	130	0	0	0	1	1	0	0	0	0	0	0	0	0
	27	252	251	0	0	0	0	0	0	1	0	0	0	0	0	0
	28	123	123	0	0	0	0	0	0	0	0	0	0	0	0	0
	29	61	61	0	0	0	0	0	0	0	0	0	0	0	0	0
	30	118	117	0	1	0	0	0	0	0	0	0	0	0	0	0
	32	23	23	0	0	0	0	0	0	0	0	0	0	0	0	0
	37	23	23	0	0	0	0	0	0	0	0	0	0	0	0	0
	38	22	22	0	0	0	0	0	0	0	0	0	0	0	0	0
	41	22	21	0	0	0	0	0	0	0	0	0	0	1	0	0
	43	76	74	2	0	0	0	0	0	0	0	0	0	0	0	0
	44	39	39	0	0	0	0	0	0	0	0	0	0	0	0	0
	62	11	11	0	0	2	0	0	2	0	0	1	2	1	3	0

Total male	1309	1290	2	1	2	1	2	2	1	0	2	7	2	11	0
	% of total #	98.55	0.15	0.08	0.15	0.08	0.15	0.15	0.08	0.00	0.15	0.53	0.16	0.85	0.00
	Incidence per 1000	985.5	1.5	0.8	1.5	0.8	1.5	1.5	0.8	0.0	1.5	5.3	1.6	8.5	0.0
Total Beagles	2559	2506	3	5	2	1	4	4	1	2	4	10	2	15	6
% of total #		97.93	0.12	0.20	0.08	0.04	0.16	0.16	0.04	0.08	0.16	0.39	0.08	0.60	0.23
Incidence per 1000		979.3	1.2	2.0	0.8	0.4	1.6	1.6	0.4	0.8	1.6	3.9	0.8	6.0	2.3

[a]Data contributed from CRL-Reno, MPI Research, CRL-Wil Ohio

Laboratory Minipigs

Although use of pigs in ophthalmic research has increased in recent years, we were not able to obtain sufficient incidence data for this manuscript. In the literature, there are several reports of the spontaneous incidence of lesions, including ocular lesions. In one source, the most common spontaneous lesions in Göttingen minipigs were found to be hyaloid artery remnants (76.5%), lens opacities (41.8%), and persistent pupillary membranes (21.4%) [53]. Optic nerve cupping has been reported in Göttingen minipigs; however, the incidence of the defect was not reported [54, 55]. Two reports retrospectively review the spontaneous histologic incidence of ocular lesions. In one of these reviews [56], ocular lesions of Göttingen minipigs consisted of inflammatory cell infiltrate in nearly 3% of minipigs, and greater than 4% of the pigs had inflammatory cell infiltrate in the lacrimal gland. Hanford minipigs were reported to have lacrimal inflammatory cell infiltrates in 1.7% of animals and chronic inflammation in 3.4% of Yucatan minipigs [56]. In another review of histologic data from 417 male and 418 female Göttingen minipigs, only 3 animals were noted to have ocular lesions [57]. One animal was noted to have a cataract, two animals were noted to have "corneal hyperplasia, and one animal had mild limbal inflammation [57].

Yucatan micropigs are another species used in laboratory studies. In one survey of 112 animals, a large proportion of these 7–12-month-old pigs had hyaloid remnants (82.1%), pupillary membrane remnants (66.1%), or incomplete pigmentation of the fundus (50.0%), findings consistent with immature and incomplete development. Posterior cortical lens opacities were seen in 20.5% [58].

Cynomolgus Monkeys

In our dataset of 3728 cynomolgus monkeys (*Macaca fascicularis*) ranging from 107 to 618 weeks of age, the most common ocular lesions were either unilateral (1.4%) or bilateral (1.3%) cataract and optic disc hypoplasia/optic disc atrophy (1.1%), followed in frequency by unilateral chorioretinitis (0.6%) and uveitis (0.3%) (Table 4.8). In four studies evaluating the incidence of spontaneous disease in laboratory cynomolgus monkeys, ocular lesions were not mentioned suggesting the relatively low incidence of spontaneous ocular disease in this species [59–62].

Conclusions

After evaluation of the records of a large number of selected common laboratory animals from contract research organizations in North America, we present the incidence of ocular findings by age and gender as observed by veterinary ophthalmologists of

Table 4.8 Incidence of spontaneous ocular lesions in cynomolgus monkeys[a]

			Number of animals examined with lesion													
Sex	Age (week)	Total # examined	No ocular lesions (bilateral)	Cataract (bilateral)	Cataract (unilateral)	Corneal opacity (unilateral or bilateral)	Eyelid defect (unilateral)	Persistent pupillary membrane (bilateral)	Iris coloboma (bilateral)	Uveitis (unilateral)	Persistent hyaloid (unilateral)	Vitreous opacity (bilateral)	Retinal degeneration (unilateral or bilateral)	Retinal detachment (unilateral)	Chorioretinitis (unilateral)	Optic disc hypoplasia/atrophy (bilateral)
Female	107–135	205	196	0	0	0	1	1	0	0	1	0	0	1	4	1
	136–156	343	334	1	0	0	0	0	0	5	1	0	0	0	1	1
	157–168	620	586	7	7	3	1	0	1	0	0	2	2	0	1	10
	169–176	142	138	1	1	0	0	0	0	0	0	0	0	0	2	0
	177–189	184	184	0	0	0	0	0	0	0	0	0	0	0	0	0
	190–230	193	193	0	0	0	0	0	0	0	0	0	0	0	0	0
	230–618	74	72	0	1	0	0	0	0	0	0	0	0	1	0	0
Total female		1761	1703	9	9	3	2	1	1	5	2	2	2	2	8	12
	% of total #		96.71	0.51	0.51	0.17	0.11	0.06	0.06	0.28	0.11	0.11	0.11	0.11	0.47	0.68
	Incidence per 1000		967.1	5.1	5.1	1.7	1.1	0.6	0.6	2.8	1.1	1.1	1.1	1.1	4.7	6.8

(continued)

Table 4.8 (continued)

Sex	Age (week)	Total # examined	Number of animals examined with lesion No ocular lesions (bilateral)	Cataract (bilateral)	Cataract (unilateral)	Corneal opacity (unilateral or bilateral)	Eyelid defect (unilateral)	Persistent pupillary membrane (bilateral)	Iris coloboma (bilateral)	Uveitis (unilateral)	Persistent hyaloid (unilateral)	Vitreous opacity (bilateral)	Retinal degeneration (unilateral or bilateral)	Retinal detachment (unilateral)	Chorioretinitis (unilateral)	Optic disc hypoplasia/atrophy (bilateral)
Male	107–135	267	255	3	1	1	0	0	0	1	0	0	0	0	6	0
	136–156	396	368	5	9	1	0	0	0	4	0	0	0	0	8	1
	157–168	851	759	27	31	2	1	2	0	0	0	0	3	0	1	25
	169–176	136	132	0	1	0	0	0	0	0	0	0	0	0	1	1
	177–189	117	115	1	0	0	0	0	0	0	1	0	0	0	0	0
	190–230	141	138	2	1	0	0	0	0	0	0	0	0	0	0	0
	230–618	59	58	0	1	0	0	0	0	0	0	0	0	0	0	0
Total male		1967	1825	38	44	4	1	2	0	5	1	0	3	0	16	27
	% of total #		92.78	1.93	2.24	0.20	0.05	0.10	0.00	0.25	0.05	0.00	0.15	0.00	0.81	1.37
	Incidence per 1000		927.8	19.3	22.4	2.0	0.5	1.0	0.0	2.5	0.5	0.0	1.5	0.0	8.1	13.7
Total cynomologous		3728	3528	47	53	4	3	3	1	10	3	2	5	2	24	39
% of total #			94.64	1.26	1.42	0.11	0.08	0.08	0.08	0.27	0.08	0.05	0.14	0.05	0.64	1.05
Incidence per 1000			946.4	12.6	14.2	1.1	0.8	0.8	0.8	2.7	0.8	0.5	1.4	0.5	6.4	10.5

[a]Data contributed from CRL-Wil Ohio; CRL-Reno, MPI Research

animals during routine pre-study examinations and in control groups. With this information, lesions associated with test article administration can be differentiated from spontaneous lesions. In general, the information provided in our analysis is similar to that reported in most species, but our data represents a much larger dataset compared to that previously reported.

Acknowledgments The authors thank the following contract research organizations and individuals for assistance in collection of the data for this chapter:

Charles River Laboratories, Wil Research, Ashland, Ohio. Robert Wally, Brian Ronk and Jeanette Howell

Charles River Laboratories, Reno, Nevada. Dr. Margaret Collins

Charles River Laboratories, Horsham, Pennsylvania. Dr. Douglas Learn

Envigo, East Millstone, New Jersey. Christopher Blum

MPI Research, Mattawan, Michigan

Powered Research, Research Triangle Park, North Carolina. Dr. David Culp, Justin Prater

References

1. Reduce, refine, replace. Nat Immunol. 2010;11(11):971. https://doi.org/10.1038/ni1110-971.
2. Aldinger KA, Sokoloff G, Rosenberg DM, Palmer AA, Millen KJ. Genetic variation and population substructure in outbred CD-1 mice: implications for genome-wide association studies. PLoS One. 2009;4(3):e4729. https://doi.org/10.1371/journal.pone.0004729.
3. Chia R, Achilli F, Festing MFW, Fisher EMC. The origins and uses of mouse outbred stocks. Nat Genet. 2005;37(11):1181–6. https://doi.org/10.1038/ng1665.
4. Mukaratirwa S, Petterino C, Naylor SW, Bradley A. Incidences and range of spontaneous lesions in the eye of Crl:CD-1(ICR)BR mice used in toxicity studies. Toxicol Pathol. 2014;43:530–5.
5. Hubert M, Gerin G, Durand-cavagna G. Spontaneous ophthalmic lesions in young swiss mice. Lab Anim Sci. 1999;49(3):232–40.
6. Van Winkle TJ, Balk MW. Spontaneous corneal opacities in laboratory mice. Lab Anim Sci. 1986;36(3):248–55.
7. Williams DL. Ocular disease in rats: a review. Vet Ophthalmol. 2002;5(3):183–91. https://doi.org/10.1046/j.1463-5224.2002.00251.x.
8. Kuno H, Usui T, Eydelloth RS, Wolf ED. Spontaneous ophthalmic lesions in young Sprague-Dawley rats. J Vet Med Sci. 1991;53(4):607–14. https://doi.org/10.1292/jvms.53.607.
9. Wegener A, Jochims K. Clinical, histological and ultrastructural characteristics of a spontaneous corneal opacity in Sprague-Dawley rats. Ophthalmic Res. 1994;26(5):296–303.
10. Taradach C, Regnier B, Perraud J. Eye lesions in Sprague-Dawley rats: type and incidence in relation to age. Lab Anim. 1981;15(3):285–7.
11. Hubert MF, Gillet JP, Durand-Cavagna G. Spontaneous retinal changes in Sprague Dawley rats. Lab Anim Sci. 1994;44(6):561–7.
12. Lin WL, Essner E. An electron microscopic study of retinal degeneration in Sprague-Dawley rats. Lab Anim Sci. 1987;37(2):180–6.
13. White WJ, Lee CS. The development and maintenance of the Crl:CD(SD) IGS BR rat breeding system. Charles River Lab. 1998;8:8–14.
14. Pettersen JC, Morrissey RL, Saunders DR, et al. A 2-year comparison study of Crl:CD BR and Hsd:Sprague-Dawley SD rats. Toxicol Sci. 1996;33(2):196–211. https://doi.org/10.1093/toxsci/33.2.196.

15. Wojcinski ZW, Houston B, Gragtmans B, Rogers J, Piscopo I, Baker K. A spontaneous corneal change in juvenile Wistar rats. J Comp Pathol. 1999;120(3):281–94. https://doi.org/10.1053/jcpa.1998.0276.
16. Eiben R. Frequency of spontaneous opacities in the cornea and lens observed in chronic toxicity studies in Wistar rats: experience with a standardized terminology glossary (Hattersheimer Kreis). Res Commun Pharmacol Toxicol. 2001;6(3-4):238–45.
17. Inagaki K, Koga H, Inoue K, Suzuki K, Suzuki H. Spontaneous intraocular hemorrhage in rats during postnatal ocular development. Comp Med. 2014;64(1):34–43.
18. Turner PV, Albassam MA. Susceptibility of rats to corneal lesions after injectable anesthesia. Comp Med. 2005;55(2):175–82.
19. Lavail MM, Sidman RL. C57BL/6J mice with inherited retinal degeneration. Arch Ophthalmol. 1974;91(5):394–400. https://doi.org/10.1001/archopht.1974.03900060406015.
20. Cook CS, Sulik KK. Sequential scanning electron microscopic analyses of normal and spontaneously occurring abnormal ocular development in C57B1/6J mice. Scan Electron Microsc. 1986;3:1215–27.
21. Tyndall DA, Cook CS. Spontaneous, asymmetrical microphthalmia in C57Bl/6J mice. J Craniofac Genet Dev Biol. 1990;10(4):353–61.
22. Smith RS, Roderick TH, Sundberg JP. Microphthalmia and associated abnormalities in inbred black mice. Lab Anim Sci. 1994;44(6):551–60.
23. Kohale K, Ingle A, Kelkar A, Parab P. Dense cataract and microphthalmia—new spontaneous mutation in BALB/c mice. Comp Med. 2004;54(3):275–9.
24. Park K, Seo JH. Study on the ophthalmic diseases in ICR mice and BALB/c mice. Exp Anim. 2006;55(2):83–90.
25. Bakthavachalu B, Kalanke S, Galande S, et al. Dense cataract and microphthalmia (dcm) in BALB/c mice is caused by mutations in the GJA8 locus. J Genet. 2010;89(2):147–54.
26. Losco PE, Troup CM. Corneal dystrophy in Fischer 344 rats. Lab Anim Sci. 1988;38(6):702–10.
27. Bruner RH, Keller WF, Stitzel KA, et al. Spontaneous corneal dystrophy and generalized basement membrane changes in Fischer-344 rats. Toxicol Pathol. 1992;20:357–66. https://doi.org/10.1177/019262339202000306.
28. Okano T, Uga S, Ishikawa S, Shumiya S. Histopathological study of hereditary cataractous lenses in SCR strain rat. Exp Eye Res. 1993;57(5):567–76. https://doi.org/10.1006/exer.1993.1161.
29. Komich RJ. Anophthalmos: an inherited trait in a new stock of guinea pigs. Am J Vet Res. 1971;32(12):2099–105.
30. Wander AH, Bubel HC, McDowell SG. The pathogenesis of herpetic ocular disease in the guinea pig. Arch Virol. 1987;95(3-4):197–209. https://doi.org/10.1007/BF01310780.
31. Williams D, Sullivan A. Ocular disease in the guinea pig (cavia porcellus): a survey of 1000 animals. Vet Ophthalmol. 2010;13(Suppl 1):54–62. https://doi.org/10.1111/j.1463-5224.2010.00812.x.
32. Otto G, Lipman NS, Murphy JC. Corneal dermoid in a hairless guinea pig. Lab Anim Sci. 1991;41(2):171–2.
33. Wappler O, Allgoewer I, Schaeffer EH. Conjunctival dermoid in two guinea pigs: a case report. Vet Ophthalmol. 2002;5(3):245–8. https://doi.org/10.1046/j.1463-5224.2002.00242.x.
34. Bettelheim FA, Churchill AC, Zigler JS. On the nature of hereditary cataract in strain 13/N guinea pigs. Curr Eye Res. 1997;16(9):917–24. https://doi.org/10.1076/ceyr.16.9.917.5047.
35. Lu F, Zhou X, Jiang L, et al. Axial myopia induced by hyperopic defocus in guinea pigs: a detailed assessment on susceptibility and recovery. Exp Eye Res. 2009;89(1):101–8. https://doi.org/10.1016/j.exer.2009.02.019.
36. Brooks DE, McCracken MD, Collins BR. Heterotopic bone formation in the ciliary body of an aged guinea pig. Lab Anim Sci. 1990;40(1):88–90.
37. Griffith JW, Lang CM. Vitamin E and selenium status of guinea pigs with myocardial necrosis. Lab Anim Sci. 1987;37:776–9.

38. Schaffer EH, Pfleghaar S. Secondary open angle glaucoma from osseous choristoma of the ciliary body in guinea pigs. Tierarztl Prax. 1995;23(4):410–4.
39. Racine J, Behn D, Simard E, Lachapelle P. Spontaneous occurrence of a potentially night blinding disorder in guinea pigs. Doc Ophthalmol. 2003;107:59–69. https://doi.org/10.1023/A:1024435911882.
40. Ninomiya H, Inomata T. Microvasculature of the mouse eye: scanning electron microscopy of vascular corrosion casts. J Exp Anim Sci. 2006;43(3):149–59. https://doi.org/10.1016/j.jeas.2006.05.002.
41. Schiavo DM. Multifocal retinal dysplasia in the Syrian hamster LAK:LVG (SYR). J Environ Pathol Toxicol. 1980;3(5-6):569–76.
42. Asher JH, James SC. The primary ultrastructural defect caused by anophthalmic white (Wh) in the Syrian hamster. Proc Natl Acad Sci U S A. 1982;79(14):4371–5.
43. Atkinson M. Suspected keratitis sicca in a Syrian hamster. Vet Rec. 2000;146(23):680.
44. Rajaei SM, Sadjadi R, Sabzevari A, Ghaffari MS. Results of phenol red thread test in clinically normal Syrian hamsters (Mesocricetus auratus). Vet Ophthalmol. 2013;16(6):436–9. https://doi.org/10.1111/vop.12024.
45. Hausler HR, Sibay TM, Stachowska B. Observations of retinal microaneurysms in a metahypophyseal diabetic Chinese hamster. Am J Ophthalmol. 1963;56(2):242–4. https://doi.org/10.1016/0002-9394(63)91857-9.
46. Holve DL, Mundwiler KE, Pritt SL. Incidence of spontaneous ocular lesions in laboratory rabbits. Comp Med. 2011;61(5):436–40.
47. Jeong MB, Kim NR, Yi NY, et al. N Z White Rabbits. 2005;54:395–402.
48. Munger RJ, Langevin N, Podval J. Spontaneous cataracts in laboratory rabbits. Vet Ophthalmol. 2002;5(3):177–81. https://doi.org/10.1046/j.1463-5224.2002.00245.x.
49. Peng X, Roshwalb S, Cooper TK, Zimmerman H, Christensen ND. High incidence of spontaneous cataracts in aging laboratory rabbits of an inbred strain. Vet Ophthalmol. 2015;18(3):186–90. https://doi.org/10.1111/vop.12203.
50. Morishima H, Nonoyama T, Sasaki S, Miyajima H. Spontaneous lesions in beagle dogs used in toxicity studies. Jikken Dobutsu. 1990;39(2):239–48.
51. Barnes J, Cotton P, Robinson S, Jacobsen M. Spontaneous pathology and routine clinical pathology parameters in aging beagle dogs: a comparison with adolescent and young adults. Vet Pathol. 2016;53(2):447–55. https://doi.org/10.1177/0300985815610390.
52. Hottendorf GH, Hirth RS. Lesions of spontaneous subclinical disease in beagle dogs. Vet Pathol. 1974;11(3):240–58. https://doi.org/10.1177/030098587401100306.
53. Loget O. Spontaneous ocular findings and esthesiometry/tonometry measurement in the Göttingen minipig (conventional and microbiologically defined). In: Weisse I, Hockwin O, Green K, Tripathi R, editors. Ocular toxicology. Boston: Springer; 1994. p. 351–402.
54. McInnes EF, McKeag S. A brief review of infrequent spontaneous findings, peculiar anatomical microscopic features, and potential artifacts in Göttingen minipigs. Toxicol Pathol. 2016;44(3):338–45. https://doi.org/10.1177/0192623315622423.
55. McInnes EF. Minipigs. In: Background lesions in laboratory animals. Edinburgh: Elsevier; 2011. p. 81–5. https://doi.org/10.1016/B978-0-7020-3519-7.00006-1.
56. Helke KL, Nelson KN, Sargeant AM, et al. Background pathological changes in minipigs. Toxicol Pathol. 2016;44(3):325–37. https://doi.org/10.1177/0192623315611762.
57. Jeppesen G, Skydsgaard M. Spontaneous background pathology in Göttingen minipigs. Toxicol Pathol. 2015;43(2):257–66. https://doi.org/10.1177/0192623314538344.
58. Saint-Macary G, Berthoux C. Ophthalmologic observations in the young Yucatan micropig. Lab Anim Sci. 1994;44(4):334–7.
59. Ito T, Chatani F, Sasaki S, Ando T, Miyajima H. Spontaneous lesions in cynomolgus monkeys used in toxicity studies. Jikken Dobutsu. 1992;41(4):455–69.
60. Drevon-Gaillot E, Perron-Lepage MF, Clément C, Burnett R. A review of background findings in cynomolgus monkeys (Macaca fascicularis) from three different geographical origins. Exp Toxicol Pathol. 2006;58(2-3):77–88. https://doi.org/10.1016/j.etp.2006.07.003.

61. Chamanza R, Marxfeld HA, Blanco AI, Naylor SW, Bradley AE. Incidences and range of spontaneous findings in control cynomolgus monkeys (Macaca fascicularis) used in toxicity studies. Toxicol Pathol. 2010;38(4):642–57. https://doi.org/10.1177/0192623310368981.
62. Sato J, Doi T, Kanno T, Wako Y, Tsuchitani M, Narama I. Histopathology of incidental findings in cynomolgus monkeys (Macaca fascicularis) used in toxicity studies. J Toxicol Pathol. 2012;25(1):63–101. https://doi.org/10.1293/tox.25.63.

Chapter 5
Standardized Scoring of Ocular Findings in the Context of Drug and Device Development Programs

J. Seth Eaton, Paul E. Miller, Ellison Bentley, Sara M. Thomasy, and Christopher J. Murphy

Abstract This chapter presents a comprehensive review of the approaches and methods used to perform clinical ocular scoring of the anterior and posterior segment in laboratory animals in toxicologic and preclinical drug development studies. It represents a distillation and integration of two recent publications from our group with expanded commentary (Eaton et al., J Ocul Pharmacol Ther 33:707–717, 2017; 718–734). The reader is introduced to the indications and features of the most commonly used semi-quantitative scoring systems in laboratory studies, as well as important limitations and considerations for each. The reader is also introduced to the ocular scoring systems employed by the clinical team at Ocular Services On Demand (OSOD), which modify many criteria from previous systems and introduce novel scoring elements to improve the applicability and predictive value of clinical observations made in

---

Endorsed by the American College of Veterinary Ophthalmologists (ACVO).

J. S. Eaton (✉) · S. M. Thomasy
Ocular Services on Demand (OSOD), LLC, Madison, WI, USA

Department of Surgical and Radiological Sciences, School of Veterinary Medicine, University of California - Davis, Davis, CA, USA
e-mail: seaton@ocularservices.com

P. E. Miller · E. Bentley
Ocular Services on Demand (OSOD), LLC, Madison, WI, USA

Department of Surgical Sciences, School of Veterinary Medicine, University of Wisconsin – Madison, Madison, WI, USA

C. J. Murphy (✉)
Department of Surgical and Radiological Sciences, School of Veterinary Medicine, University of California - Davis, Davis, CA, USA

Department of Ophthalmology and Vision Science, School of Medicine, University of California - Davis, Sacramento, CA, USA

Ocular Services on Demand (OSOD), LLC, Madison, WI, USA
e-mail: cjmurphy@ucdavis.edu

B. C. Gilger et al. (eds.), *Standards for Ocular Toxicology and Inflammation*, https://doi.org/10.1007/978-3-319-78364-2_5

support of modern preclinical ocular drug and device development programs. Species considerations pertinent to ocular examination and clinical scoring in general toxicology and ocular drug/device development are also discussed.

Keywords Slit lamp · Scoring · Semi-quantitative · Toxicology · Preclinical

Introduction and Background

Slit lamp biomicroscopy and ophthalmoscopic examination are integral components of complete clinical evaluation of the eye in humans and animals. Performed in tandem, these techniques permit the trained clinician to (1) assess all ocular structures and clear ocular media in the anterior and posterior segment of the eye, (2) accurately identify and localize opacities in the optical pathway, (3) characterize ocular inflammation and other structural lesions, and (4) characterize the appearance and spatial location of test articles or implanted devices in preclinical toxicologic studies. Interpretation of biomicroscopic and ophthalmoscopic findings provides the foundation for clinical characterization of ocular disease and formulation of clinical diagnoses. In ocular toxicology, accurate interpretation of clinical ophthalmic observations requires the examiner to have a comprehensive knowledge of the diagnostic instrumentation used as well as detailed ocular information regarding the species/strain of laboratory animal being examined. The residency-trained veterinary ophthalmologist can serve as a key expert in clinical comparative ophthalmology and welfare assurance of laboratory animals used in in vivo preclinical ocular drug and device development studies, as well as assessment of "off-target" ocular adverse events (e.g., ocular findings arising in the context of a development program for a systemically administered agent). Knowledge required for expert assessment of ocular findings includes but is not limited to (1) the functional ocular morphology and normal variations of the species/strain of laboratory animal being evaluated; (2) species differences in ocular responses to anesthetic events, invasive procedures, and (in some cases) classes of drugs; and (3) anticipated background lesions of the species/strain of laboratory animal being examined.

When performing ophthalmic examinations in the preclinical setting, it is critical that the examiner employs a defined ocular scoring system to record their observations. Like those used in other medical and surgical fields, ocular scoring systems provide semi-quantitative criteria to assist diagnosis, determine prognosis, assess response to treatment, and guide clinical decision-making. In ocular toxicology and preclinical drug/device safety evaluation, these systems offer similar advantages. Sequential scorings specify the structures affected, define severity and changes over time of adverse events, allow accurate comparison between study groups, assist in dose optimization, and help to identify findings that may adversely impact the welfare of laboratory animals. In the identification and advancement of lead investigational drugs or devices into agency-regulated clinical trials, sound semi-quantitative preclinical data are also critical in ensuring the safety of the human patients or other target species enrolled in those studies. N.B.: When multiple examiners are engaged sequentially in a single study/program, it is imperative that the examiners be harmonized in the use of any particular scoring system.

When interpreting the results obtained using any ocular scoring system, the veterinary ophthalmologist must be aware of the features, advantages, and inherent limitations of the system utilized. It should be noted that the great majority of scoring systems were developed for application to a specific species and, in some cases, strain of laboratory animal. As a result, applying a scoring system to a species/strain for purposes other than that for which it was originally developed can complicate interpretation of the data obtained and diminish its utility [3]. Furthermore, a published system's criteria may be skewed or oriented to meet study-specific objectives or even to specific institutional biases, which can complicate applicability when used in other studies or programs [4]. Many ocular scoring systems have been published, describing a variety of criteria for clinical ocular scoring in human patients and animals. OSOD recently published a comparative review of 138 published slit lamp-based systems for scoring of anterior segment observations, identifying noteworthy limitations to each, including those used commonly in the context of preclinical and toxicologic research [1]. Currently, no single system published for the scoring of ocular findings in animals provides a full complement of criteria required to accurately evaluate the full range of laboratory strains and species. Therefore, use of modified or combined scoring systems is commonly practiced. Furthermore, the great majority of these systems lack standardized slit lamp settings; and many of the published schemes lack scoring criteria applicable to studies investigating the test materials or routes of intraocular administration very commonly evaluated in modern preclinical drug development.

The chapter herein summarizes the features of the most commonly employed scoring systems for clinical evaluation of the eye (both the anterior and posterior segments) in laboratory species. Particular emphasis is placed upon the respective ocular structures and parameters assessed by these systems and the limitations that clinicians should be mindful of when applying their scoring criteria to different laboratory species. The reader will also be introduced to the Semi-quantitative Preclinical Ocular Toxicology Scoring (SPOTS) systems used by the veterinary ophthalmologists at Ocular Services On Demand (OSOD) which modify many criteria of previously published systems [2]. These systems introduce novel scoring criteria to improve applicability and predictive value over a wider range of laboratory strains and species and for the investigational methods used in modern preclinical ocular drug and device development.

Scoring of the Anterior Segment

In toxicologic and preclinical drug development studies, routine scoring of the anterior segment should comprise slit lamp evaluation of the following structures: the conjunctival membranes, the cornea, the anterior chamber and aqueous humor, the

Table 5.1 Anterior segment structures and parameters commonly scored by published slit lamp-based systems in toxicologic and preclinical studies involving laboratory species

Structure	Parameter scored
Conjunctiva	Hyperemia (congestion, injection)
	Swelling (chemosis)
	Discharge
Cornea	Opacity
	Fluorescein staining (fluorescein stain retention)
	Vascularization (neovascularization, pannus)
Aqueous humor/anterior chamber	Aqueous/anterior chamber flare
	Aqueous/anterior chamber cell
Iris	Congestion (hyperemia, involvement)
Lens	Opacity (cataract)

Synonymous terminology is presented in parentheses

iris, and the lens. The parameters scored by published slit lamp-based ocular scoring systems commonly used in preclinical studies are presented in Table 5.1. While not commonly scored by published slit lamp-based systems, the anterior vitreous can also be evaluated and scored for inflammatory cells or opacities, and notations can be made (depending on spatial location and extent) as to test article size, appearance, density, and distribution. Drug-related adverse effects involving the periocular and orbital structures, eyelids, nictitating membrane, and nasolacrimal puncta should be identified and recorded, though observations involving these structures are typically descriptive and not assigned semi-quantitative scores unless dictated by a modified or novel study-specific system (see *Scoring System Modifications*).

In studies conducted using laboratory species, slit lamp biomicroscopic evaluation of the anterior segment (including the anterior vitreous) can be performed using either table-mounted or handheld instruments. While table-mounted slit lamps may offer comparatively superior optics, handheld instruments (e.g., Kowa™ SL Series, Keeler™ Classic PSL Portable Slit Lamp, Reichert™ PSL Portable Slit Lamp, Haag-Streit™ 904 Portable Slit Lamp, Zeiss™ HSO-10) offer ergonomic advantages for the efficient evaluation of the full range of laboratory species [5].

The Standardization of Uveitis Nomenclature (SUN) System

The Standardization of Uveitis Nomenclature (SUN) System Working Group published the SUN system in 2005 to provide consensus methods and scoring schemes for the classification and reporting of clinical data in human patients with naturally occurring uveitis [6]. While other groups have published scoring and classification schemes for similar purposes [7, 8], the SUN system remains widely used. SUN's scoring criteria for aqueous or anterior chamber (AC) cells and flare are also very commonly used in preclinical studies involving laboratory animals [5, 9]. This adaptation is likely due to the lack of a scoring scheme for aqueous cells in historically popular scoring systems designed for laboratory species (Table 5.2).

Table 5.2 Comparison of semi-quantitative parameters and species assessed by common slit lamp-based scoring systems in toxicology and drug development (✓ indicates that the above system contains scoring criteria for the corresponding parameter at the left)

	McDonald-Shadduck	Hackett-McDonald	Draize	Standardization of uveitis nomenclature (SUN)
Conjunctival congestion	✓	✓	✓	
Conjunctival swelling	✓	✓	✓	
Conjunctival discharge	✓	✓	✓	
Corneal opacity (severity)	✓	✓	✓	
Corneal opacity (area)	✓	✓	✓	
Fluorescein stain (severity)	✓	✓		
Fluorescein stain (area)	✓	✓		
Pannus (corneal vascularization)	✓	✓		
Aqueous (anterior chamber) flare	✓	✓		✓
Aqueous (anterior chamber) cell				✓
PLR (pupillary light reflex)		✓		
Iris involvement/iritis	✓	✓	✓	
Lens		✓		
Vitreous cells				
Original species described	Albino rabbit	Albino rabbit	Albino rabbit	Human patient

The SUN's scheme for scoring of AC cells and flare specifies that the examiner assess the anterior segment using a slit beam measuring 1 mm height × 1 mm width. Semi-quantitative criteria (Table 5.3) are then used to assign a score based on the cell density or flare characteristics observed within that beam as it illuminates the anterior chamber which, in the human eye, equates to an optical section volume of approximately 3.5 mm^3 [10]. Despite its straightforward methodology, however, there are inherent challenges associated with adoption and use of the SUN system in laboratory species.

Precise recreation of SUN's beam dimensions using a handheld slit lamp is problematic and limits the applicability of SUN's specified technique. A 1 mm-diameter *circular* beam has recently become available on the Kowa™ SL-17, but we note that a 1 mm circular beam geometry samples a different aqueous volume than the 1 × 1 mm square specified by SUN (see inset). This is very relevant as all cell scoring systems are based on estimating the *total number* of cells present in the entire volume of the beam traversing the anterior chamber.

Table 5.3 Scoring schemes for aqueous (anterior chamber) cells and flare according to the standardization of uveitis nomenclature (SUN) system

Scheme for anterior chamber cells	
Grade (score)	Cells in field (field size is a 1 mm × 1 mm slit beam)
0	<1
0.5+	1–5
1+	6–15
2+	16–25
3+	26–50
4+	>50
Scheme for anterior chamber flare	
Grade (score)	Description
0	None
1+	Faint
2+	Moderate (iris and lens details clear)
3+	Marked (iris and lens details hazy)
4+	Intense (fibrin or plastic aqueous)

Assuming an anterior chamber depth of 1.5 mm:
A 1 mm circular beam would sample a cylinder volume ($V = \pi r^2 h$) of 1.18 mm^3
A 1 mm square beam would sample a rectangular prism volume ($V = whl$) of 1.5 mm^2

In addition to technical challenges, the inherent geometric variations of the species being examined will also influence the use of SUN's scoring criteria [10] (see *Aqueous (Anterior Chamber) Cell* in *The SPOTS Scoring System – Anterior Segment*). It is also known that ocular inflammatory reactivity is highly species-dependent [11] and, in some laboratory species, may reach levels of severity that exceed SUN's criteria for human patients with naturally-occurring disease. When using the SUN system, the combined effect of having a profound cellular response and an increased volume of aqueous being sampled in animals with deep chambers can result in premature "topping out" of the maximum score assigned, and prevent identification of meaningful differences in response to a test article or device. This discrepancy is particularly relevant in the context of investigating biologic agents under development for the treatment of ocular disease and the immune-mediated inflammatory responses that may be elicited by their use in nonhuman species.

The McDonald-Shadduck and Hackett-McDonald Systems

While recognizing there is a lack of a designated "standard" system in preclinical studies, the systems of McDonald-Shadduck [12] and Hackett-McDonald [13] are perhaps the most widely used for scoring of slit lamp biomicroscopic findings in laboratory species [5, 9]. These two systems expanded upon the early ocular scoring systems reported by Friedenwald [14] and Draize [15] whose criteria were principally used to assess the ocular irritancy profiles of non-therapeutic substances (organic and inorganic) in albino rabbits. The McDonald-Shadduck and Hackett-McDonald systems' criteria, presented together in Table 5.4, provide scoring schemes for parameters essential for evaluation of ocular irritation of topical agents including conjunctival congestion, conjunctival swelling and discharge, and corneal opacification. Unlike the systems of Friedenwald and Draize, these systems also incorporate intraocular inflammatory parameters such as aqueous flare and iris congestion, expanding their applicability in safety and efficacy assessment of topical therapeutic drugs or devices. The Hackett-McDonald system also presents a qualitative scheme for description of lens opacities (Table 5.5). Furthermore, both systems were published in tandem with validation metrics for intra- and interobserver reproducibility.

Since the publication of these slit lamp-based systems, however, approaches to ocular drug delivery have expanded beyond topical administration. Currently, the landscape of ocular drug and device development comprises an expanding list of intraocular drug administration routes and implantable biomaterials and devices. Therefore, the application of previously published systems in modern preclinical efficacy and safety studies may be met with certain limitations. Current regulatory requirements dictate that, with few exceptions, preclinical evaluation of ocular drugs must be conducted in at least two nonhuman species, one of which must be pigmented, given the potential influence of melanin on drug pharmacokinetics and pharmacodynamics, distribution, and efficacy [10, 16–18]. Like most scoring systems published for the evaluation of laboratory species, however, the systems of McDonald-Shadduck and Hackett-McDonald describe scoring criteria that were specifically developed for application to the albino rabbit [1]. The morphologic features of the anterior segment in albino rabbits pertinent to clinical observation and scoring (e.g., lack of perilimbal and iridal pigmentation) differ from pigmented rabbit strains and from other laboratory species. Furthermore, the McDonald-Shadduck or Hackett-McDonald systems do not specify standard instrument settings for slit lamp examination. Use of non-standardized settings can heavily influence the reproducibility of scoring outcomes (both intra- and interobserver), particularly for aqueous and vitreous cells. As neither system incorporates a scoring scheme for aqueous cells (see Table 5.2), elements of the SUN system are often incorporated into scoring protocols for preclinical studies, despite its inherent limitations in preclinical studies using laboratory species (see *The Standardization of Uveitis Nomenclature (SUN) System above*).

Table 5.4 Complete anterior segment scoring criteria for the semi-quantitative preclinical ocular toxicology scoring (SPOTS) and original McDonald-Shadduck and Hackett-McDonald scoring systems

Observation/lesion	Score	SPOTS system scoring criteria	Original McDonald-Shadduck/ Hackett-McDonald criteria
Pupillary light reflex (PLR)	0	Normal, brisk pupillary reflex	Normal pupillary response
	1	Pupil is relatively dilated and/or dyscoric with a sluggish pupillary reflex	Sluggish pupillary response
	2	Pupil is fully dilated and/or dyscoric with no detectable pupillary reflex	Maximally impaired (i.e., fixed) pupillary response
	3	Miotic pupil. Pupillary light reflex is difficult to evaluate, due to the small pupil size	
Conjunctival hyperemia	0	Bulbar conjunctiva is normal in appearance for the species. Small, pale pink vessels may be observed, primarily at, or adjacent to, the limbus. In rabbits, small perilimbal vessels associated with the dorsal and ventral rectus muscles may be seen at 12 and 6 o'clock, respectively	Normal. May appear blanched to reddish pink without perilimbal injection (except at 12:00 and 6:00 o'clock positions) with vessels of the palpebral and bulbar conjunctiva easily observed
	1	Pink-to-red bulbar conjunctival vessels with minimal branching are visible extending 1–3 mm posteriorly from the limbus toward the conjunctival fornix. In rabbits, pink-to-red perilimbal vessels are visible primarily at the upper and lower aspects of the perilimbal region	A flushed, reddish color predominately confined to the palpebral conjunctiva with some perilimbal injection but primarily confined to the lower and upper parts of the eye from the 4:00 and 7:00 and 11:00 to 1: 00 o'clock positions
	2	Prominent red bulbar conjunctival vessels with multiple branches are visible extending from the limbus to the conjunctival fornix. In rabbits, prominent red perilimbal vessels are visible involving at least 75% of the circumference of the perilimbal region	Bright red color of the palpebral conjunctiva with accompanying perilimbal injection covering at least 75% of the circumference of the perilimbal region
	3	Red-to-dark red, engorged bulbar conjunctival vessels with extensive branching and/or tortuosity are visible extending from the limbus to the conjunctival fornix. The conjunctiva between large vessels may have a flushed pink-to-red appearance. In rabbits, red-to-dark red engorged perilimbal vessels are visible, with pink-to-red flushing of the adjacent bulbar conjunctiva. In any species, bulbar and/or palpebral conjunctival petechia may be present	Dark, beefy red color with congestion of both the bulbar and the palpebral conjunctiva along with pronounced perilimbal injection and the presence of petechiae on the conjunctiva. The petechiae generally predominate along the nictitating membrane and the upper palpebral conjunctiva

(continued)

Table 5.4 (continued)

Observation/lesion	Score	SPOTS system scoring criteria	Original McDonald-Shadduck/ Hackett-McDonald criteria
Conjunctival swelling	0	No abnormal swelling of the conjunctival tissue	Normal or no swelling of the conjunctival tissue
	1	Bulbar conjunctival swelling above normal is observed focally, most commonly in the perilimbal region with no eversion of the eyelid(s) or change in eyelid margin contour	Swelling above normal without eversion of the lids (can be easily ascertained by noting that the upper and lower eyelids are positioned as in the normal eye); swelling generally starts in the lower cul-de-sac near the inner canthus, which needs slit lamp examination
	2	Bulbar conjunctival swelling above normal is observed diffusely but with no eversion of the eyelid(s) or change in eyelid margin contour	Swelling with misalignment of the normal approximation of the lower and upper eyelids; primarily confined to the upper eyelid so that in the initial stages the misapproximation of the eyelids begins by partial eversion of the upper eyelid. In this stage, swelling is confined generally to the upper eyelid, although it exists in the lower cul-de-sac (observed best with the slit lamp)
	3	Bulbar and palpebral conjunctival swelling is observed, resulting in eyelid eversion and/or misalignment. The eyelid margin(s) may appear swollen and/or have an irregular, "undulating" contour but can still be closed completely	Swelling definite with partial eversion of the upper and lower eyelids essentially equivalent. This can be easily ascertained by looking at the animal head-on and noticing the positioning of the eyelids; if the eye margins do not meet, eversion has occurred
	4[a]	Bulbar and palpebral conjunctival swelling is severe, partially or completely obscuring examination of the rest of the ocular surface and globe. Eyelid closure is incomplete with exposed bulbar and/or palpebral conjunctiva protruding between the eyelid margins	Eversion of the upper eyelid is pronounced with less pronounced eversion of the lower eyelid. It is difficult to retract the lids and observe the perilimbal region
Conjunctival discharge	0	No abnormal discharge	Normal. No discharge
	1	Discharge is above normal and present on the surface of the eye or in the medial canthus but not on the lids or hairs of the eyelids	Discharge above normal and present on the inner portion of the eye but not on the lids or hairs of the eyelids. One can ignore the small amount that is in the inner and outer canthus if it has not been removed prior to starting the study
	2	Discharge is abundant, easily observed, and has accumulated on the lids and around the hairs of the eyelids	Discharge is abundant, easily observed, and has collected on the lids and around the hairs of the eyelids
	3	Discharge has been flowing over the eyelids so as to wet or accumulate on the hairs of the eyelids and the skin around the eyes, past the orbital rim	Discharge has been flowing over the eyelids so as to wet the hairs substantially on the skin around the eye

(continued)

Table 5.4 (continued)

Observation/lesion	Score	SPOTS system scoring criteria	Original McDonald-Shadduck/ Hackett-McDonald criteria
Corneal opacity (severity)[b,c]	0	Normal cornea. Appears with the slit lamp as having a bright gray line on the epithelial surface and a bright gray line on the endothelial surface with a marble-like gray appearance of the stroma	Normal cornea. Appears with the slit lamp as having a bright gray line on the epithelial surface and a bright gray line on the endothelial surface with a marble-like gray appearance of the stroma
	1	Minimal loss of corneal transparency. With diffuse illumination, the underlying anterior segment structures are clearly visible, although corneal opacity is apparent to an experienced observer	Some loss of transparency. Only the anterior half of the stroma is involved as observed with an optical section of the slit lamp. The underlying structures are clearly visible with diffuse illumination, although some cloudiness can be readily apparent with diffuse illumination
	2	Mild loss of corneal transparency. With diffuse illumination, the underlying anterior segment structures are visible, although there is a reduction in the ability to appreciate their detail	Moderate loss of transparency. In addition to involving the anterior stroma, the cloudiness extends all the way to the endothelium. The stroma has lost its marble-like appearance and is homogeneously white. With diffuse illumination, underlying structures are clearly visible
	3	Moderate loss of corneal transparency. With diffuse illumination, there is a greater inability to see the details of the underlying anterior segment structures than with a score of 2, but the observer is still able to grade flare, iris vessel congestion, observe for pupillary response, and note lenticular changes	Involvement of the entire thickness of the stroma. With optical section, the endothelial surface is still visible. However, with diffuse illumination the underlying structures are just barely visible (to the extent that the observer is still able to grade flare, iritis, observe for pupillary response, and note lenticular changes)
	4	Severe loss of corneal transparency. With diffuse illumination, the underlying anterior segment structures cannot be seen so that the evaluation of aqueous flare, iris vessel congestion, pupillary response, and lenticular changes is not possible	Involvement of the entire thickness of the stroma. With the optical section, cannot clearly visualize the endothelium. With diffuse illumination, the underlying structures cannot be seen. Cloudiness removes the capability for judging and grading aqueous flare, iritis, lenticular changes, and pupillary response
Corneal opacity (area)[c,d]	0	Normal cornea with no area of corneal opacity	Normal cornea with no area of cloudiness
	1	1–25% area of corneal opacity	1–25% area of corneal opacity
	2	26–50% area of corneal opacity	26–50% area of corneal opacity
	3	51–75% area of corneal opacity	51–75% area of corneal opacity
	4	76–100% area of corneal opacity	76–100% area of corneal opacity
Corneal vascularization	0	No corneal vascularization	No pannus
	1	Vascularization is present, but vessels have not penetrated beyond 2 mm axially	Vascularization is present, but vessels have not invaded the entire corneal circumference. Where localized vessel invasion has occurred, they have not penetrated beyond 2 mm
	2	Vascularization is present, and vessels have penetrated beyond 2 mm axially	Vessels have invaded 2 mm or more around the entire corneal circumference

(continued)

Table 5.4 (continued)

Observation/lesion	Score	SPOTS system scoring criteria	Original McDonald-Shadduck/ Hackett-McDonald criteria
Anterior chamber (aqueous) flare	0	No protein is visible in the anterior chamber when viewed by an experienced observer using slit lamp biomicroscopy; a small, bright, focal slit beam of white light; and high magnification	Absence of visible light beam light in the anterior chamber (no Tyndall effect)
	0.5	Trace amount of protein is detectable in the anterior chamber. This protein is only visible with careful scrutiny by an experienced observer using slit lamp biomicroscopy; a small, bright, focal slit beam of white light; and high magnification	
	1	Mild amount of protein is detectable in the anterior chamber. The presence of protein in the anterior chamber is immediately apparent to an experienced observer using slit lamp biomicroscopy and high magnification, but such protein is detected only with careful observation with the naked eye and a small, bright, focal slit beam of white light	The Tyndall effect is barely discernible. The intensity of the light beam in the anterior chamber is less than the intensity of the slit beam as it passes through the lens
	2	Moderate amount of protein is detectable in the anterior chamber. These grades are similar to grade 1, but the opacity would be readily visible to the naked eye of an observer using any source of a focused beam of white light. This is a continuum of moderate opacification, with grade 2 less apparent than grade 3	The Tyndall beam in the anterior chamber is easily discernible and is equal in intensity to the slit beam as it passes through the lens
	3	Moderate amount of protein is detectable in the anterior chamber. These grades are similar to grade 1, but the opacity would be readily visible to the naked eye of an observer using any source of a focused beam of white light. This is a continuum of moderate opacification, with grade 2 less apparent than grade 3	The Tyndall beam in the anterior chamber is easily discernible; its intensity is greater than the intensity of the slit beam as it passes through the lens
	4	Large (severe) amount of protein is detectable in the anterior chamber. Similar to grade 3, but the optical density of the protein approaches that of the lens behind it. Additionally, frank fibrin deposition is frequently seen in acute circumstances. It needs to be noted that because fibrin may persist for a period of time after partial or complete restoration of the blood-aqueous barrier, it is possible to have resorbing fibrin present with lower numeric assignations for flare (e.g., grade 1 flare with fibrin)	

(continued)

Table 5.4 (continued)

Observation/lesion	Score	SPOTS system scoring criteria	Original McDonald-Shadduck/ Hackett-McDonald criteria
Anterior chamber (aqueous) cells[e]	0	No cells in field	No scores for anterior chamber (aqueous) cells
	0.5	1–5 cells in field	
	1	6–25 cells in field	
	2	26–50 cells in field	
	3	51–100 cells in field	
	4	>100 cells in field	
Iris involvement[f]	0	Normal iris without any hyperemia of the iris vessels	Normal iris without any hyperemia of the iris vessels. Occasionally around the 12:00 to 1:00 o'clock position near the pupillary border and the 6:00 and 7:00 o'clock position near the pupillary border, there is a small area around 1–3 mm in diameter in which both the secondary and tertiary vessels are slightly hyperemic
	1	Minimal injection of secondary vessels but not tertiary	Minimal injection of secondary vessels but not tertiary. Generally, it is uniform but may be of greater intensity at the 1:00 or 6:00 o'clock position. If it is confined to the 1:00 or 6:00 o'clock position, the tertiary vessels must be substantially hyperemic
	2	Minimal injection of the tertiary vessels and minimal to moderate injection of the secondary vessels	Minimal injection of tertiary vessels and minimal to moderate injection of the secondary vessels
	3	Moderate injection of the secondary and tertiary vessels with a slight swelling of the iris stroma (this gives the iris surface a slightly rugose appearance)	Moderate injection of the secondary and tertiary vessels with slight swelling of the iris stroma (this gives the iris surface a slightly rugose appearance, which is usually most prominent near the 3:00 and 9:00 o'clock positions)
	4	Severe injection of the secondary and tertiary vessels with marked swelling of the iris stroma. The iris appears rugose and may be accompanied by hemorrhage in the iris or anterior chamber (hyphema)	Marked injection of the secondary and tertiary vessels with marked swelling of the iris stroma. The iris appears rugose and may be accompanied by hemorrhage (hyphema) in the anterior chamber
Anterior vitreous cells[e]	0	≤1 cell in field	No scores for anterior vitreous cells
	0.5	1–5 cells in field	
	1	6–25 cells in field	
	2	26–50 cells in field	
	3	51–100 cells in field	
	4	>100 cells in field	

(continued)

Table 5.4 (continued)

Observation/lesion	Score	SPOTS system scoring criteria	Original McDonald-Shadduck/ Hackett-McDonald criteria
Fluorescein staining (severity)[c,g]	0	Absence of fluorescein staining	Absence of fluorescein staining
	1	Slight multifocal punctate fluorescein staining	Slight fluorescein staining confined to a small focus. With diffuse illumination the underlying structures are easily visible. (The outline of the pupillary margin is as if there was no fluorescein staining)
	2	Distinct multifocal to coalescent punctate fluorescein staining	Moderate fluorescein staining confined to a small focus. With diffuse illumination the underlying structures are clearly visible, although there is some loss of detail
	3	Frank fluorescein staining associated with focal or multifocal epithelial loss, but no stromal loss	Marked fluorescein staining. Staining may involve a larger portion of the cornea. With diffuse illumination underlying structures are barely visible but are not completely obliterated
	4	Frank fluorescein staining associated with focal or multifocal epithelial and stromal loss	Extreme fluorescein staining. With diffuse illumination the underlying structures cannot be observed
Fluorescein staining (area)[c,h]	0	No area of fluorescein staining	No area of fluorescein staining
	1	1–25% area of fluorescein staining	1–25% area of fluorescein staining
	2	26–50% area of fluorescein staining	26–50% area of fluorescein staining
	3	51–75% area of fluorescein staining	51–75% area of fluorescein staining
	4	76 to 100% area of fluorescein staining	76–100% area of fluorescein staining

Footnotes for the SPOTS scoring system:

[a]Conjunctival swelling scored as "4" may present with varying degrees of severity, primarily depending on the degree of conjunctival exposure

[b]If multiple areas of opacity with varying scores are observed in an eye, the assigned score should correspond to the most severely affected area

[c]Using either the SPOTS or McDonald-Shadduck/Hackett-McDonald system, two scores (severity and area) are assigned for corneal opacity and fluorescein staining

[d]If multiple corneal opacities are observed in an eye, diagramming of the lesions' characteristics is recommended in lieu of a corneal opacity (area) score

[e]All aqueous (AC) and anterior vitreous cell scores should be accompanied by one of the following notations for cell color: predominantly (~75%) white, mixed color (~50% white, 50% brown and/or red), predominantly (~75%) brown, or predominantly (~75%) red

[f]In pigmented strains/species, visibility of secondary and tertiary iridal vessels may be obscured

[g]If multiple fluorescein stain severity scores are observed in an eye, the assigned score should correspond to the most severely affected area

[h]If multiple fluorescein staining lesions are observed in an eye, diagramming of staining distribution is recommended in lieu of a fluorescein staining (area) score

Table 5.5 Criteria for description of lens opacity (cataract) using the Hackett-McDonald and semi-quantitative preclinical ocular toxicology scoring (SPOTS) systems

Lens opacity[a]
The lens should be evaluated routinely during ocular evaluations and graded as 0 (normal) or 1 (abnormal). The presence of lenticular opacities should be described and the location noted as defined below
The crystalline lens is readily observed with the aid of the slit lamp biomicroscope, and the location of lenticular opacity can readily be discerned by direct and retroillumination. The location of lenticular opacities can be arbitrarily divided into the following lenticular regions beginning with the anterior capsule:
·Anterior capsule ·Anterior subcapsular ·Anterior cortical ·Nuclear ·Equatorial cortical ·Posterior cortical ·Posterior subcapsular ·Posterior capsule
• *Punctate*: A focal or multifocal, discrete, dot-like lens opacity that is visible only to a trained observer with a SL-15 or SL-17 slit lamp biomicroscope (or equivalent) at 10× to 16× magnification
• *Incipient*: A focal lens opacity that is visible upon gross inspection of the eye with an indirect ophthalmoscope or other focal light source and retroillumination. The view of the fundus is minimally impaired by the opacity. Upon slit lamp biomicroscopy, the opacity can be localized to a specific region of the lens, and other regions of the lens appear normal
• *Incomplete*: A diffuse lens opacity visible upon gross inspection of the eye with an indirect ophthalmoscope or other focal light source and retroillumination. The view of the fundus is significantly impaired, but a red reflex can still be obtained. Upon slit lamp biomicroscopy, the opacity involves multiple regions of the lens
• *Complete*: A diffuse lens opacity visible upon gross inspection of the eye with an indirect ophthalmoscope or other focal light source. The fundus cannot be seen, and a red reflex cannot be elicited. Upon slit lamp biomicroscopy, the entire lens is opaque
• *Resorbing*: A diffuse lens opacity visible upon gross inspection of the eye with an indirect ophthalmoscope or other focal light source. The fundus may or may not be visible, and a red reflex may or may not be elicited. The lens capsule may be wrinkled, and the lens itself is dehydrated and flattened or liquid and soft in appearance. Upon slit lamp biomicroscopy, the entire lens is involved in the opacity

[a]Diagramming of lens opacities is recommended using the SPOTS system to facilitate localization and longitudinal monitoring

The Semi-quantitative Preclinical Ocular Toxicology Scoring (SPOTS) System: Anterior Segment

The recently published SPOTS system [2] developed by Ocular Services On Demand (OSOD) evolved from the iterative collaborative engagement of the group's board-certified veterinary ophthalmologists over the execution of hundreds of preclinical drug safety evaluations and general and ocular toxicology studies; these studies involved myriad test articles and novel material platforms, administered via a comprehensive list of routes and drug delivery systems, in all relevant laboratory species. Its semi-quantitative criteria for the anterior segment expand upon those described by McDonald-Shadduck and Hackett-McDonald and introduce novel scoring schemes for AC and vitreous cells. These elements, presented alongside those of the McDonald-Shadduck and Hackett-McDonald Systems in Table 5.4, address many of the limitations of previously published systems, expanding slit lamp-based scoring criteria to improve applicability to the full range of species and strains used and to drug delivery approaches investigated in modern ocular drug development studies. Furthermore, the SPOTS system specifies standard slit lamp settings that can be applied to both table-mounted and handheld instruments.

Scoring of the anterior segment is performed using a Kowa™ SL-15 or SL-17 handheld slit lamp (or equivalent). Examinations are performed using high beam illumination (as tolerated by the animal) and magnification that permits optimized viewing of aqueous or anterior vitreous cells (10× or 16×, depending on the species being examined). Initially, diffuse illumination is used to evaluate the pupillary light reflex (PLR) and to survey the adnexa and ocular surface. Thereafter, a slit beam with a width of 0.2 mm and height of 12 mm is used to illuminate the anterior structures and clear anterior media (aqueous humor, lens, and anterior vitreous). In addition, the beam should be consistently set to an angle of 30–45° to the eye's vertical axial (90°) meridian. The examiner should remember, though, that he or she will not see the full beam height at maximal magnification, unless the species being examined has a vertical corneal diameter (VCD) ≥12 mm. In species with smaller limbal diameters, the effective beam height is decreased accordingly.

Pupillary Light Reflex (PLR)

Evaluation of the pupillary light reflex (PLR) is an important parameter in ocular toxicology. After topical or intraocular administration of a drug or test material, abnormalities in the briskness and/or completeness of the PLR may indicate adverse effects on efferent pupillary function (neurological or structural) or afferent input from the retina or optic nerve. McDonald-Shadduck (M-S) and Hackett-McDonald (H-M) score PLR as a normal reflex ("0") to maximal impairment "2," with an intermediate score ("1") indicating a sluggish PLR. The SPOTS system utilizes similar criteria but also includes dyscoria as a possible accompanying finding, as post-inflammatory structural iridal changes (e.g., synechiae) are commonly observed in toxicologic studies and lead to the impairment of the PLR. Additionally, the SPOTS system incorporates a third score ("3") to designate pupillary miosis, commonly observed with anterior segment inflammation or in association with administration of certain drugs (e.g., topical prostaglandin analogs in dogs [19–21]), complicating evaluation of the PLR.

Conjunctiva

Conjunctival hyperemia, swelling (chemosis), and discharge are critical parameters in the preclinical evaluation of the irritancy potential of topically applied ophthalmic drugs and formulations, ocular surface devices (e.g., contact lenses), and subconjunctival drug formulations or implants. Conjunctival hyperemia may also develop secondary to anterior segment inflammation associated with intraocular drug and device administration. Early ocular scoring systems described for laboratory species like the Draize system [15] provided a tool for rational assessment of conjunctival manifestations of inflammation in the albino rabbit. The criteria of this system and similar ones, however, were largely developed to accommodate toxicity evaluation of non-pharmaceutical compounds [22]. The systems of M-S and H-M improved upon earlier ones, enhancing applicability in preclinical drug evaluation, but similarly their systems were also developed specifically for documenting findings in albino rabbits. The spatial distribution of the conjunctival vasculature of the rabbit has a characteristic perilimbal anatomical distribution, and the clinical manifestations of conjunctival irritation or inflammation are not necessarily shared by other species like the dog or NHP. To extend the applicability of conjunctival hyperemia scoring to multiple species, the SPOTS scoring system provides criteria for both rabbits and non-rabbit species (Fig. 5.1). In addition, scoring criteria for conjunctival swelling have been refined to more closely assimilate the features of reactive chemosis more commonly observed in modern ocular drug development. Scoring criteria for conjunctival discharge remain largely similar to those of M-S and H-M.

Corneal Opacity and Fluorescein Staining

The original systems of M-S and H-M specified a "two-score" format for corneal opacity and fluorescein staining with the first score indicating lesion severity and the second score indicating the area of the cornea affected. However, the original

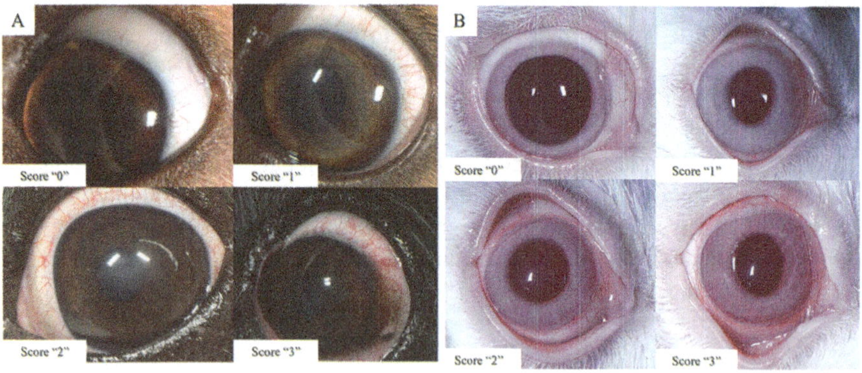

Fig. 5.1 (**a** and **b**). Photographic exemplars demonstrating conjunctival hyperemia scoring criteria using the SPOTS system in (**a**) a non-rabbit species (canine images presented) and (**b**) rabbits (albino strain images presented). Note the more radial distribution of hyperemic conjunctival vessels with extension toward the conjunctival fornix in the canine images and the primarily perilimbal distribution of hyperemic conjunctival vessels in the rabbit images. Figure reprinted with permissions from Eaton, J. S., et al. The SPOTS system:An ocular scoring system optimized for use in modern preclinical drug development and toxicology. *J Ocul Pharm Ther* **33**, 718–34 (2017)

scoring criteria for corneal opacity severity described ascending semi-quantitative scores corresponding to both increasing loss of transparency and anterior to posterior (A-P) lesion distribution. This can prove problematic when conducting sequential scoring within a drug/device development program since the specific attributes that are combined to arrive at a single integrated score may not be observed as described and hinder the examiner's ability to identify and assign a single score; and this also introduces the possibility at arriving at the same score but with different distinct attributes. Furthermore, while the attributes of A-P distribution used in scoring corneal opacity may be easily applied in the evaluation of topically applied substance or drugs, their characteristics may not correlate with the range of ocular responses and opacifying corneal lesions observed following intraocular injections or via other modern routes of drug administration. The SPOTS scheme for scoring the severity of corneal opacity uses semi-quantitative scores solely accounting for opacity density, namely, loss of corneal transparency and obscuration of underlying anterior segment structures. This facilitates longitudinal monitoring both within and between observers in a given study.

Similarly, McDonald-Shadduck and Hackett-McDonald scoring criteria for fluorescein staining severity incorporated elements of both intensity of staining as well as distribution. As for corneal opacity severity, the SPOTS system has refined these criteria, incorporating severity descriptions that more accurately reflect retention patterns observed with increasing severity of corneal surface disease or ulceration, and provides a clearer distinction between minor clinical corneal epithelial toxicity (Fig. 5.2) from more severe forms.

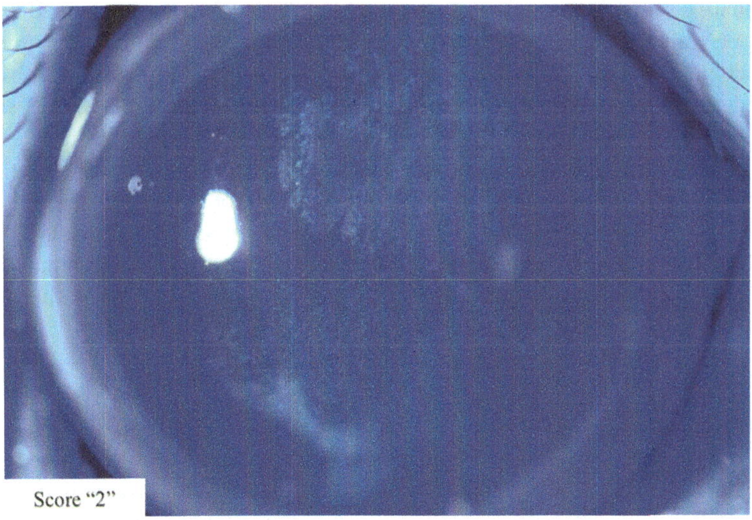

Fig. 5.2 Photographic exemplar demonstrating criteria characteristic of a score "2" for fluorescein staining severity using the SPOTS system (nonhuman primate image presented). Figure reprinted with permissions from Eaton, J. S., et al. The SPOTS system: An ocular scoring system optimized for use in modern preclinical drug development and toxicology. *J Ocul Pharm Ther* **33**, 718–34 (2017)

The SPOTS system also advocates the use of diagrams to describe and capture important features of corneal opacities (e.g., location, stromal distribution) and other aspects of anterior segment lesions that are not easily numerically scored but which provide valuable information in drug and device development programs. Furthermore, diagrammatic documentation of lesions improves accurate capture of longitudinal findings for a single observer and improves correspondence between sequential observers which may be necessary in longer or more complex preclinical investigations. Use of a standard or modified lesion color-coding scheme as previously published [23] can also improve the sequential documentation of both background and important ocular findings (Fig. 5.3a).

The SPOTS system also specifies that the assigned severity score for corneal opacity or fluorescein staining in an eye with lesions of varying severity should correspond to the most severely affected area (e.g., the highest score observed across the cornea). Furthermore, an accompanying diagram should be made to accurately record the appearances and distribution of those lesions. Scoring schemes for designating lesion area (size) are the same as those described by M-S and H-M.

Corneal Vascularization

Corneal vascularization (synonymous with "corneal neovascularization" or "pannus") can be a useful indicator of ocular inflammation, particularly ocular surface inflammation in eyes treated with topical agents or topical applied or implanted devices. The systems of M-S and H-M use criteria that define a single semi-quantitative score that integrates both vessel length and distribution around the cornea. As with scoring of corneal opacity and fluorescein staining, however, the distinct attributes used to arrive at a single score may not be consistently observed in tandem across sequential evaluations. To minimize ambiguity, the SPOTS system scores corneal vascularization only on the basis of vessel length. Lesion diagramming is also recommended to provide qualitative features of corneal vascularization. The veterinary ophthalmologist must also take note that in many preclinical scoring systems, "corneal vascularization" is synonymous with "pannus," though the clinical definition in human patients is non-specific [29], unlike its typical use in veterinary ophthalmology to denote a specific immune-mediated infiltrative disease described in dogs [30].

Aqueous (Anterior Chamber) Flare

Aqueous flare is indicative of blood-aqueous barrier (BAB) breakdown and therefore a hallmark attribute of anterior segment inflammation [31]. Aqueous flare lends itself well to semi-quantitative scoring, as higher degrees of aqueous flare generally correlate with greater degrees of anterior segment inflammation. Depending on the scoring system, however, the criteria that distinguish aqueous flare severity may be described differently. The systems of M-S and H-M designate 4 scores for aqueous

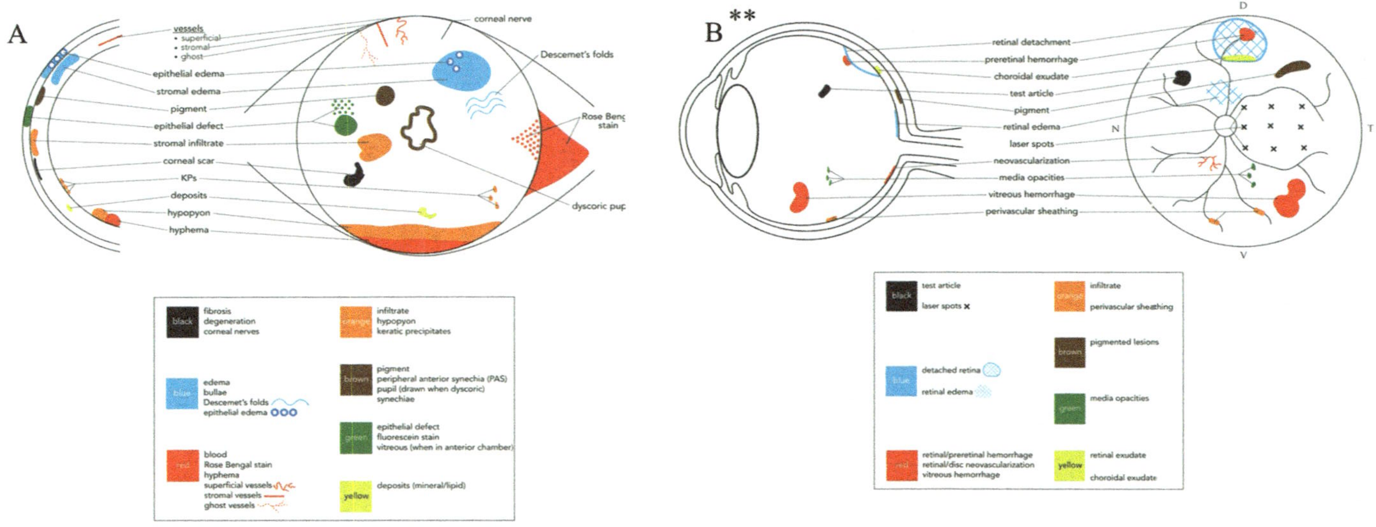

Fig. 5.3 (**a** and **b**). Examples of diagrams modified from standardized color-coding systems [23, 24] for illustrating lesions involving (**a**) the anterior segment and (**b**) the posterior segment. Figures reprinted with permissions from Eaton, J. S., et al. The SPOTS system: An ocular scoring system optimized for use in modern preclinical drug development and toxicology. *J Ocul Pharm Ther* **33**, 718–34 (2017). **The en face diagram presents lesions in the context of anatomical features of the nonhuman primate (NHP) fundus (e.g., holangiotic retinal vascular pattern and macula). Lesions depicted comprise those typically observed in preclinical studies involving the posterior segment, including the grid of macular/perimacular laser-induced lesions observed in animal models of choroidal neovascularization [25–28]. Diagrammatic features may vary depending on the anatomical variations and specializations in fundus anatomy of the species being examined (e.g., merangiotic vascular pattern in rabbits, presence of a tapetum lucidum in dogs, and lack of a true macula in most laboratory species). While green is conventionally used by vitreoretinal physicians and surgeons to represent vitreous hemorrhage, our system has adopted red instead to disambiguate documentation of the lesion in different laboratory species (*D* dorsal [interchangeable with superior], *V* ventral [interchangeable with inferior], *T* temporal, *N* nasal)

flare ranging from no flare ("0") to a high score of "3," based on the visibility of a Tyndall effect within the AC (scattering of incident light due to increased protein in the normally optically clear aqueous humor). In these systems, scoring of the Tyndall effect is also defined against the background of the optical density of the lens. The SUN system describes 5 scores for flare, comprising less granular descriptions of flare severity ranging from none ("0") to intense (fibrin or plastic aqueous) ("4"), and scores corresponding to faint ("1"), moderate ("2"), and marked ("3") in between.

In the preclinical setting, refined scoring criteria for aqueous flare enable the identification of often subtle differences in ocular inflammation associated with different test materials. In our collective experience, the optical density of the lens provides a helpful benchmark for scoring of aqueous flare. The SPOTS scoring criteria for aqueous flare provides 6 scores with a maximal aqueous flare score ("4") designated as "approaching the optical density of the lens." Similar to the systems of M-S and H-M, scoring criteria are based upon Tyndall effect visibility in the AC. The scores used are absence of flare ("0"), trace ("0.5"), mild ("1"), moderate ("2–3"), and severe ("4"). Trace (minimal) aqueous flare ("0.5") indicates a Tyndall effect that is visible only with careful scrutiny with a slit lamp in a darkened room by a highly experienced examiner. The SPOTS system's criteria also clarify that the observation of AC fibrin is not unequivocally linked to a maximal flare score as indicated by SUN, since resorbing fibrin can be found in association with lower scores for flare in the anterior chamber.

Aqueous (Anterior Chamber) Cell

The presence of cells in the aqueous of the anterior chamber (AC) is also an important marker of anterior segment inflammation, and precise and accurate semi-quantitative scoring of this finding is critical in safety evaluations of modern ophthalmic pharmaceuticals [10]. However, scoring schemes for this finding are not included in the systems of M-S and H-M. Therefore, the AC cell scheme of the SUN system, widely used for clinical assessment of human patients, is often adopted for scoring in laboratory animals. As previously mentioned, however, replication of SUN's 1 × 1 mm slit beam may be difficult to impossible to achieve using a specific handheld instrument, and the applicability and predictive value of its scoring schemes in laboratory species may be also confounded by differences in ocular reactivity between humans and laboratory species [11]. In light of this, as well as the larger slit beam employed (0.2 mm width × 12 mm height), the cell densities corresponding to scores "1" through "4" in the SPOTS system are comparatively greater. As mentioned previously, use of the SUN system has the caveat that it can result in "topping out" of scores for AC cell prematurely when examining species with deeper anterior chambers and concomitant greater aqueous volume sampling by the slit beam. The SPOTS system enables examiners to better stratify the data and distinguish inflammatory responses based on severity between different drug formulations or when assessing for dose-responsiveness and across the entire spectrum of laboratory species.

When using any system's AC cell scoring scheme, the examiner must also recognize the inherent influence of species-related variations in anterior segment geometry on scoring of AC cells. As recently reported by our group [10], differences in geometric attributes of anterior segment anatomy such as AC depth, corneal curvature, and iris/lens curvature heavily influence the volume (and percentage of total AC volume) that is "sampled" by a slit beam of defined dimensions. Using geometric and mathematical modeling, this analysis showed that application of semi-quantitative scoring schemes (including the SUN and OSOD scoring criteria) yields dramatic differences in actual cell counts for a given cell density, depending on the species being evaluated. For example, in cats and dogs with comparatively deeper AC depths than humans, the scoring criteria of SUN and an OSOD scheme that preceded the SPOTS system yielded cell counts that overestimated those of humans, and the inverse was demonstrated for rodent species like rats and mice, yielding counts that dramatically underestimated those of human patients. This report also provided correction factors, when using the aforementioned systems to score AC cells, useful for consideration when comparing results obtained between different species and for attempting to ascertain the predictive value of preclinical studies with regard to human clinical trials.

When assigning a score for AC cells in any species, the examiner should also include a description of the predominant cell color observed as this may provide important information regarding the source and nature of the cells (i.e., leukocytes, erythrocytes, melanocytes, etc.). The SPOTS system notes cell color as (1) predominantly white, (2) predominantly brown, or (3) predominantly red, with the term "predominant" indicating that the color represents approximately 75% of the cells observed. The term "mixed color" is used if no cell color predominates.

Iris Involvement

The SPOTS scheme for recording effects on iridal vasculature (synonymous with "iris congestion" or "iridal vessel injection") is similar to those previously published, ranging from "0" to "4" depending on the severity of vessel injection. Additional attributes considered in scoring include iris swelling or rugosity. The examiner should be aware, however, that the descriptions of iris congestion used by M-S and H-M include some vascular features that are either highly specific to rabbits or only visible in nonpigmented strains. For example, the aforementioned systems indicate that the normal iris (score of "0") may include the ability to visualize secondary and tertiary vessels "occasionally around the 12:00 to 1:00 o'clock position near the pupillary border and the 6:00 to 7:00 o'clock position near the pupillary border." The criteria in the SPOTS System, therefore, have been simplified, distinguishing iris involvement using descriptions of vessel involvement and iris swelling only.

Anterior Vitreous Cell

The slit lamp biomicroscope can be used to illuminate the anterior vitreous, permitting the examiner to locate and describe opacities or cells. While scoring schemes for vitreous cells are not commonly published in the preclinical literature, identification of the character and severity of anterior vitreous infiltrates is essential when examining the eyes of animals receiving intraocular drugs or devices, especially those administered to the posterior segment. The SPOTS scheme for anterior vitreous cells employs the same six semi-quantitative designations used for AC cells (ranging from "0" to "4," including trace ("0.5")). Cell color should also be noted and recorded using the same terminology described for AC cells.

Lens Opacity

The SPOTS scheme for scoring of lens opacities is similar to that described by Hackett-McDonald, differentiated according to location within the lens (e.g., anterior or posterior, capsular or cortical, nuclear, equatorial, etc.). In addition, the SPOTS scheme recommends that the examiner provide a description of lens opacity size, ranging from punctate to resorption of a complete cataract (see Table 5.5). Furthermore, the SPOTS system advocates that the examiner diagram lens opacities, particularly when multiple lesions are observed, to facilitate longitudinal monitoring and interpretation.

The SPOTS - Modified SUN System

The SUN scoring scheme is commonly adopted in preclinical and toxicologic studies involving laboratory species. Since the SUN system is commonly used in human clinical trials, study sponsors and drug development professionals may promote its use in preclinical studies with the intention of maintaining consistency of methods within a department or company and enhancing translatability between preclinical and clinical programs.

The SUN scoring scheme for AC cells and aqueous flare requires the examiner to use a 1 mm × 1 mm slit beam, which is easily performed using table-mounted instruments. Creating these precise beam dimensions using most available handheld units, however, is difficult. A 1 mm diameter circular beam is available on the newer Kowa™ SL-17 instrument, but these beam dimensions do not exactly mimic the 1 mm diameter square beam specified by SUN. To geometrically mimic the optical section created using SUN's beam settings, the SPOTS—Modified SUN system—specifies settings that create a beam measuring 0.1 mm width and 10 mm height (as determined by measuring the beam's height when imaged at the plane of focus), angled at 30–45° to the eye's vertical axial (90°) meridian. Using a beam with these dimensional values provides the same sampling volume as a 1 × 1 mm square beam. SUN's semi-quantitative scores (Table 5.3) can then be employed as originally described. It needs to be noted that using a beam with these dimensions is not possible in species possessing a vertical corneal diameter (VCD) <10 mm. Depending on the species, accurate examination and scoring of aqueous and anterior vitreous cells requires a high magnification setting, typically 10× or 16× on most handheld instruments.

Scoring of the Posterior Segment

Compared to the numerous semi-quantitative slit lamp-based systems published for assessment of the anterior segment [1], those published for the posterior segment (vitreous, retina, optic disk) are less common, particularly in the preclinical literature. Like the SUN system, the majority of posterior segment systems reported in humans are designed for the clinical evaluation of naturally occurring human inflammatory diseases or retinopathies [32–34]. Therefore, these systems are often difficult to apply directly to laboratory species in preclinical studies using investigational drugs or devices. Furthermore, the range of different retinal vascular patterns across the most commonly used laboratory species and other anatomical variations like the presence or absence of a tapetum lucidum complicate the adaptation of such systems for use in animals in preclinical studies. Some systems, however, like the National Eye Institute's Scoring System for Vitreous Inflammation reported by Nussenblatt et al. [35], describe semi-quantitative scoring criteria based on photographic standards for vitreous haze that may be applicable to laboratory species. The veterinary ophthalmologists in OSOD have developed a scoring system based on the criteria reported by Nussenblatt and have also incorporated additional scoring parameters for posterior segment findings that have particular relevance in modern ocular toxicology and preclinical drug development.

Indirect ophthalmoscopy using a condensing lens and binocular ophthalmoscopic headset (like those made by Keeler™, Heine™, and Welch-Allyn™) is the preferred technique for posterior segment evaluation in the laboratory setting. Compared to direct ophthalmoscopy, this approach provides the examiner with a larger field of view and enhanced depth perception. If a finding warrants closer scrutiny, a specialized indirect macular lens (like the Volk™ Macula Plus 5.5), a PanOptic™ (Welch Allyn) ophthalmoscope, and/or direct ophthalmoscope can be used to achieve higher magnification and improve detail.

The National Eye Institute (NEI) Scoring System for Vitreous Inflammation

Nussenblatt and his colleagues at the National Eye Institute (NEI) published their photograph-based scoring system for vitreous haze in human patients in 1985 [35]. The system (Table 5.6) requires the examiner to perform indirect ophthalmoscopy

Table 5.6 Scoring criteria for vitreous haze in the semi-quantitative preclinical ocular toxicology scoring (SPOTS) and national eye institute (NEI) systems

Observation/lesion	Score	SPOTS scoring criteria	Original scoring criteria of Nussenblatt et al.[a]
Vitreous haze	0	No vitreous haze	No vitreous haze
	0.5	Minimal vitreous haze with only slight blurring of the margins of the optic disk and retinal vasculature	Slight blurring of the optic disk is observed, and the normal striations and reflex of the retinal nerve fiber layer cannot be visualized. The retinal vessels are blurred but visible
	1	Mild vitreous haze with slight blurring of the margins of the optic disk. View of the retinal vasculature is partially obscured but still visible from the disk to the periphery	The optic disk and retinal vessels are both blurred but visible
	2	Moderate vitreous haze with blurring of the optic disk margins. The retinal vasculature is nearly completely obscured	The optic disk is blurred, and the retinal vessels are markedly obscured
	3	Marked vitreous haze in which the optic disk can be viewed but is nearly obscured; and the retinal vasculature is completely obscured	The optic nerve head can be seen, but the disk borders are quite blurry. The retinal vessels are barely visible
	4	Severe vitreous haze in which the details of all structures, including the optic disk, are obscured	The optic nerve head and retinal vessels are obscured

[a]Paraphrased based upon text descriptions and photographic standards published in the original source reference

and assign a score based upon the clarity of three fundic structures: the optic nerve head (disk), retinal vasculature, and nerve fiber layer (NFL). Compared to previous scoring systems that used specialized contact lenses and scoring schemes for vitreous opacities [36], use of the photographic standards in Nussenblatt's system was easier and faster to perform and was associated with less interobserver variability [35, 37]. This system has been widely used and also designated as the standard scheme for scoring of vitreous haze by the SUN working group [38] and has been cited as a system with utility in preclinical examination of laboratory animals [5]. As indicated in the original publication of the NEI system, however, this system is more ideally suited when diffuse vitreous inflammation is present. Furthermore, poor pupil dilation and opacification of the clear media can obscure view of the posterior segment and complicate scoring.

The SPOTS Scoring System: Posterior Segment

The SPOTS system does not specify instrument settings for examination and scoring of the posterior segment. However, indirect ophthalmoscopic examination using an adjustable headset and condensing lens is strongly advocated for effective and efficient evaluation of the ocular fundus and posterior segment structures. The OSOD examiners recommend a Volk 2.2 PanRetinal™ or 20D lens for NHPs; a 28D lens for dogs, pigs, and rabbits; a 40D lens for rats; and a 60D lens for mice. When lesions are identified, additional lesion detail and characterization can be achieved using indirect lenses with lower dioptric power and greater magnification (e.g., 14D or Volk™ Macula Plus 5.5 lens), as well use of a Welch Allyn PanOptic™ ophthalmoscope (or equivalent) and/or direct ophthalmoscope. When describing the characteristics of any lesion(s), the examiner should keep in mind that the lateral and axial magnification perceived is heavily influenced by the dimensions and optical properties of the eye being examined [39]. The lower magnification of larger eyes, for example, will artifactually "flatten" the appearance of a lesion's ophthalmoscopic height; therefore, this lesion should be considered more clinically significant when compared to a lesion with similar characteristics in a small eye with much higher axial magnification.

Similar to OSOD's anterior segment scoring system, it is recommended that posterior segment lesions be captured using a clinical diagram (see Fig. 5.3b). Additional information can be captured through incorporation of published standard color-coding schemes [24]. In addition to diagramming of retinal lesions en face, diagramming of lesions or intravitreal (IVT) test articles in cross section provides more accurate illustration of lesion shape, size, and location within the vitreous. When diagramming lesions observed using indirect ophthalmoscopy, examiners must also ensure that all pertinent features are drawn in their normal anatomic orientation, correcting for the reversed and inverted image viewed by the clinician when employing indirect ophthalmoscopy.

Vitreous Haze

As observed by Nussenblatt and his NEI colleagues in human patients, vitreous haze can provide a useful indicator of posterior segment inflammation in preclinical studies involving laboratory species [35]. The SPOTS scheme for vitreous haze adopts with slight modification Nussenblatt's criteria using 6 scores, ranging from no haze ("0") to severe "4," including a score for minimal or trace vitreous haze ("0.5"), corresponding to increasing obscuring and blurring of the optic disk and retinal vasculature (Table 5.6 and Fig. 5.4). The original NEI system also used the clarity of the nerve fiber layer in its scoring criteria. While the "sheen" of the nerve fiber layer and retinal inner limiting membrane (ILM) is easily observed on fundus examination in NHPs and radiating myelinated nerve fibers are often observed in the pig fundus and along the rabbit's merangiotic medullary rays, the ILM is not

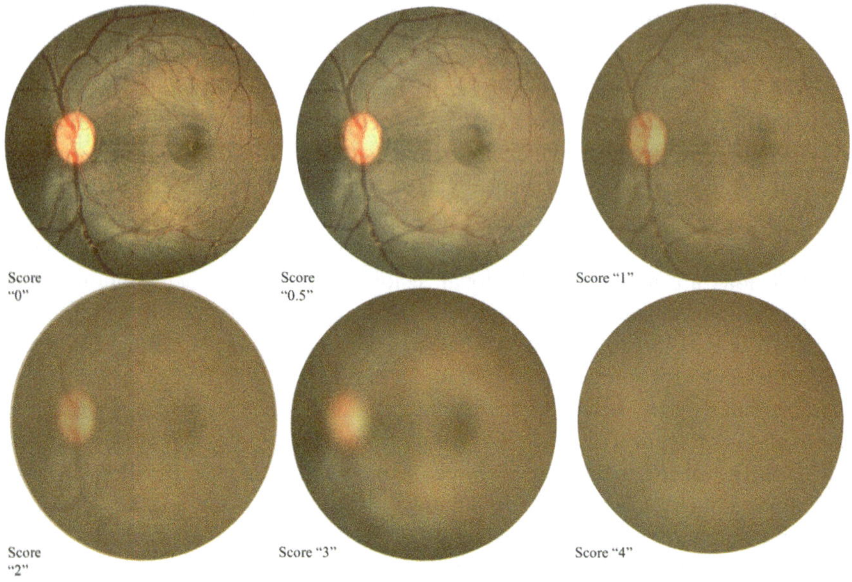

Fig. 5.4 Photographic images simulating vitreous haze scoring criteria using the SPOTS system (NHP presented). Figure reprinted with permissions from Eaton, J. S., et al. The SPOTS system: An ocular scoring system optimized for use in modern preclinical drug development and toxicology. *J Ocul Pharm Ther* **33**, 718–34 (2017)

ophthalmoscopically clearly visible in all laboratory species and strains. Therefore, it is not included in SPOTS scoring criteria.

Degraded Fundus View

Scoring for degradation of fundus view allows examiners to communicate general loss of visible detail when examining the posterior segment. The SPOTS system employs an "area under the curve" approach, integrating a decrement in transparency of all elements included in the optical path (cornea/anterior chamber/lens/vitreous). This differs from the system of Nusenblatt described above wherein loss of ophthalmoscopic detail is strictly attributable to adverse events affecting the vitreous. The SPOTS system's scores range from "0" to "3," corresponding to increasing obscuration of details of fundus anatomy (Table 5.7). Attributable causes include aqueous cells and flare, AC fibrin, lens opacities, vitreous haze and/or floaters, IVT test articles, or any combination thereof as contributing factors. Given the cumulative nature of this observation, scoring of degraded fundus view is not specific for any single finding. In our collective experience, this parameter serves as a useful general indicator of the occurrence, progression, and resolution of ocular adverse events. Additionally, it may serve as a predictor of visual compromise with conduction of human clinical trials.

Table 5.7 Posterior segment scoring criteria for the semi-quantitative preclinical ocular toxicology scoring (SPOTS) system

Observation/lesion	Score	Description
Degraded fundus view	0	Normal, unobstructed fundus view
	1	Mildly degraded view. Details of fundus anatomy are visible but slightly dulled
	2	Moderately degraded view. Normal features of fundus anatomy can be identified, but details cannot be discerned
	3	Severely degraded view. Normal features of fundus anatomy cannot be identified
Retinal perivascular sheathing	0	Normal. No perivascular sheathing
	1	Mild perivascular sheathing. Focal perivascular haze/infiltrate is visible, but faint/barely discernible and confined to one quadrant of the fundus when viewed with an indirect ophthalmoscope
	2	Moderate perivascular sheathing. White perivascular haze/infiltrate is clearly visible and involves multiple vessels in >1 fundus quadrant
	3	Severe perivascular sheathing. Dense white perivascular infiltrate is visible (often resembling human frosted branch angiitis) with segmental or confluent distribution involving most vessels of the fundus. In some cases, hemorrhage may accompany severe perivascular sheathing

Retinal Perivascular Sheathing

Perivascular sheathing (sometimes referred to as "cuffing") describes the presence of hazy- to dense-white infiltrates surrounding segments of retinal arterioles and/or venules (Fig. 5.5). Perivascular sheathing is considered indicative of retinal vasculitis and generally reflective of posterior segment inflammation in any species. This observation is not, however, considered specific for a particular etiology or inflammation type although it is commonly observed when anti-drug antibodies develop after intravitreal injection of a biologic. Regardless of its cause, sheathing can vary in its distribution and severity and can be transient or progressive in nature. The SPOTS system describes scores ranging from "0" to "3," with descriptive criteria corresponding to density of sheathing as well as area affected (Table 5.7). For reference, the clinical appearance of human frosted branch angiitis provides an excellent exemplar for the features of moderate to severe perivascular sheathing in laboratory species [40, 41]. OSOD clinicians have also found this finding to be particularly prominent in the preclinical assessment of intravitreal biologics and the use of a semi-quantitative scoring system to be very useful in recording longitudinal findings.

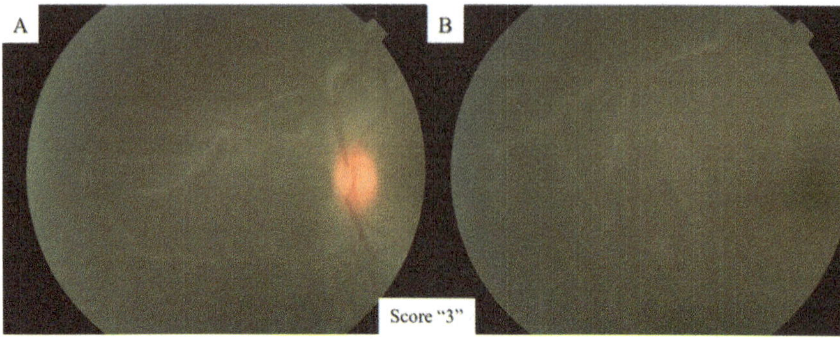

Fig. 5.5 Photographic exemplars demonstrating severe (Score "3") perivascular sheathing of the peripapillary and nasal fundus (**a**) and temporal fundus (**b**) in a nonhuman primate (NHP) using the SPOTS system. Figure reprinted with permissions from Eaton, J. S., et al. The SPOTS system: An ocular scoring system optimized for use in modern preclinical drug development and toxicology. *J Ocul Pharm Ther* **33**, 718–34 (2017)

Intravitreal Test Articles

Intravitreal delivery is now widely used in the administration of agency-approved ocular drugs, and in the ongoing development of novel drugs, devices, and sustained-release biomaterial platforms that target diseases of the posterior segment [42]. As such, in studies using IVT test articles and delivery systems, it is often desirable to record their appearance, spatial distribution, and degradation profiles in vivo. To facilitate this, clinical members of the OSOD group have found semi-quantitative scoring and diagrammatic documentation of IVT test articles to be exceptionally valuable (Table 5.8). Observation of dispersion or migration of these test materials within the vitreous and potentially the anterior chamber is important as they may provide a harbinger of risk to vision when used in human patients; and AC migration may represent a risk for impaired aqueous outflow. Clinical assessment of IVT test articles is most commonly performed with indirect ophthalmoscopy, but slit lamp biomicroscopy is often complimentary for documentation of test articles in the anterior vitreous and aqueous. Fundus photography can also be a valuable complimentary endpoint, though any clinical scoring should ultimately be based upon examination characteristics which are observed in three dimensions and recorded in the room at the time of examination.

The SPOTS scheme for IVT test articles comprises 2 scores: the first for appearance, corresponding to a test article's general optical density, and the second corresponding to its general shape, profile, and spatial distribution on ophthalmoscopic observation. Diagramming of test article features is also considered essential as this qualitative information can greatly facilitate accurate monitoring (especially between two different observers), as well as identification and documentation of in vivo properties of a test article, particularly in the context of ophthalmic examination findings.

Table 5.8 Intravitreal (IVT) test article scoring criteria for the semi-quantitative preclinical ocular toxicology scoring (SPOTS) system

Observation/lesion	Score	Description
Test article appearance[a]	1	The test article is transparent but may create refractive shift when viewing underlying fundus structures
	2	The test article is translucent, permitting only a hazy view of underlying fundus structures
	3	The test article is opaque, obscuring view of underlying fundus structures
Test article distribution[b]	1	Test article is a focal mass/depot or an intact solid implant
	2	Test article is a focal mass/depot with adjacent strands/wisps, or the implant has fragmented
	3	Test article is a focal mass/depot with adjacent strands/wisps and some diffusion
	4	Test article is a focal mass/depot with some diffusion
	5	Test article is dispersed throughout vitreous

[a]Diagramming of test article appearance and location is recommended to facilitate characterization, localization, and longitudinal monitoring
[b]Diagramming of test article distribution is recommended to facilitate characterization, localization, and longitudinal monitoring

Scoring System Modifications

Cumulatively, the scoring systems presented in this chapter provide robust guidelines and semi-quantitative scoring criteria necessary for a veterinary ophthalmologist to thoroughly and critically evaluate the spectrum of biomicroscopic and ophthalmoscopic observations and findings observed in preclinical studies. However, it must be acknowledged that, depending on the species being examined and the drug or device being evaluated, program- or study-specific modifications to any system may be necessary. Modified versions of the McDonald-Shadduck and Hackett-McDonald systems have been published [9, 43]; and while the SPOTS systems are used as the default semi-quantitative systems among all OSOD veterinary ophthalmologists and vision scientists, the specific needs or goals of a particular study or program may require modifications and/or alterations to be applied to any of the scoring schemes or criteria.

Species-Specific Considerations for Ocular Scoring

A significant challenge to veterinary ophthalmologists engaged in preclinical and toxicological studies is the clinical examination of relatively unfamiliar laboratory species, as well as the interpretation of clinical findings between different strains and species that may be involved in assessment of a specific test material or device. The scoring systems presented in this chapter enable the examiner to translate qualitative biomicroscopic and ophthalmoscopic observations into semi-quantitative measurements of severity. No single system, however, accounts for or encompasses all of the diverse and variable features of ocular morphology and physiology in different species or the differences in ocular inflammatory responses that exist between different species and strains. As the industry expert in the clinical ophthalmic evaluation of laboratory animals, the veterinary ophthalmologist must be able to apply the scoring methods and techniques presented here, must maintain a keen awareness of how the diverse features of different species' eyes influence semi-quantitative scoring, and ultimately must be able to provide guidance when interpreting study results. While a comprehensive presentation of comparative anatomical features and reported ocular background lesions is beyond the scope of this chapter, we provide in the following some important species-specific considerations for the veterinary ophthalmologist engaged in preclinical studies and ocular scoring in laboratory animals.

Rodents (Mice and Rats)

In addition to the challenges associated with examining the smaller eyes of rodents, there are several unique and important attributes that the veterinary ophthalmologist should be aware of when performing clinical examinations and scoring. Spontaneous corneal dystrophy is a well-characterized incidental finding in mice and rats [5, 44–49]. Lesions are typically observed as bilateral anterior stromal/subepithelial multifocal punctate opacities in the nasal and/or axial palpebral fissure that tend to increase in incidence and severity (size and density) as affected rodents age [5]. Furthermore, these lesions can be associated with keratitis and exacerbated or elicited by sedation, anesthesia, or corneal desiccation [50]. In our collective experience, corneal dystrophy is particularly prevalent in rats, with nearly 100% incidence in the Wistar strain, and a much more variable incidence in the Sprague-Dawley. The lesions of corneal dystrophy, especially if progressive in severity, can confound assessment and scoring of ocular surface findings like fluorescein staining, complicate semi-quantitative scoring of aqueous flare and cells, and obscure viewing of the fundus.

The anterior chamber is markedly narrow in mice and rats (~0.45 mm and 0.71 mm, respectively), delimited posteriorly by a large lens with a steep anterior and posterior curvature [51], which challenges identification and scoring of findings such as aqueous flare and cells. Similarly, the large anterior-posterior lens diameter to axial globe length ratio in these species [52–55], creates a comparatively narrow vitreous depth. Therefore, induced lens pathology is common in studies involving intravitreal injections or other dosing routes involving the posterior segment.

When examining and scoring the rodent posterior segment, the veterinary ophthalmologist must be familiar with the inherent optical magnification created by their small eyes [34]. When performing indirect ophthalmoscopy using a 40D condensing lens in the rat, for example, lateral and axial magnification are 3.68 and

18.06, respectively. Ophthalmoscopically, this inherent magnification can result in the retinal vessels appearing to "float" above the deeper retinal and choroidal structures, creating the illusion of detachment. In albino strains, there also is a considerable variability in the normal appearance and distribution of the choroidal vasculature. Therefore, examiners must become familiar with the vasculature of the rodent posterior segment to prevent normal variations from being mistaken as adverse events associate with a given test material.

Despite being relatively easy to examine without sedation or anesthesia, certain restraint techniques (particularly "scruffing") can have a remarkable effect on choroidal and retinal perfusion. Excessive restraint can lead to remarkable blanching of the choroidal and retinal vasculature and be easily mistaken for a degenerative change, especially in albino animals where choroidal vessels are more easily observed. Excessive traction on the eyelids and globe proptosis to facilitate examination can also produce similar changes. If blanching of the posterior segment vasculature is observed, the veterinary ophthalmologist should request that the restrainer alter their technique and reexamine the fundus before diagnosing degeneration or loss of vasculature.

Rodents are also the most commonly employed species in general toxicity studies investigating possible off-target ocular toxicity following systemic drug administration. As most general toxicity studies involve a large number of animals (frequently exceeding 100), some have advocated use of an indirect ophthalmoscope for evaluation of both the anterior and posterior segment to enhance the speed and efficiency of examinations. While the indirect ophthalmoscope may be able to identify large lesions of the cornea or anterior segment (e.g., large corneal dystrophic lesions or large cataracts), the slit lamp is still considered the gold standard for evaluation of the anterior segment in rodents.

Rabbits

As a large-eyed species that is relatively easy to handle and examine unanesthetized, the rabbit is one of the most commonly used species in ocular drug and device safety evaluation. While the majority of ocular scoring systems published for laboratory species describe criteria for the rabbit, the vast majority of these describe criteria for albino strains like the New Zealand white [1]. Therefore, anatomical and physiological variations attributable to pigmentation can complicate use of these scoring criteria in pigmented species like the Dutch Belted. For example, hyperemia of the perilimbal bulbar conjunctival vasculature characteristic of the species is more difficult to observe in pigmented strains with perilimbal pigment, particularly at lower score severities. The same challenge is relevant when scoring iris involvement, as congestion or tortuosity of the small secondary and tertiary iridal vessels used to assign semi-quantitative scores may be masked by iridal pigment. There is also evidence supporting a possible effect of background stress (e.g., associated with multiple consecutive anesthetic/clinical procedures, husbandry changes, rehousing, etc.) on the conjunctiva in albino rabbits, leading to comparatively higher amounts of conjunctival hyperemia [56].

Rabbits are also commonly used as models in preclinical studies of topically applied drugs and as animal models for dry eye [57–61]. Compared to humans and other species, however, there are differences in the constituents of the precorneal tear film and chemistry of the ocular surface cells which can, in turn, yield differences in interfacial attributes of the ocular surface and tear film dynamics [62–64]. Of particular importance in scoring of the ocular surface, investigation has also shown that focal, superficial punctate fluorescein staining (comparable to a score of "1" in the OSOD scoring system) can be a background finding in normal, healthy rabbits [65]. Like rodents, corneal dystrophy can also be observed in rabbits [66, 67]. In the experience of OSOD examiners, dystrophic lesions tend to be observed in the nasal and inferior region of the cornea in Dutch Belted rabbits, though the incidence of this observation is variable across studies.

The merangiotic fundus of rabbits may also create challenges in preclinical studies. In species with holangiotic retinal vascular patterns, identification and monitoring of structural retinal abnormalities such as perivascular sheathing and retinal detachment is facilitated by the numerous vessels present in all regions of the fundus, including the periphery. However, in the rabbit whose retinal vasculature is confined to the superior fundus immediately medial and lateral to the optic disk, observation of retinal pathology in the remainder of the largely avascular retina may be more difficult, particularly in albino strains. Furthermore, the absence of a tapetum lucidum in rabbits precludes the observation of changes in reflectivity associated with retinal lesions. Instead, localized retina toxicity in albino rabbits may be represented by a much more subtle change in color, appearing as focal or multifocal pallor or "whitening."

Dogs

Like rabbits, dogs are commonly used as animal models and in safety and efficacy evaluation of ocular drug and devices. Furthermore, this species is generally easy to handle and examine without anesthesia or sedation, and veterinary ophthalmologists tend to have much more experience examining this species, compared to others used in the laboratory setting. There are still, however, some unique challenges in the examination and scoring of ocular findings in dogs. For example, while the miotic effect of drugs like the prostaglandin analogs in dogs is well known to veterinary ophthalmologists, this may not be known to study teams involved in toxicologic study planning and execution. Therefore, indirect ophthalmoscopy and evaluation of the posterior segment will be difficult to perform in dogs dosed with drugs in this class, as the pupil in affected eyes is typically subsequently poorly responsive to mydriatic agents.

Veterinary ophthalmologists should also screen all dogs in laboratory studies for imperforate inferior puncta which are commonly observed in laboratory Beagles.

While this may not cause clinically observable abnormalities, the impaired lacrimal drainage in these eyes can considerably alter the distribution and exposure time of topically applied drugs and therefore alter scores recorded for features of the ocular surface and anterior segment. Another consideration in dogs is the presence of the cellular tapetum lucidum. The reflective nature of this structure may alter the appearance of fundus lesions and may "wash out" smaller and/or more subtle lesions such as mild perivascular sheathing. Altering the intensity of ophthalmoscopic illumination should be performed when evaluating subtle findings.

Pigs

Pigs, specifically minipigs such as the Göttingen and Yucatan, are becoming popular animal models in ocular drug efficacy and safety evaluation, not only because of their anatomical similarities to the human eye but also because of the increasing cost and welfare concerns regarding the use of NHPs in drug development. Anatomically, the pigmented, atapetal pig eye poses few challenges in examination and scoring. This species, however, is known for being a challenge to handle and examine when unanesthetized. This species also possesses thicker eyelids and periocular cutaneous tissue and, with relatively deep set eyes, can be a challenge when it comes to assessment and scoring of the conjunctiva. Some normal animals will develop accumulation of a thick yellow-orange waxy or greasy discharge on their eyelids and periocular area, and the tear film can be particularly viscous which may impact examination and scoring, ease of acquiring tonometry readings, and could theoretically influence pharmacokinetics and drug delivery via the topical route.

Nonhuman Primates

While numerous species of NHP have been used in vision science, the predominant species currently used in ocular toxicology and drug development are rhesus macaques and the smaller cynomolgus macaques. These species do, however, require the handler and examiner to be familiar with safe husbandry and handling practices and also require anesthesia for safe and effective ocular examination. There are also several noteworthy anatomical features of the NHPs that bear relevance in the context of clinical examination and ocular scoring.

Anatomically, the macaques have a prominent brow ridge and comparatively deep-set eyes which can make examination of the conjunctiva more difficult. Many macaques will also have heavy pigmentation of their bulbar conjunctiva which can complicate scoring of conjunctival hyperemia. Of the routinely used laboratory species, the NHPs are also the only ones with a true macula and fovea, and the examiner must be familiar with the normal appearance and features of this specialized region of the retina. The retinal inner limiting membrane and nerve fiber layer in macaques are also particularly prominent on ophthalmic examination, particularly adjacent to the retinal vasculature, and can be mistaken for perivascular sheathing or other forms of retinal pathology if the examiner is not familiar with its appearance. Normal young, healthy macaques may also possess focal variations in fundus color associated with variations in pigmentation of the retinal pigment epithelium. These normal variations do not have any known functional consequence.

Qualitatively, inflammatory responses involving the anterior segment in macaques are often characterized by high numbers of anterior chamber cells. Furthermore, on slit lamp examination, the inflammatory cells observed in the aqueous humor of NHPs tend to be much finer and granular in appearance and are typically white in color. Also, unlike most other animal species, NHPs possess an analog to the human Schlemm's canal for aqueous outflow [68]. The presence of this anatomical feature may predispose macaques with severe ocular inflammation or ocular hypertension to reflex the blood into the anterior chamber, which has been commonly observed by members of the clinical team at OSOD.

Conclusion

Veterinary ophthalmologists are experts whose knowledge and skills in ocular examination and assessment are critical to the responsible conduction of preclinical ocular drug and device development and toxicology studies. The veterinary ophthalmologist engaged in such studies must also have a complete understanding of the importance of semi-quantitative scoring, using a system that is appropriate to the species and strain being examined. Systems like SUN and those developed by McDonald-Shadduck and Hackett-McDonald provide scoring criteria for a number of important clinical parameters but were designed with respect to human patients and albino rabbits, respectively. Systems like the SPOTS system modify and expand upon many of these criteria to expand system applicability and predictive value in other laboratory strains and species and also provide standardized slit lamp settings to improve reproducibility between examiners and between studies. Regardless of which scoring system is used, the veterinary ophthalmologist must be aware of the limitations of each when interpreting study results and must also have a keen knowledge of species-specific considerations relevant to examination in the context of ocular drug and device development programs.

References

1. Eaton JS, Miller PE, Bentley E, Thomasy SM, Murphy CJ. Slit lamp-based ocular scoring systems in toxicology and drug development: a literature survey. J Ocul Pharmacol Ther. 2017;33:707–17.
2. Eaton JS, Miller PE, Bentley E, Thomasy SM, Murphy CJ. The SPOTS system: an ocular scoring system optimized for use in modern preclinical drug development and toxicology. J Ocul Pharmacol Ther. 2017;33:718–34.

3. Singer M. Oxford textbook of critical care. New York: Oxford University Press; 2016.
4. Barbini P, Cevenini G, Furini S, Barbini E. A naive approach for deriving scoring systems to support clinical decision making. J Eval Clin Pract. 2014;20:1–6. https://doi.org/10.1111/jep.12064.
5. Wilkie DA. The ophthalmic examination as it pertains to general ocular toxicology: basic and advanced techniques and species-associated findings. In: Ocular pharmacology and toxicology. Totowa: Humana Press; 2014. p. 143–203.
6. Jabs DA, Nussenblatt RB, Rosenbaum JT. Standardization of uveitis nomenclature for reporting clinical data. Results of the First International Workshop. Am J Ophthalmol. 2005;140:509–16.
7. BenEzra D, Forrester JV, Nussenblatt RB, Tabbara K, Timonen P. Uveitis scoring system. Berlin: Springer; 1991. p. 1–2.
8. Deschenes J, Murray PI, Rao NA, Nussenblatt RB. International Uveitis Study Group (IUSG) clinical classification of uveitis. Ocul Immunol Inflamm. 2008;16(1-2):1.
9. Munger RJ. Veterinary ophthalmology in laboratory animal studies. Vet Ophthalmol. 2002;5:167–75.
10. Thomasy SM, et al. Species differences in the geometry of the anterior segment differentially affect anterior chamber cell scoring systems in laboratory animals. J Ocul Pharmacol Ther. 2016;32:28–37. https://doi.org/10.1089/jop.2015.0071.
11. Bito LZ. Species differences in the responses of the eye to irritation and trauma: a hypothesis of divergence in ocular defense mechanisms, and the choice of experimental animals for eye research. Exp Eye Res. 1984;39:807–29.
12. McDonald TO, Shadduck JA. In: Marzulli FN, Maibach HI, editors. Dermatotoxicology and pharmacology, Advanced in modern toxicology, vol. 4. Washington, DC: Hemisphere; 1977. p. 139–91.
13. Hackett RB, McDonald TO. Assessing ocular irritation. In: Dermatotoxicology. Washington, DC: Hemisphere; 1996. p. 557–67.
14. Friedenwald J, Hughes W, Herrmann H. Acid-base tolerance of the cornea. Arch Ophthalmol. 1944;31:279–83.
15. Draize JH, Woodard G, Calvery HO. Methods for the study of irritation and toxicity of substances applied topically to the skin and mucous membranes. J Pharmacol Exp Ther. 1944;82:377–90.
16. Sasaki H, Yamamura K, Nishida K, Nakamura J, Ichikawa M. Delivery of drugs to the eye by topical application. Prog Retin Eye Res. 1996;15:583–620.
17. Salminen L, Urtti A, Periviita L. Effect of ocular pigmentation on pilocarpine pharmacology in the rabbit eye. I. Drag distribution and metabolism. Int J Pharm. 1984;18:17–24.
18. Urtti A, Salminen L, Kujari H, Jäntti V. Effect of ocular pigmentation on pilocarpine pharmacology in the rabbit eye. II. Drug response. Int J Pharm. 1984;19:53–61.
19. Studer ME, Martin CL, Stiles J. Effects of 0.005% latanoprost solution on intraocular pressure in healthy dogs and cats. Am J Vet Res. 2000;61:1220–4.
20. Gelatt KN, MacKay EO. Effect of different dose schedules of latanoprost on intraocular pressure and pupil size in the glaucomatous Beagle. Vet Ophthalmol. 2001;4:283–8.
21. Gelatt KN, MacKay EO. Effect of different dose schedules of bimatoprost on intraocular pressure and pupil size in the glaucomatous Beagle. J Ocul Pharmacol Ther. 2002;18:525–34.
22. Wilhelmus KR. The Draize eye test. Surv Ophthalmol. 2001;45:493–515. https://doi.org/10.1016/S0039-6257(01)00211-9.
23. Waring GO, Laibson PR. A systematic method of drawing corneal pathologic conditions. Arch Ophthalmol. 1977;95:1540–2.
24. Friberg TR, Jenny YY. Chapter 156, Choroidal and retinal folds. In: Albert and Jakobiec's principles and practice of ophthalmology. 3rd ed. Philadelphia: Elsevier Inc; 2008. p. 2039–48.
25. Krzystolik MG, Afshari MA, Adamis AP, et al. Prevention of experimental choroidal neovascularization with intravitreal anti-vascular endothelial growth factor antibody fragment. Arch Ophthalmol. 2002;20:338–46.
26. Nork TM, Dubielzig RR, Christian BJ, et al. Prevention of experimental choroidal neovascularization and resolution of active lesions by VEGF trap in nonhuman primates. Arch Ophthalmol. 2001;129:1042–52.

27. Ryan SJ. Subretinal neovascularization: natural history of an experimental model. Arch Ophthalmol. 1982;100:1804–9.
28. Ohkuma H, Ryan SJ. Experimental subretinal neovascularization in the monkey: permeability of new vessels. Arch Ophthalmol. 1983;101:1102–10.
29. Jakobiec FA, Stacy RC, Mendoza PR, Chodosh J. Hyperplastic corneal pannus: an immunohistochemical analysis and review. Surv Ophthalmol. 2014;59:448–53.
30. Williams D. Histological and immunohistochemical evaluation of canine chronic superficial keratitis. Res Vet Sci. 1999;67:191–5.
31. Gelatt KN, Gilger BC, Kern TJ. Veterinary ophthalmology. Ames: Wiley; 2012.
32. Dumonde D, et al. Anti-retinal autoimmunity and circulating immune complexes in patients with retinal vasculitis. Lancet. 1982;320:787–92.
33. Lee EK, Lee S-Y, Yu HG. A clinical grading system based on ultra-wide field retinal imaging for sunset glow fundus in Vogt-Koyanagi-Harada disease. Graefes Arch Clin Exp Ophthalmol. 2015;253:359–68.
34. Seddon JM, Sharma S, Adelman RA. Evaluation of the clinical age-related maculopathy staging system. Ophthalmology. 2006;113:260–6.
35. Nussenblatt RB, Palestine AG, Chan C-C, Roberge F. Standardizatlon of vitreal inflammatory activity in intermediate and posterior uveitis. Ophthalmology. 1985;92:467–71.
36. Kimura SJ, Thygeson P, Hogan MJ. Signs and symptoms of uveitis. II. Classification of the posterior manifestations of uveitis. Am J Ophthalmol. 1959;47:171.
37. Kempen JH, Ganesh SK, Sangwan VS, Rathinam SR. Interobserver agreement in grading activity and site of inflammation in eyes of patients with uveitis. Am J Ophthalmol. 2008;146:813–8.
38. Sen HN, et al. A standardized grading system for scleritis. Ophthalmology. 2011;118:768–71. https://doi.org/10.1016/j.ophtha.2010.08.027.
39. Murphy CJ, Rowland HC. The optics of comparative ophthalmoscopy. Vis Res. 1987;27:599–607.
40. Agarwal M, Malathi J, Biswas J. Frosted branch angiitis in a patient with typhoid fever. Ocul Immunol Inflamm. 2016:1–3. https://doi.org/10.1080/09273948.2016.1265654.
41. Wood EH, Wong RW. Bilateral frosted branch angiitis as the presenting sign of antiphospholipid antibody syndrome. J Ophthalmic Inflamm Infect. 2016;6:20.
42. Short BG. Safety evaluation of ocular drug delivery formulations: techniques and practical considerations. Toxicol Pathol. 2008;36:49–62.
43. Hosseini A, et al. Efficacy of a phosphorodiamidate morpholino oligomer antisense compound in the inhibition of corneal transplant rejection in a rat cornea transplant model. J Ocul Pharmacol Ther. 2012;28:194–201.
44. Taradach C, Greaves P, Rubin LF. Spontaneous eye lesions in laboratory animals: incidence in relation to age. CRC Crit Rev Toxicol. 1984;12:121–47.
45. Taradach C, Regnier B, Perraud J. Eye lesions in Sprague-Dawley rats: type and incidence in relation to age. Lab Anim. 1981;15:285–7.
46. Wegener A, Kaegler M, Stinn W. Frequency and nature of spontaneous age-related eye lesions observed in a 2-year inhalation toxicity study in rats. Ophthalmic Res. 2002;34(5):281–7.
47. Eiben R. Frequency of spontaneous opacities in the cornea and lens observed in chronic toxicity studies in Wistar rats: experience with a standardized terminology glossary (Hattersheimer Kreis). Res Commun Pharmacol Toxicol. 2001;6(3/4):238–51.
48. Bruner RH, Keller WF, Stitzel KA, Sauers LJ, Reer PJ, Long PH, Bruce RD, Alden CL. Spontaneous corneal dystrophy and generalized basement membrane changes in Fischer-344 rats. Toxicol Pathol. 2016;20(3–1):357–66.
49. Van TW, Balk MW. Spontaneous corneal opacities in laboratory mice. Lab Anim Sci. 1986;36(3):248–55.
50. Koehn D, Meyer KJ, Syed NA, Anderson MG. Ketamine/xylazine-induced corneal damage in mice. PLoS One. 2015;10:e0132804.
51. Bawa G, Tkatchenko TV, Avrutsky I, Tkatchenko AV. Variational analysis of the mouse and rat eye optical parameters. Biomed Opt Express. 2013;4:2585–95.

52. Massof RW, Chang FW. A revision of the rat schematic eye. Vis Res. 1972;12:793–6.
53. Pe'er J, Muckarem M, Zajicek G. Epithelial cell migration in the normal rat lens. Ann Anat. 1996;178:433–6.
54. Remtulla S, Hallett P. A schematic eye for the mouse, and comparisons with the rat. Vis Res. 1985;25:21–31.
55. Mailankot M, et al. Indoleamine 2, 3-dioxygenase overexpression causes kynurenine-modification of proteins, fiber cell apoptosis and cataract formation in the mouse lens. Lab Investig. 2009;89:498.
56. Sharif NA, et al. Preclinical pharmacology of AL-12182, a new ocular hypotensive 11-oxa prostaglandin analog. J Ocul Pharmacol Ther. 2006;22:291–309.
57. Barabino S, Dana MR. Animal models of dry eye: a critical assessment of opportunities and limitations. Investig Ophthalmol Vis Sci. 2004;45:1641–6.
58. Burgalassi S, Panichi L, Chetoni P, Saettone MF, Boldrini E. Development of a simple dry eye model in the albino rabbit and evaluation of some tear substitutes. Ophthalmic Res. 1999;31:229–35.
59. Guo Z, et al. Autologous lacrimal-lymphoid mixed-cell reactions induce dacryoadenitis in rabbits. Exp Eye Res. 2000;71:23–31. https://doi.org/10.1006/exer.2000.0855.
60. Li N, et al. Establishment of the mild, moderate and severe dry eye models using three methods in rabbits. BMC Ophthalmol. 2013;13:50. https://doi.org/10.1186/1471-2415-13-50.
61. Toshida H, Nguyen DH, Beuerman RW, Murakami A. Neurologic evaluation of acute lacrimomimetic effect of cyclosporine in an experimental rabbit dry eye model. Investig Ophthalmol Vis Sci. 2009;50:2736–41.
62. Yañez-Soto B, et al. Interfacial phenomena and the ocular surface. Ocul Surf. 2014;12:178–201.
63. Yánez-Soto B, Leonard BC, Raghunathan VK, Abbott NL, Murphy CJ. Effect of stratification on surface properties of corneal epithelial cells. Invest Ophthalmol Vis Sci. 2015;56:8340–8.
64. Leonard BC, Yañez-Soto B, Raghunathan VK, Abbott NL, Murphy CJ. Species variation and spatial differences in mucin expression from corneal epithelial cells. Exp Eye Res. 2016;152:43–8.
65. Kikkawa Y. Normal corneal staining with fluorescein. Exp Eye Res. 1972;14:13–20.
66. Moore C, Dubielzig R, Glaza S. Anterior corneal dystrophy of American Dutch belted rabbits: biomicroscopic and histopathologic findings. Vet Pathol. 1987;24:28–33.
67. Port C, Dodd D. Two cases of corneal epithelial dystrophy in rabbits. Lab Anim Sci. 1983;33:587–8.
68. Holmberg ÅS. Schlemm's canal and the trabecular meshwork. An electron microscopic study of the normal structure in man and monkey (Cercopithecus ethiops). Doc Ophthalmol. 1965;19:339–73.

Index

B. C. Gilger et al. (eds.), *Standards for Ocular Toxicology and Inflammation*,
https://doi.org/10.1007/978-3-319-78364-2